THE FAMILY GENETIC SOURCEBOOK

Benjamin A. Pierce

WILEY

John Wiley & Sons, Inc.

New York • Chichester • Brisbane • Toronto • Singapore

Library of Congress Cataloging-in-Publication Data

Pierce, Benjamin A.
    The family genetic sourcebook / Benjamin A. Pierce.
      p. cm.
    Includes bibliographical references (p.   )
    ISBN 0-471-61709-1
    1. Medical genetics—Popular works.   I. Title.
RB155.P54   1990
616'.042—dc20   89-24884
                                              CIP

Printed in the United States of America

90 91 10 9 8 7 6 5 4 3 2 1

To Marlene, Sarah, and Michael

PREFACE

During the past decade, incredible advances in the study of genetics have transformed our understanding of human heredity. Scientists have identified scores of new genes, genes that influence our appearance, our biochemistry, our health, and even our behavior. Powerful new techniques in molecular genetics are altering the way biologists study heredity and are providing detailed information about the mechanisms of gene action. Perhaps the most important theme to emerge from this work is that genes are central to who and what we are.

In spite of recent advances in the study of genetics and the growing importance of human heredity, the average person knows little about the nature of genes or how they work. This lack of understanding is not because people are disinterested in their heredity. On the contrary, as a professional geneticist I am continually approached by parents, students, and friends who ask: "How is red hair inherited?" or "My father has heart disease; am I likely to inherit it?" or "Is obesity genetic?" Geneticists have detailed answers to many of these questions; yet, little of the information has been available to the average person. My goal in writing this book is to provide such information to the layperson in a direct, clear, and nontechnical style.

The Family Genetic Sourcebook is divided into two parts. The first half consists of seven chapters that provide an introduction to the principles of heredity. Chapter 1 discusses the importance of heredity and provides a brief history of the study of genetics; I emphasize a number of recent advances that have revolutionized the field of human genetics. Chapter 2 focuses on basic concepts: What a gene is, how genes determine our traits, how genetic information is encoded, the structure of a chromosome, and how chromosomes are inherited. Chapter 3 explains the inheritance of simple genetic traits, and Chapter 4 discusses the inheritance of more complicated multifactorial traits. Chapter 5 touches on chromosome disorders. Chapter 6 explains genetic counseling, prenatal diagnosis, and treatment of genetic diseases. Chapter 7 contains detailed instructions for charting your own family history.

The second part of the book, entitled "The Catalog of Genetic Traits" is an alphabetical listing of over 100 human traits, diseases, and disorders that have a genetic basis. Each entry in the catalog contains a brief description of the trait or disease and an explanation of its inheritance. Flipping through the catalog, the reader encounters discussions of how genes influence alcoholism, the genetic basis of diabetes, and how reading disabilities are inherited. The genetics of height, weight, eye color, hair color, intelligence, and many other human traits are explained. Cross-listings and references to relevant sections in the introductory chapters facilitate easy use of the catalog and enable the reader to acquire an understanding of the principles of human heredity.

The Family Genetic Sourcebook is not a book written primarily for physicians or geneticists; however, I think many physicians and geneticists will find it a useful guide for explaining inheritance and a handy reference to human genetic traits. Rather, my intended audience consists of people with little or no formal training in genetics but with an interest in heredity; this will include parents and prospective parents, teachers, social workers, nurses, biology students, and any reader with an interest in their own heredity. I have tried to keep that audience firmly in mind as I explain how heredity works and how human traits are inherited. I have attempted to clarify complex processes and, wherever possible, to use nontechnical terms. But I have avoided simplification. Too often, human inheritance is explained to the layperson only in terms of simple patterns of inheritance—autosomal dominant, autosomal recessive, or X-linked inheritance. Thus, many people believe (incorrectly) that blue eyes is a simple recessive trait or that left-handedness is inherited in a straightforward fashion. Unfortunately, the inheritance of most human traits is more complex. Even the layperson must master the concepts of penetrance, genetic heterogeneity, and multifactorial interactions to understand his or her own inheritance. One of the themes that I hope the book conveys is that many human traits are genetic, but few have a simple genetic basis.

The book should not be used as a "do-it-yourself" guide to genetic counseling. I have attempted to help the reader understand how inheritance works and to appreciate that many common traits and diseases are influenced by genes. Where possible, I have attempted to give a brief account of the genetics of human traits, and some idea of the chances of passing the traits on. However, I have repeatedly emphasized the complexities of many genetic diseases and the importance of seeking counsel from a physician or genetic counselor when such a disorder runs in the family. At the back of the book I have provided an extensive list of genetic centers where genetic counseling and prenatal diagnosis are available.

The Family Genetic Sourcebook can be a valuable companion for genetic counseling, but should not serve as a substitute for it.

"The Catalog of Genetic Traits" is far from a complete listing of all human traits and diseases with a genetic basis; thousands of human traits and disorders are influenced by genes, but only a few could be included. I have omitted many classical genetic diseases because they are rare and will be of little interest to the average reader. I have tried to discuss traits that many people have questions about and traits that I think the reader will find interesting. In addition, my hope is that the traits included will convey to the reader a sense of the diversity of human traits that are influenced by genes. There are hundreds of other genetic traits that I would have liked to discuss, but limitations of space prevented their inclusion.

This book has been made possible by the contributions of numerous people. Ray Canham and Jeffry Mitton stimulated my initial interest in heredity and helped shape my professional development as a population geneticist. Tom Hanks and members of the Baylor Scholarly Writing Workshop assisted in the improvement of my writing skills. Sharon Conry, George Hudock, Ricki Lewis, Amanda Pierce, J. Rush Pierce Sr., and J. Rush Pierce Jr. read initial drafts of the book and made valuable suggestions on content, organization, style, and clarity. J. Rush Pierce Sr. and J. Rush Pierce Jr. shared with me their medical expertise concerning many of the diseases included in the catalog. Marlene Tyrrell carefully edited the entire book, greatly improving its readability. Ted Scheffler, David Sobel, Nancy Woodruff at John Wiley & Sons, and Bob Cooper at Spectrum Publisher Services expertly guided the book through its inception, development, and publication. Finally, I wish to thank my family—Marlene, Sarah, and Michael—for their encouragement, their patience, their unending support.

Benjamin A. Pierce

CONTENTS

Chapter 1

GENES, HEREDITY, AND HUMAN AFFAIRS

Albinism in the Hopi Indians

On the edge of the Painted Desert in northern Arizona rises a large flat-topped mountain called Black Mesa, the home of the Hopi Indian tribe. Fingerlike projections of the mesa extend down into the surrounding desert, and perched alongside and on top of the barren mesa rocks are 11 Hopi villages. In spite of their small size and isolation, many of the villages are quite old. One village, Oraibi, was established in 1150 A.D. and is one of the oldest continually occupied settlements in North America.

Ales Hrdlička, a physician and anthropologist, visited the Hopi villages of Black Mesa in 1900 and made a startling observation: Among the normally dark-skinned inhabitants of the villages were 11 white people —not fair-skinned Caucasians, but white Hopis. These peculiar Indians were albinos; they suffered from a disorder that prevents the formation of pigment in the skin, hair, and eyes. Albinism is a genetic disorder, a disease caused by a defective gene. Genes are the fundamental units of heredity, consisting of pieces of chemical information that determine our traits, and they pass from parent to offspring at the moment of conception. No one knows exactly how many genes we possess, but a rough estimate is around 100,000. Among this vast inventory of genetic information is a gene that codes for pigmentation. In an albino, that gene is defective.

Albinism actually comes in several varieties. In the most severe form, pigment is never produced. Albinos with this condition possess completely white skin and hair, lacking even a trace of pigment. In another type, the genetic defect greatly reduces pigmentation, but slight coloring of the skin, hair, and eyes frequently occurs with age; this less severe form of albinism is the type found among the Hopis. Besides influencing pigmentation, the gene that causes albinism produces other effects. For example, nystagmus, a condition that involves jerky movements of the eyeballs, is common, and many albinos are legally blind. The skin of an albino is also extremely sensitive to sunlight, so sunburning is a constant problem, and skin cancer occurs frequently.

Albinism is not unique to the Hopis. In fact, albinos occur in all human races, and human albinos are mentioned in ancient writings. The Hopis are remarkable, not because albinos are present among members of the tribe, but because this genetic trait occurs in incredibly high frequency among the inhabitants of certain Hopi villages. In 1900, when Hrdlička visited Black Mesa, the frequency of albinos was 1 out of every 182 Hopis. Almost 70 years later, in 1969, 26 albinos were found on the reservation, giving a frequency of 1 in 231 inhabitants. The incidence of albinism among other human groups is much lower: only about 1/40,000 in North American whites, or 200 times less frequent than in the Hopi Indians. The frequency in other races varies somewhat, but albinism is usually quite rare. Why is this genetic trait so much more common in the Hopis than among other people? Studies carried out in the 1960s by Charles Woolf and Frank Dukepoo of Arizona State University suggest that the answer to this question lies in the unique place that albinos occupy in the Hopi culture and heritage.

Unlike people with genetic defects in many societies, albinos have always been given high regard in the Hopi community. Traditionally, the tribe completely accepted the albinos and considered them to be smart, clean, and pretty. Many Hopis associated the whiteness of an albino with purity. Albinos performed in Hopi ceremonies and, in the past, assumed positions of leadership as chiefs and priests. They were seen as a special part of the Hopi heritage—the presence of many albinos in one's village was regarded as a desirable sign of racial purity.

In the hot arid environment of the Southwest, sensitivity to the sun can be an incapacitating trait, and albinos are extremely vulnerable to sunburning. However, albinos in the Hopi community received special consideration. The Hopis have farmed for centuries, working fields of corn and vegetables below the mesa. Traditionally, all the Hopi men and boys would leave the villages each day and go to the fields to work, returning only after sundown. Because of their sensitivity to the sun, male albinos were apparently excused from this labor. Instead of working the fields, they remained behind with the women of the village, performing tasks such as weaving, cooking, and cleaning. Woolf and Dukepoo suggest that by remaining in the village during the day, albino men had more opportunities for sexual activity with the women of the tribe. Perhaps in this way the genes for albinism were spread throughout the village and reached such a high frequency. We cannot be certain that this is the sole reason that albinos are so common among the Hopi people, but the facts

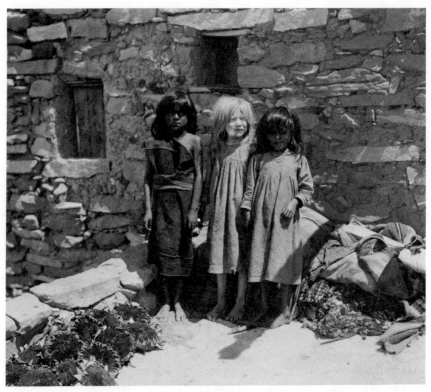

Figure 1.1.   Three Hopi Indian girls, taken about 1900. The girl in the center is an albino. (Field Museum of Natural History [Neg# 118], Chicago.)

are consistent with this explanation. Even if other factors are involved, there is little doubt that the special status accorded the albino in Hopi culture has contributed to the high frequency of albino genes in that culture.

How Genes Influence Our Lives

Albinism in the Hopi Indians illustrates how possessing a single gene can profoundly affect one's life. In the Hopi culture, an albino was set apart, given special status, and provided with a different role in society—all because of a single genetic difference. Of course, most of us are not albinos. Nevertheless, the genes we do possess mark us in ways that may have just as great an impact. Genes determine our height, our weight, and our looks—all of which influence how others react to us and how we view ourselves. Genes influence our physical strength, and they affect our susceptibility to many diseases and psychiatric disorders. They even play a role in shaping our intelligence.

To be sure, genes don't completely run our lives; we are not simply robots blindly following the programmed instructions of our genes. There is little doubt that genes do point us in certain directions, however, making us more susceptible to some influences and less susceptible to others. Consider hereditary predisposition to alcoholism. A large number of studies demonstrate that genes influence addiction to alcohol, and alcoholism tends to run in families. If your father was an alcoholic, you are more likely to become an alcoholic yourself, even if you were adopted into a foster home at birth and never met your father. In fact, sons of hospitalized alcoholic fathers are four times more likely to become alcoholic than those without an alcoholic father, even when both groups are reared by nonalcoholic foster parents. So genes affect alcoholism, but there is no gene that forces anyone to drink. Genes may make us susceptible to alcohol abuse; they may increase or decrease our "risk" of becoming an alcoholic. Our free will is also involved, however, and the vast majority of sons and daughters of alcoholic fathers never become alcoholics themselves. We don't yet know *how* genes affect our susceptibility to alcoholism. Perhaps the genes promote certain personality types, and these personalities are more likely to become dependent on alcohol. Perhaps genes influence how we metabolize alcohol, which in turn affects our tendency to overdrink. It doesn't really matter how genes do this, although the question is certainly interesting; more important is recognizing that our susceptibility to alcoholism is influenced by our genes.

Heredity and Health

One way genes affect us is by influencing our health. Most of us will personally suffer from several major diseases during our lifetime, and disease constantly touches those around us. However, few of us think much about genetic diseases. We may know someone who has a child with Down syndrome or a child with a birth defect, but, in general, we think of genetic diseases as rare disorders that affect other people. To some extent this notion is true. Many genetic diseases are rare, particularly those with devastating effects in newborns and children. Down syndrome, the most common of the chromosomal disorders, occurs with a frequency of only about 1 in 800 births (though the frequency in older mothers is considerably higher). Phenylketonuria (PKU) is one of the more common inborn errors of metabolism, and most states require testing of newborns for this genetic disease. Yet the occurrence of PKU is only about 1 in 11,000 births among whites in the United States, and the frequency in blacks is even less. Most of the other classic genetic diseases that we hear about also occur at low frequencies: sickle cell disease arises in 1 out of 600 black births in this country; cystic fibrosis occurs in 1 in 2,000 to 1 in 6,000 white births; hemophilia, or bleeder's disease, appears in 1 out of every 10,000 male births; Tay-Sachs disease has a frequency of only about 1 in 360,000 births in the general population. (But the frequency of these diseases may be much higher in certain ethnic groups; for example, Tay-Sachs disease is about 100 times more common in Ashkenazi Jews, occurring with a frequency of 1 in 3,600 births.)

These classic hereditary diseases, all with a simple genetic basis, are uncommon. Without a family history of the disease, their occurrence in our own children is very unlikely. What is seldom recognized is that many common diseases, including some of the leading causes of death in modern society, are also influenced by our genes. For example, many types of heart disease have a genetic basis. Predispositions to diabetes and to some forms of cancer are inherited. Depression, schizophrenia, and manic-depressive illness are partly genetic. Even obesity, one of the major health problems of our culture, is influenced by genes. The hereditary basis of these diseases is more complicated than that of the classical genetic disorders, and environmental factors are also important. There is little doubt, however, that our susceptibility to these medical problems is affected by our genetic constitution.

Let us consider the genetic history of disease in a typical American family. John and Cathy live in a large midwestern city and are in their middle thirties. John has a degree in business; Cathy is a computer programmer. They have two children: Michael, who is four and Amanda, two. John and Cathy are in good health and both of their children were born with no major medical problems. John and Cathy recently visited their family physician. In discussing their medical histories, the doctor asked whether any genetic diseases occurred in their families. Cathy and John quickly answered no.

However, upon examination of their family histories, we find evidence of a number of genetically influenced diseases and disorders. John has two brothers, both of whom are asthmatics; asthma has a hereditary component. John's father suffers from high blood pressure, and John's uncle died at age 42 of a heart attack following a history of high blood pressure. Several of John's relatives have been hospitalized for depression. Cathy's grandfather developed a hereditary tremor, an uncontrollable shaking of the hands, late in his life, and this trait is already apparent in two of Cathy's brothers. Her father suffers from glaucoma; Cathy's sister and mother both have thyroid diseases. All of these diseases and disorders found in Cathy and John's families are partly hereditary in nature.

John and Cathy might be dismayed by this information, and they might feel that they are particularly unlucky in regard to the genes they carry. However, these are all common medical problems, and we could probably find a similar list of genetic diseases in nearly everyone's family. The point is that all of us carry genes that will affect our health and all of us are susceptible to some genetic diseases. This does not mean that we will develop the diseases or that our children will have them; we simply have a greater chance of getting the diseases than does the average person in the general population. A geneticist would say that John and Cathy, along with their children, are at "greater risk" for developing some of these diseases.

We cannot change the genes we inherit, but we can recognize our susceptibility to certain traits and act to minimize the chance of developing problems. Most of the common genetic diseases—heart disease, cancer, diabetes, alcoholism, psychiatric illnesses—are influenced by environmental factors as well as genes. Although we cannot alter our genetic predisposition, frequently we can change some of the environmental contributors. For example, if you have a long family history of alcoholism, you would do well to limit your alcohol consumption; if high blood pressure runs in your family, you should have regular physical checkups and follow your physician's advice concerning diet and exercise.

Hemophilia in European Royalty

Genes not only shape our personal lives; sometimes they influence the course of history as well. The appearance of hemophilia in the royal families of Europe illustrates the importance of heredity in the course of human events. Hemophilia, or bleeder's disease, is a rare disorder in which the blood fails to clot—even a bruise can lead to internal bleeding and death. Several forms of hemophilia exist; the one appearing among European royalty was X-linked, which means that the gene causing the disease is located on a particular structure called the X chromosome.

At this point, I need to digress briefly and discuss how we inherit a gene like the one causing hemophilia. The genes we possess come in pairs—each of us actually has two genes for each genetically determined trait. The reason for this is obvious after a moment's reflection: One gene of the pair is inherited from our mother and the other from our father. The two genes that we inherit for a trait may be alike or they may differ, but together they determine the trait. Consider the genes that cause hemophilia. All females have a pair of genes that normally produce a substance required for blood clotting. (Actually a number of gene pairs are involved in different aspects of the clotting process, but for simplicity I will consider only a single pair.) Most women have two normal genes and produce plenty of the blood-clotting factor. Occasionally, a female is born with one gene that codes for the clotting substance and one defective gene that fails to produce the substance (the hemophilia gene). In this case, the woman produces less of the blood-clotting substance, since she has only one functional gene, but that one gene still produces enough of the substance to prevent hemophilia. Thus, the woman with one normal gene and one hemophilia gene will not have hemophilia, but she can still pass the defective gene on to her children; such a person is called a *carrier*. For a female to have hemophilia, she must possess two defective hemophilia genes: one inherited from her mother and one from her father. With two defective genes, no clotting substance is produced, and the woman is a bleeder. When two copies of the gene are required for the trait to be expressed, the gene is said to be *recessive*.

Up to this point, I have purposely confined our discussion of genes and hemophilia to females, because the situation is more complicated in males. The genes are located on structures called *chromosomes*. Most cells of the human body possess 46 chromosomes (notable exceptions are the eggs and sperm), which come in 23 pairs. One of the pairs consists of the sex chromosomes, so called because the sexes are different at this chromosome pair: females have two X-shaped chromosomes, which are appropriately called X chromosomes, and males possess one X chromosome and a smaller chromosome called the Y. Recall that hemophilia is X-linked, meaning that the gene for blood clotting is located on the X chromosome. The X chromosome carries genes that are important in both males and females, but the inheritance of these genes differs between the sexes, because males and females have different numbers of X chromosomes. All females possess two X chromosomes, one inherited from the mother and one from the father, and thus in females, X-linked genes come in pairs. However, males have only a single X chromosome, which they always inherit from their mother; in order to be male they must inherit their father's Y chromosome. The point I want to emphasize, is that because males have only a single X chromosome, they possess only a single gene for X-linked traits such as hemophilia. If that single gene produces the clotting substance, the male will be free of hemophilia; on the other hand, if the gene is defective, no clotting substance is produced and he will be hemophilic. Although two defective genes must be present for a female to have hemophilia, only a single gene is required in the male; consequently, hemophilia is more common in males than females. In the chapters that follow, I will present a more detailed explanation of how sex is determined and how X-linked traits are inherited. For now, let us return to the history of hemophilia in European royalty.

Most likely, a gene for hemophilia first appeared in the English royal family in 1819, when Victoria Alexandrina was born to the Duke of Kent and the Princess of Saxe-Coburg. Victoria, later Queen of England and ruler of the British Empire for over 60 years, was a carrier of hemophilia; that is, she carried a defective gene for hemophilia, but did not have the disease herself, because she also carried a normal gene for the blood-clotting factor. Victoria bore nine children. One, Leopold, was hemophilic and died at age 31; before his death, he passed on the gene for hemophilia to his daughter. At least two of Victoria's daughters also inherited the gene, but like their mother were unaffected carriers. Through intermarriage of the royal families of Europe, the gene was eventually passed into the royal houses of Germany, Russia, and Spain. In all, ten male descendants of Victoria suffered from hemophilia, and most bled to death at an early age.

The most famous of the royal hemophiliacs was Alexis, born to the Russian Tsar Nicholas II and Alexandra, granddaughter of Queen Victoria. Unknowingly, Alexandra was a carrier of the hemophilia gene. Alexis was her first-born son and male heir to the Russian throne: When he was born in 1904 there was great rejoicing throughout the royal family. Almost immediately, however, Nicholas and Alexandra learned that their son possessed hemophilia—an incurable hereditary disease. The child suffered terribly from the disorder: Minor injuries frequently produced internal hemorrhaging and excruciating pain. His parents for-

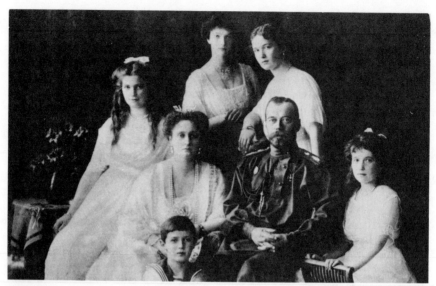

Figure 1.2.   Tsar Nicholas II and Alexandra of Russia and their children. Alexis, seated beneath Alexandra, suffered from hemophilia, a genetic disease. (The Bettmann Archive.)

bade him to participate in sports and other physical activities that might endanger his life, but scrapes and bruises were inevitable. Alexis went through one crisis after another, and his physicians were frequently helpless to stop his bleeding.

Like most parents with a seriously ill child, Nicholas and Alexandra worried constantly about Alexis and were greatly distressed by his illness and suffering. Alexandra experienced tremendous guilt, and she and Nicholas felt powerless in his bleeding crises. In desperation, they turned to a mystic and monk named Rasputin. Under Rasputin's care, Alexis recovered from several serious bleeding episodes, and Rasputin consequently gained considerable influence over the royal family. At this time, the Russian people revolted, eventually overthrowing the Tsar and ushering in a Marxist state in Russia. Nicholas, Alexandra, and the entire royal family, including Alexis, were executed by the Bolsheviks on July 17, 1918.

Historians have argued that Rasputin's influence on the royal family and the Tsar's distraction with his son's hemophilia paved the way for the Russian Revolution. Perhaps a more peaceful transfer of power might have taken place had Alexis not been sick. Undoubtedly numerous factors, many of them deeply embedded in the fabric of Russian culture and history, contributed to the uprising of the Russian people. It would be wrong to attribute the Russian Revolution entirely to the presence of one sick child. Nevertheless, a gene for hemophilia, passed down four generations from Queen Victoria to Alexis, deeply affected the lives of Nicholas and Alexandra and played a significant role in the history of world events.

The Historical Roots of Genetics

Heredity in Early Human Cultures

The study of genetics and human heredity is a very young science, being entirely a product of the twentieth century. In fact, the word *gene* did not appear until 1909. Nevertheless, human understanding of heredity and the use of genetic principles extends back more than 10,000 years, to when the first plants and animals were being domesticated for agricultural purposes. The process of domestication required an understanding of heredity. Among the wild plants and animals of nature, many individual differences occurred. Early humans selected those individual plants and animals with desirable traits, and by interbreeding them, they produced offspring with more of the same traits. Continuing this process for many generations, they gradually converted wild plants and animals into the domesticated varieties that made agriculture possible. The success of domestication indicates that early human cultures understood a simple, but important rule of heredity: "like breeds like."

Ancient writings provide evidence that early societies also displayed a keen interest in human heredity and that people recognized the genetic nature of human traits thousands of years ago. Hindu sacred books dating back 2,000 years attribute the characteristics of children primarily to the father, but differences between a son and his father were thought to result from the influence of the mother. These writings also provide rules for choosing a spouse, suggesting that women from a family with undesirable traits should be avoided. The ancient Greeks displayed a thorough knowledge of human heredity, evidence of which permeates their poetic and philosophical literature. The Talmud, a book of Jewish civil and religious laws based on oral traditions going back thousands of years, describes in some detail the pattern of inheritance for hemophilia. It states that if a woman bears two sons who died of bleeding following circumcision, any additional sons should not be circumcised. Furthermore, the sons of her sisters must not be circumcised, but the sons of her brothers should. This is sound genetic advice based on the X-linked inheritance of hemophilia.

Gregor Mendel, Father of Genetics

Although the notion that traits are inherited has been an essential part of agriculture for thousands of years, and even though ancient civilizations recognized that human characteristics were passed from parent to child, the precise mechanism of inheritance remained unknown until 1865. On February 8 of that year a young Augustinian monk named Gregor Mendel stood before the Natural Science Society of Brünn (now Brno in Czechoslovakia) and described a series of genetic experiments he had conducted on pea plants grown in the monastery garden. With elegance and simplicity, Mendel outlined his conclusion that traits in pea plants were determined by two factors, one inherited from the female parent and one from the male parent. He explained how these two factors separated when the sex cells (eggs and pollen in plants) were formed, one factor going into each sex cell. When sex cells fused in the process of fertilization, the factor from the pollen united with the factor from the egg, and together they determined the trait of the offspring. Mendel also recognized that chance determined which one of the two factors an offspring inherited from its mother and which one of the two factors it inherited from its father; this role of chance produced distinctive ratios of traits in the offspring.

Mendel spoke again of his work at the next meeting of the society on March 8; following that meeting the secretary of the Natural Science Society asked Mendel to publish the text of his report in the journal of the society's proceedings. The article appeared in print the following year, in 1866. There was considerable interest in his work among those who heard the lectures, but, surprisingly, none of the participants recognized the far-reaching implications of his conclusions. Even more puzzling was the minimal response by the scientific community to the publication of his results. The journal containing his report was sent to 133 other associations of scientists in a number of different countries, and many scientists at that time were conducting experiments on plant breeding.

Nevertheless, no one seemed to notice that Mendel had discovered the key to inheritance.

Mendel continued his genetics experiments for several years, publishing another paper on the subject in 1870. He also carried out a number of other scientific investigations, including horticultural studies of flowers and fruit trees, research with honey bees, and extensive weather observations. In 1868 Mendel was elected abbot of the monastery at Brünn, and his ecclesiastical and administrative duties increased. Several years later, the government increased the tax levied on the monastery property, and, on principle, Mendel refused to pay. The ensuing controversy drained away Mendel's time and health, and he died in his sleep on January 6, 1884.

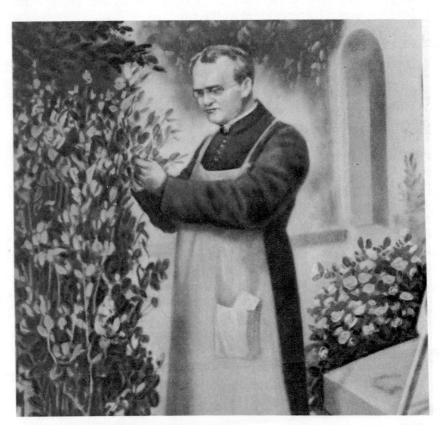

Figure 1.3. Gregor Mendel, an Augustinian monk, who first discovered the principles of heredity.

Mendel's discovery remained buried in the scientific literature for 35 years. Around the turn of the century, three botanists—Hugo de Vries, a Dutch scientist; Erich von Tschermak, working in Vienna; and Carl Correns, in Tubingen—all began to conduct breeding experiments on plants. Working independently of one another, they repeated experiments of the type that Mendel had carried out 35 years earlier, and they observed the same characteristic ratios in the offspring of their crosses that Mendel had seen. In the process of analyzing and writing up their results, they happened to locate Mendel's 1866 paper on inheritance in pea plants. All three scientists immediately interpreted their own results in terms of Mendel's rules of inheritance and published their results in 1900 with reference to Mendel's work. With the appearance of these three papers in 1900, Mendel's pioneering work in genetics was finally appreciated; today he is generally recognized as the father of genetics.

Archibald Garrod and Genetic Diseases

Following the rediscovery of Mendel's work in 1900, a growing number of biologists began to study heredity. They applied his principles to the inheritance of other organisms, demonstrating that Mendel's rules worked not just for pea plants, but also for mice, fruit flies, chickens, guinea pigs, corn, wheat, and virtually every organism studied. The first person to apply Mendel's principles to human traits was Sir Archibald Garrod, an English physician and biochemist. Garrod had been interested in a peculiar disease called *alkaptonuria*. Individuals with alkaptonuria are easily recognized, for their urine turns black upon exposure to air. They also suffer from arthritis, particularly in the spine, but this fact was not recognized in Garrod's time. Garrod became intrigued with the biochemistry of this disorder. What caused the urine of an alkaptonuric to turn black? In the course of his studies he noticed that although the disease is rare, several children of a single family were often affected with alkaptonuria. Furthermore, the parents of such children were always free from the disease, but frequently were first cousins. Garrod recognized that these observations were consistent with Mendel's theory, and he concluded in 1902 that alkaptonuria was a genetic disease.

Later, Garrod observed the same pattern of inheritance in three other human disorders: albinism, which involves a defect in the pigmentation (discussed earlier in this chapter); *cystinuria*, a disorder in which an amino acid called cystine is excreted in the urine, forming crystals and stones in the urinary tract; and *pentosuria*, a harmless metabolic disorder characterized by excretion of a special sugar in the urine. Garrod went on to suggest that each of these genetic diseases results from a defect in a specific protein. Far ahead of his time, Garrod proposed that each gene codes for a protein, and if a *mutation* (a genetic accident) occurs in the gene, then the protein will be absent and the disease symptoms will result. His idea that genes code for proteins turned out to be correct, and of fundamental importance, but like Mendel's his contribution was not appreciated for many years.

During the first half of the twentieth century, geneticists working on fruit flies, corn, bacteria, and other organisms made great strides in our understanding of genes and heredity. There was considerable interest in the chemical structure of genes, and several studies hinted that a substance called *DNA* was the source of all genetic information. DNA is shorthand for deoxyribonucleic acid, a long, elegantly spiraled molecule that is found in all living cells. Although DNA appeared to be important to heredity, the physical structure of the DNA molecule remained unknown, and so molecular studies of genes were impossible. Over the years, researchers had unearthed a number of important clues about the chemistry of DNA, but no one knew exactly how to fit these clues together into a coherent model of DNA structure.

The Rise of Molecular Genetics

The science of molecular genetics was born in 1953, when James Watson, a postdoctoral student from the United States, and Francis Crick, a graduate student at Cambridge University in England, unraveled the structure of the DNA molecule. Using intuition and creativity, these two scientists put together the available information about the chemistry of DNA to produce a molecular model of DNA that turned out to be correct in almost all aspects. Watson and Crick showed that DNA consisted of a long series of units, called *nucleotides*, linked end to end. The nucleotides came in four types, which are now commonly abbreviated by the letters A, T, G, and C. Watson and Crick proposed that genetic information was encoded within the sequence of nucleotides, with the four types of nucleotides (A,T,G, and C) serving as code letters. Scientists now understood what genetic information looked like at the molecular level, and they began to study the molecular biology of the gene.

At first, advances in molecular genetics occurred at a modest rate. How genetic information was encoded in the DNA had yet to be worked out. The processes involved in transmitting the DNA to future generations were unknown, and exactly how the DNA determined a trait was still a mystery. All these problems required new techniques and procedures for manipulating and observing the genes at the molecular level. As new techniques developed, and as more information about the molecular nature of genes accumulated, the pace of new discoveries and insights quickened.

Recombinant DNA

In 1973, 20 years after Watson and Crick's landmark discovery, four scientists working in a laboratory in California conducted an experiment that would fundamentally alter the way genetic research was conducted. Stanley Cohen and Annie Chang, from Stanford University School of Medicine, and Herbert Boyer and R. B. Helling, at the University of California School of Medicine at San Francisco, constructed a novel form of DNA by splicing together two pieces of DNA from different sources. They then implanted this new DNA molecule into a bacterial cell. What they created was a genetically distinct organism that had never before existed. Very quickly, the researchers succeeded in using these same techniques to transfer genes between two different forms of bacteria, and they then transferred genes from a frog into a bacterial cell. They called their new DNA molecules *chimeras*, after the mythological Chimera, which possessed the head of a lion, the body of a goat, and the tail of a serpent.

These techniques for splicing DNA and transferring genes rapidly attained widespread use and have proven to be among the most powerful experimental tools in all of science. Usually called *recombinant DNA* by scientists, but also referred to as *gene cloning, gene transfer,* or *genetic engineering,* the methods involve cutting the DNA apart at specific places, modifying and reassembling it, and then placing it back into a cell. In many cases a gene is placed inside bacterial cells, and the bacteria are then used as gene factories to mass-produce a specific fragment of the DNA. With large quantities of a gene, scientists can examine its structure, study the way it functions, and transfer it into cells of other organisms.

The ability to carry out genetic manipulations allowed scientists directly to alter the DNA—in essence, to create artificially designed genes. With this capability, questions in genetic research previously impossible to address could now be studied with relative ease. Within a few years, information about the nature of genetic information was pouring forth at an incredible rate, and the new findings changed some of our most fundamental concepts about genes and how they work. In addition to using these techniques in genetic research, biologists began to apply them to problems in other fields of biology, such as development, evolution, physiology, and neurobiology. In these areas, recombinant DNA has also yielded spectacular advances; the new technology is currently revolutionizing the entire field of biology.

Recombinant DNA technology also promises to be a major economic force. In 1976 the first biotechnology company, Genentech, was formed to develop commercial applications from recombinant DNA methods; now, 350 to 400 biotech companies are in business. Many pharmaceutical, oil, chemical, agricultural, and food-processing companies are currently using recombinant DNA techniques to develop new products, such as crops that produce their own pesticides, bacteria that consume toxic wastes, and vaccines against malaria. Several products produced by these methods are already on the market, and sales in the field are projected to exceed one billion dollars annually by 1990. John Naisbitt, author of *Megatrends* (a best-selling book on future economic and social trends), predicts that biotechnology will be to the coming twenty years what electronics has been for the past twenty years.

A Revolution in Human Genetics

While developments in molecular genetics and genetic engineering have been attracting public attention, a quieter but perhaps more significant transformation has been taking place in the science of human heredity. New techniques in molecular genetics have certainly contributed much to this revolution, yet important developments in several other areas have also made significant contributions. Diagnostic procedures, such as ultrasound technology, biochemical assays, hormone tests, and chorionic villus sampling, have greatly improved our ability to detect genetic diseases. Microscopic study of chromosomes has now reached a fine art, and computer-driven machines are used to quickly analyze large numbers of chromosomes. Powerful computer programs have been developed that analyze patterns of inheritance in families, a technique called *complex segregation analysis.*

Let's consider complex segregation analysis. This technique has recently been used to study the inheritance of a number of diseases and disorders. For example, leprosy is an age-old disease caused by a bacterium. The disease was well known in biblical times and even today it affects about 13 million people worldwide. In its severest form, leprosy can produce paralysis, disfigurement, and blindness, but people infected with leprosy exhibit a variety of responses. Some people have no obvious symptoms, some are mildly affected, and others are grossly disfigured by the disease. Physicians have noticed that members of some families are vulnerable to leprosy infection, whereas members of other families appear to be relatively immune. This observation suggests that genes play some role in susceptibility to the leprosy bacteria. However, no specific pattern of inheritance is obvious. Geneticists have recently applied complex segregation analysis to leprosy in an attempt to determine if genes are involved in the disease. One such study was conducted on 27 families from the island of Desirade. This small Caribbean island has one of the highest frequencies of leprosy in the world. For over 200 years, all people with leprosy from a number of surrounding islands were deported to Desirade. When the leper colony was closed in 1959, most of the leprosy patients remained on the island. In 1984, 53 islanders with leprosy were examined, and their family histories were recorded. Complex segregation analysis using computers was then applied to the information. The results indicated that genes are important to leprosy infection; susceptibility to the disease is probably controlled by a single gene. Although genes may influence one's susceptibility to leprosy, leprosy should not be considered a genetic disease—it is caused by bacteria, and one cannot contract leprosy unless exposed to the bacteria.

The technique of complex segregation analysis, which was impossible before the advent of modern computers, is now providing valuable insight into the genetic basis of breast cancer, colon cancer, heart disease, birth defects, depression, and numerous other diseases and disorders.

Complex segregation analysis is just one of many new developments that are rapidly expanding our knowledge of human heredity. Advances in molecular genetics are also being applied to problems in human genetics. Along with numerous other applications, molecular techniques are helping to determine where genes are located on the chromosomes; using this approach a number of genes for important hereditary diseases have been located within the past five years. Genes for muscular dystrophy, neurofibromatosis, chronic granulomatosis disease, Huntington's disease, polycistic kidney disease, cystic fibrosis, and Alzheimer's disease have now been mapped to specific chromosomes. Finding the particular chromosome where a gene resides is significant, because once the chromosomal location of a disease-causing gene has been established, geneticists can narrow their focus, find the gene itself, and isolate it. The gene can then be transferred to bacterial cells with recombinant DNA techniques and produced in large quantities, allowing the gene to be studied in detail. Information from such studies may eventually tell us how the symptoms of the disease arise and may suggest strategies for treatment.

Recent developments in the study of Duchenne muscular dystrophy illustrate the power of this approach. Duchenne muscular dystrophy is one of the most common of the inherited muscle disorders; it has devastating effects on the patient and his family. Like hemophilia, the disease is X-linked and therefore occurs mostly in males. A child with this disorder appears completely normal at birth; the subtle symptoms of the disease are not noticeable until about age three. At first, a boy with Duchenne muscular dystrophy may have difficulty getting up from the floor or climbing stairs. Stumbling becomes more and more frequent. The child experiences muscle weakness that gets progressively worse, and eventually he loses the ability to walk. Most boys with Duchenne muscular dystrophy die before reaching their twentieth birthday.

Duchenne muscular dystrophy was first described in 1852, but until recently the biochemical cause of the disease remained a mystery. Even today no cure or even therapy for slowing the disease is available. Within the last three years, however, rapid progress has resulted from the application of molecular techniques to the study of this disease. The gene's location on the X chromosome was recognized a number of years ago from its distinctive pattern of X-linked inheritance. Assigning it to a precise place on the X chromosome, however, was not accomplished until 1983, when molecular techniques were combined with family studies of the disease. Three years later, in 1986, DNA from the muscular dystrophy gene was isolated and cloned in a bacterial cell. With the cloned gene, scientists were able to compare the DNA of patients with Duchenne muscular dystrophy with that of normal individuals. This research quickly indicated that the muscular dystrophy gene consists of a defective piece of DNA; the corresponding DNA from a normal individual produces a protein essential for proper muscle development. Those with Duchenne muscular dystrophy have a defective copy of this normal gene and therefore fail to produce the essential protein. This much was clear from examination of the DNA itself, but the essential protein involved in the disease was still unknown. Only five months later, however, biologists had discovered the protein and named it *dystrophin*.

With dystrophin in hand, a number of important facts about Duchenne muscular dystrophy became apparent. Normal individuals have dystrophin, but the protein is absent in those with Duchenne muscular dystrophy. Even in normal individuals, dystrophin is present only in tiny

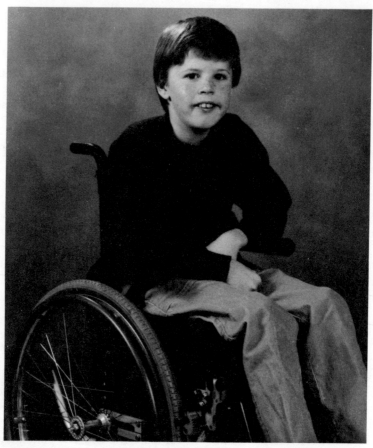

Figure 1.4.   A 15-year-old boy with Duchenne muscular dystrophy, a hereditary muscle disorder. Recent advances in molecular genetics have identified the
primary defect in this disease. (Courtesy of the Muscular Dystrophy Association.)

amounts, but this small amount of dystrophin plays a critical role in the
functioning of the muscle. Exactly how the absence of dystrophin produces the symptoms of Duchenne muscular dystrophy is not yet clear.
However, medical scientists now know the basic defect that causes the
disease, and this knowledge may suggest possible therapies for treating
patients of Duchenne muscular dystrophy.

For many diseases such as Duchenne muscular dystrophy, development of a rational therapy for coping with the disease is not possible until

the molecular basis of the disorder is known. The rapid advances in our knowledge of Duchenne muscular dystrophy were unimaginable even ten years ago. The muscular dystrophy story is not unique—similar advances are taking place in dozens of other genetic diseases, and hundreds of genetic traits in humans are now under study.

Another recent breakthrough has been the development of diagnostic tests for detecting disease-causing genes. Consider Huntington disease. Huntington disease is a severe genetic disorder that usually first appears in middle age. The disease causes progressive loss of control over muscle movement, memory, and other mental functions. It frequently lasts 15 years or more and may lead to insanity. Eventually the person with Huntington disease dies—there is no cure or even treatment for arresting the mental deterioration.

Huntington disease is named after George Huntington, a physician who gave an excellent description of its symptoms in 1872. Many families with Huntington disease in the northeastern part of the United States can be traced to two brothers and another relative who emigrated from England in 1630 and settled in New England. During colonial times, New Englanders branded a number of members of this family as witches, believing that the twitching, grimacing, and insanity produced by the disease were manifestations of the devil.

Huntington disease is a particularly tragic disorder. Because the symptoms do not usually appear until the thirties or forties, most affected individuals marry and produce children before they become aware of their disease. Each child of a person with Huntington disease has a 50 percent chance of inheriting the disorder, but the child will not know for certain whether they will develop the disease for many years. This uncertainty, coupled with the terrible course of the disease, creates anxiety for those who may have inherited the disease; it also makes family planning, career choices, and other personal decisions difficult. Many individuals at risk for developing Huntington disease have longed for some means of determining whether they have inherited the disorder.

These hopes were realized in 1983, when a genetic marker (an identifiable DNA sequence) close to the Huntington disease gene was found. Although the actual gene that causes Huntington disease has not, as of this writing, been isolated, the discovery of a genetic marker close to the disease gene created the possibility of determining which children of a person with Huntington disease are likely to have inherited the disorder. By examining the DNA of family members with new molecular techniques (see Chapter 6), geneticists can frequently determine who is likely to have inherited the disease gene. The test is not completely accurate, but with newly discovered genetic markers many individuals may learn that their chances of inheriting the disease are less than five percent; others may learn that their chances of inheriting the disease are greater than 95 percent. Furthermore, the test can also be applied to unborn babies.

Although about two thirds of those at risk have indicated a desire to know if they will develop Huntington disease, the use of this new genetic test raises a number of important issues. For example, those that learn they are free of the disease may be better off with this information; many will feel intense joy and relief. However, what about those who learn that they have inherited Huntington disease, an incurable disorder that will kill them after years of mental and physical disintegration? Will these people develop depression? Will their marriages dissolve? Will they attempt suicide?

Concerns about the effects of predictive testing are currently being addressed in several pilot studies. One such study is being conducted at the Johns Hopkins University School of Medicine in Baltimore. A small number of individuals who had requested predictive testing are carefully screened for psychiatric problems and for the ability to cope with the potentially bad news. Only those who are psychologically stable are allowed to undergo testing. Each person receives information about the test and psychological counseling before and after testing.

The initial results from the Johns Hopkins study have been encouraging. As might be expected, the reactions to the test results have varied from elation to sadness. In those people found likely to be free of the disease, many expressed emotions of joy and freedom. Several have become engaged, and one has had a baby. Of those who received the bad news that they probably carry the Huntington gene and will develop Huntington disease, all appear to be coping well. These individuals expressed shock and some experienced initial depression. However, there was no increase in major psychiatric illnesses and no suicide attempts. Other pilot studies in North America have obtained similar results. These short-term findings suggest that predictive testing for this disease may be practical on a large scale, provided stringent screening and psychological support are provided. However, at this point, the long-term effects are unknown. Also, the pilot studies do not address the social issues involved, such as the effect of predictive testing on insurability and employability.

Rapid advances in molecular genetics and our increasing knowledge of many inherited disorders makes genetic screening for many diseases likely in the near future. Genetic testing is already available for hemophilia, phenylketonuria, sickle cell disease, thalassemia, Duchenne muscular dystrophy, and scores of other classical genetic diseases. Scientists are also working on genetic tests to predict who has an inherited susceptibility to many common diseases such as heart disease, cancer, and diabetes. Colon cancer, for example, results from a number of genetic alterations occurring within a single cell. Most of these alterations occur sporadically or may be induced by cancer-causing agents we encounter in our environment. However, one or more of these genetic defects may be inherited, producing a predisposition to colon cancer. A person who inherits one genetic defect will not automatically get cancer, but for them fewer additional genetic changes are required for cancer to arise. Thus the person with an inherited genetic defect is at higher risk for eventually developing cancer. (See *Cancer* and *Colon and rectal cancer* in "The Catalog of Genetic Traits.") Scientists have begun to identify some of the genetic defects that produce a predisposition to colon cancer. Simple genetic tests may someday allow us to determine our predisposition to a large number of different cancers.

Genetic tests may also allow doctors to provide better treatment for those who already have a disease. In colon cancer, scientists are already examining the defective genes that are present in a patient's tumor. Patients whose tumors contain numerous genetic defects are more likely to develop additional tumors and are more likely to die from their cancer. Thus, knowledge of how many genetic defects have occurred in tumorous tissue can provide physicians with important information about how to treat colon cancer. For individuals with only a few genetic defects, surgical removal of the cancer may be sufficient treatment. However, if the cancer has acquired a number of genetic defects, more aggressive chemotherapy may be required in addition to surgery.

PKU is another genetic disease where knowledge of the genetic defect may allow better treatment. PKU results from a pair of defective genes that produce mental retardation; such retardation can be prevented if a child with the disease is put on a special diet during the first few months of life. Early detection of the disease is essential for preventing retardation, and most states now routinely screen all newborns for this genetic disorder. Detailed knowledge of the genetic defect causing PKU may also be useful in treating the disorder. For years, physicians have noticed that patients with PKU vary in their symptoms and in their response to treatment. A few patients develop normally even without a special diet; others become mentally retarded even when the special diet is begun immediately after birth. Recent molecular studies of the gene causing PKU indicate that there are a number of different ways the PKU gene can be defective. Defects in certain parts of the gene have relatively mild effects; defects in other parts produce severe mental retardation. By examining the type of genetic defect a person with PKU possesses, physicians may one day be able to tailor a specific treatment for the PKU patient that is most appropriate for their genetic defect. These techniques are still in the experimental stages, but there is little doubt that genetic tests will someday allow physicians to provide more specific and more effective treatments for many diseases.

Ultimately, geneticists want to harness the power of molecular genetics not merely to detect genetic diseases, but to treat these disorders by transferring healthy copies of genes into people with genetic diseases. Termed *gene therapy*, this approach would go to the heart of the problem —the genes themselves. It offers hope to thousands of those who suffer from untreatable genetic diseases. Just a few years ago, gene therapy was viewed as a distant, futuristic possibility. However, numerous advances in the techniques of gene transfer have taken place during the past three years, and now scientists are poised to begin gene therapy in humans.

The first gene transfer experiment involving a human in the United States took place on May 22, 1989. This first experiment was not actually therapeutic—it was not designed to treat a genetic disease. Rather, researchers inserted a special marker gene in normal white blood cells of a cancer patient to track the movement of the cells as they fight the cancer. Although not gene therapy, this experiment has proven that gene transfer can be carried out in humans; it paves the way for gene therapy in the near future.

The advances I have discussed—complex segregation analysis, molecular mapping of genes, genetic testing using DNA analysis—are a few examples of the rapid progress that is being made in the science of human genetics, progress that is bringing genetics out of the laboratory and into our everyday lives. These developments promise to affect us all. At the same time, they demand that we understand something about the nature of genes and how heredity works, so that we can use these new developments intelligently and constructively.

Chapter 2

THE NATURE OF HEREDITY

Six years ago, I spent a long night in October on the obstetrics ward of Lawrence and Memorial Hospital, awaiting the birth of our first child. Eight months earlier, Marlene and I learned that we would have an addition to our family. Like most prospective parents, we spent much of the pregnancy speculating about the baby: Was it a boy or a girl? What color were its eyes? Who would it look like?

Forty-five minutes before midnight, after 12 long hours of labor for Marlene, I saw our baby for the first time, or rather I saw a small part of her. That first glimpse of Sarah was a mere two inches of the top of her head when she crowned the birth canal. As I stared in surprise, the nurse announced "It's a redhead!" During all the time I spent conjuring up images of our future baby, I never once thought of red hair, for her mother and I both have black hair. I wasn't disappointed—it was, in fact, a beautiful head of red curls. I just never considered the possibility of a red-haired daughter.

Sarah's Red Hair: The Differences Between Genotype and Phenotype

How could Marlene and I conceive a child with red hair, when our own hair is black? If genes determine red hair, and they do, how could we pass on genes for red hair to Sarah, when neither of us possesses red hair? The answer to this question is that traits themselves are not inherited. What are inherited are the genes, chemical instructions that tell the body how to make a trait.

When my daughter Sarah was conceived, a sperm containing my genes fused with an egg carrying her mother's genes. At that moment Sarah was a single cell, barely five thousandths of an inch in diameter. She lacked hair, eyes, and nails; she didn't even possess a head. Her stomach, liver, heart, and lungs had not yet formed. In fact, she possessed not a single trait that we would recognize as human. However, she did possess genes for those traits. The genes that she inherited from her mother and me contained all the instructions necessary to construct every feature of her body, including those for how to make red hair. Over the next nine months those genes directed the development of my daughter, coding for muscles and bones, organs and skin. Ultimately, they fashioned a complete human, a person who is uniquely Sarah.

So Sarah did not inherit my traits or her mother's traits—what she inherited from us was a set of genes that then directed the development of her traits. The distinction between the genes we inherit and the traits we possess is an important one, so important, in fact, that geneticists have special terms to distinguish between them. The trait is called the *phenotype*. Red hair is a phenotype, for example. Having a genetic disease, such as cystic fibrosis, is also a phenotype, and not having the disease is another phenotype. Even behavioral traits, such as shy and aggressive, are phenotypes. Many of our phenotypes are encoded in the chemical instructions of our genes, but the genes are distinct from the phenotype. The genes that code for a particular phenotype are termed the *genotype,* and it is the genotype that is inherited. This distinction between genotype and phenotype is crucial for understanding how heredity works.

I should point out that although many phenotypes are genetically influenced, the word *phenotype* does not imply that the trait must be genetic. Indeed, many phenotypes are not determined by genes at all. For example, I have a scar on my left arm that I acquired from the smallpox vaccination I received as a child. That scar is one of my traits; it is my phenotype. The scar was not inherited, and I will not pass it on to my children. Only the genes are inherited. Traits that we acquire during our lifetime, like a vaccination scar, are not incorporated into our genes, and they will not become a part of the genetic legacy we transmit to our children.

I still have not completely answered the question I originally presented: How could two people with one trait, black hair to be specific, produce a child with an entirely different trait, such as red hair? As we have seen, part of the answer to this question is that no child ever inherits a phenotype; only the genes or coding instructions for the trait are passed on. The question then becomes: How could two parents possess genes for red hair, when their own phenotype is black hair? To address this question, we must look at how a genotype is inherited and how that genotype is translated into a phenotype.

How Our Genes Are Inherited

As we discussed briefly in Chapter 1, each of us possesses a pair of genes for a particular trait. One gene of the pair is inherited from our mother and the other comes from our father. These two genes constitute our genotype. Consider a pair of genes that determines red hair in humans. One kind of gene causes the production of red pigment in the hair; we will symbolize this gene with a small letter *r*. Another gene, symbolized with a capital *R*, produces no red pigment, so that the resulting hair color is not red. (In this case the color may be black, brown, or blond, depending upon other pairs of genes. We will ignore this complexity for now and assume that a single pair of genes determines the presence or absence of red hair.) Geneticists call these alternate forms of genes that code for a trait *alleles*. So little *r*, which codes for the presence of red hair, is an allele, and big *R*, which codes for nonred hair, is an allele. Each genotype consists of two such alleles. Those two alleles might be the same. For example, one individual's genotype might consist of two alleles for red hair, *rr*; because only alleles for red hair are present at this genotype, the individual would develop red hair. Alternatively, a person might possess two alleles that code for nonred hair (*RR*). Lacking even a single gene for red hair, this person would develop nonred hair. Genotypes such as these, consisting of two identical alleles, are said to be *homozygous*; thus, the individual with the genotype *rr* is homozygous for red hair, and the individual with *RR* is homozygous for nonred hair.

The two alleles that a person possesses at a genotype, however, need not be the same. An allele for red hair (*r*) might be inherited from the father, and an allele for nonred hair (*R*) might be inherited from the mother. This individual's genotype would be *Rr*. When the genotype consists of two different alleles, the individual is termed *heterozygous*. The phenotype exhibited by the heterozygote depends upon the way in which the two alleles interact. In some cases, the phenotype requires two copies of the allele to be expressed; such a trait is said to be *recessive*. If red hair is recessive, then only individuals with the genotype *rr* have red hair—the heterozygote *Rr* has nonred hair. Other traits are *dominant*, which means that the trait requires only a single copy of the allele to be expressed. In our example, the allele for nonred hair (*R*) is dominant to the allele for red hair (*r*), because the *Rr* heterozygote has nonred hair. In summary, when a single allele at the genotype causes the phenotype to appear, the trait is dominant; when two alleles are required, the trait is recessive.

In the process of reproduction, each parent passes on only one of the two alleles that comprise their genotype. Which allele is transmitted to the offspring is a matter of chance. For example, suppose that my geno-type is *Rr*. Each child I produce will inherit one of the two alleles at this genotype. On the average, half will inherit the *R* allele for nonred hair, and half will receive the *r* allele coding for red hair, as is illustrated in Figure 2.1. If my spouse is also heterozygous, some of our children may inherit a red allele from me and a red allele from her; their genotype will

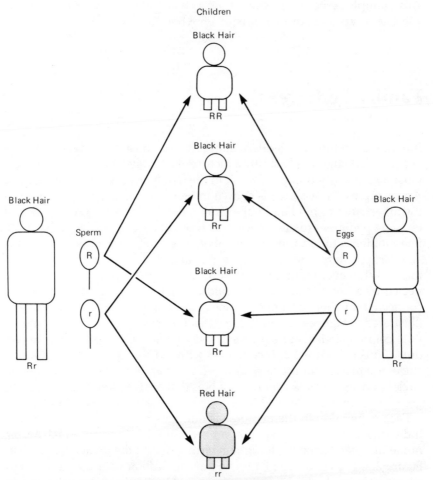

Figure 2.1.   A cross between two parents heterozygous for red hair, assuming that red hair is a recessive trait. Although both parents have black hair, an average of one out of four offspring will have red hair.

be *rr*, and they will have red hair. In this way, a child could have red hair (*rr*) and yet both parents possess nonred hair (*Rr*). Of course, other children might inherit an *R* allele from both of us, giving them the genotype *RR* with nonred hair. Our son in fact has black hair, although I have no way of knowing what his actual genotype is. Other children might receive an *R* allele from one of us and an *r* allele from the other— these children would be heterozygotes and would also possess nonred hair. The genetics of hair color is actually more complicated than I have presented here—several gene pairs are probably involved. However, this example serves to illustrate how a child's phenotype can differ from the phenotypes of both parents, even when the trait is genetic.

Family Pedigrees

Inheritance in humans is often analyzed with the aid of a device called a *pedigree*. A pedigree is basically a picture of a family history, a picture that illustrates the inheritance of a trait in the family over several generations. An example of a pedigree is shown in Figure 2.2; this pedigree outlines the inheritance of red hair in one family. In the chapters to come, we will be using pedigrees to discuss various types of inheritance, so let us take a few moments to examine the symbols used in a typical pedigree. In a standard pedigree, squares represent males, and circles represent females. Whenever mating occurs between two individuals, they are connected by a horizontal line; the children that result from the mating are connected to their parents by lines extending below the parents, as illustrated in Figure 2.2. Individuals that possess the trait are represented with colored circles and squares; those that lack the trait are left uncolored. Thus in Figure 2.2, each person with red hair is shown as a colored circle or square, and those without red hair are represented with white circles and squares. Additional symbols that are frequently used in pedigrees are shown in Figure 2.3.

Each generation in the pedigree is numbered with a Roman numeral. Individuals within each generation are numbered with normal Arabic numerals, listed from left to right in birth order. In the pedigree shown in Figure 2.2, I have included a few names to facilitate our discussion, but normally individuals are simply referenced by their numbers. For example, John is the tenth person on the third line; therefore his technical

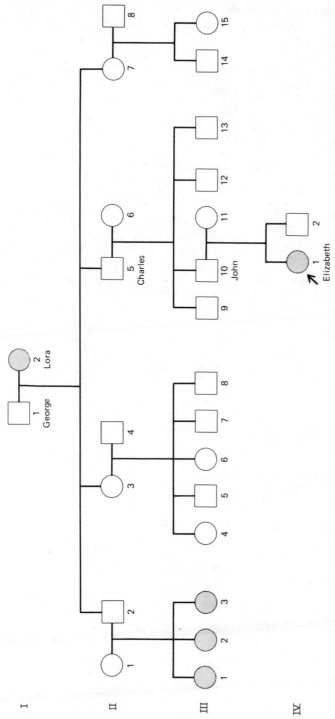

Figure 2.2. A pedigree illustrating the inheritance of red hair in one family. An explanation of the symbols used in this Figure is given in Figure 2.3.

31

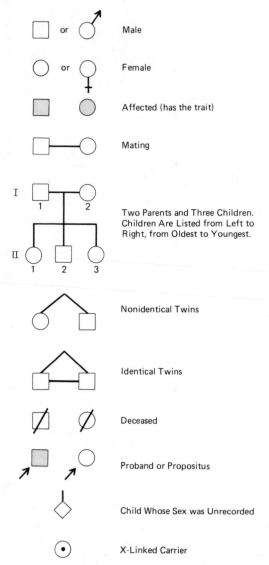

Figure 2.3.   Symbols commonly used in pedigrees.

designation within the pedigree is individual III-10. John's position in the pedigree indicates that he was the second among four boys born to his parents. The person who first prompts the creation of the pedigree is called the *proband, propositus,* or sometimes the *index case;* this person is usually indicated on the pedigree with an arrow. In Figure 2.2, Elizabeth is the proband.

Charlie Chaplin's Blood Type

Now that we understand how to read a pedigree, let's look at another example of genes that determine a phenotype. Most of us possess one of four common blood types: type A, type B, type AB, or type O. (Blood types are frequently designated as *A negative* or *O positive.* The positive and negative designations are yet another phenotype that is under separate genetic control from the ABO blood types.) What the different blood types represent are different types of chemicals, called *antigens,* that are located on the surface of our red blood cells. Blood types are important in blood transfusions because our immune system—our body's defense network—recognizes some blood types as foreign and mounts an all-out attack against any foreign antigens found in the body. The resulting immune reaction is usually severe and sometimes fatal.

The first blood transfusions involving humans were carried out in 1667 by Jean-Baptiste Denis and Paul Emmerez in Paris. On June 15, 1667, they transferred 12 ounces of blood from a lamb to a feverish young man. The man quickly recovered. Encouraged by this initial success, Denis carried out additional transfusions. His third patient, a young Swedish nobleman, received two transfusions of calf's blood and promptly died as a result of the immune reaction to the foreign animal blood. Denis's fourth patient also died, and this patient's wife charged Denis with murder. Denis was eventually cleared by the courts (it appears that the wife actually poisoned her husband with arsenic and then blamed Denis for the death), but further blood transfusions were prohibited in France and later in England.

In the 1800s, physicians began to experiment once again with blood transfusions; this time transfusions were not only attempted with animal blood, but also with human blood. However, the procedure remained risky—sometimes the patient recovered and sometimes the patient died.

Then, in 1900, an Austrian physician named Karl Landsteiner discovered the ABO blood types and showed that only certain combinations of blood were compatible. Shortly thereafter scientists discovered that the ABO blood type was a genetically determined trait.

Each person has a genotype that determines their ABO blood type. Like the previous example involving red hair, this genotype consists of two alleles. We can think of the genotype as consisting of two slots, each slot occupied by an allele. In the genotype for red hair, each slot could be occupied by either an r allele coding for red hair or an R allele coding for nonred hair. The ABO genotype is similar, except that there are more than two alleles that can potentially occupy the two slots of the genotype. In most groups of humans, three alleles are common; these are designated I^A, I^B, and i. An individual's ABO genotype would consist of any two of these alleles, so six different genotypes are possible: $I^A I^A$, $I^A i$, $I^B I^B$, $I^B i$, $I^A I^B$, and ii. Each allele consists of genetic information coding for one of the antigens, the chemical substances located on the red blood cells that determine our blood types. The I^A allele codes for a chemical called the A antigen, and likewise the I^B allele codes for a chemical called the B antigen. The i allele is different; it produces no detectable antigen. As we indicated, each individual possesses two of these three alleles at their ABO genotype. So, let us consider some possible genotypes and the blood types they produce.

If you have the genotype $I^A I^A$, you produce only A antigens—your blood type is A, as shown in Table 2.1. Similarly, if you have the genotype $I^B I^B$, you produce only B antigens, and your blood type is B. When the genotype consists of $I^A I^B$, the red blood cells possess both types of antigens—both A and B—and the blood type is called AB. Now, recall that the i allele produces no antigen. Thus, an individual homozygous for

Table 2.1 The Genetic Basis of the ABO Blood Types

Genotype	Antigen	Blood Type
$I^A I^A$	A antigen	A
$I^A i$	A antigen	A
$I^B I^B$	B antigen	B
$I^B i$	B antigen	B
$I^A I^B$	A antigen and B antigen	AB
ii	No antigen	O

i (genotype *ii*) has no ABO antigen. Their blood type is said to be O. Because *i* produces no antigen, the individual with the genotype $I^A i$ produces only A antigen and has A blood type. In the same manner, the blood type for a person with the genotype $I^B i$ is B. Because the heterozygote $I^A i$ has blood type A, we say that I^A is dominant to *i*, and by the same reasoning, I^B is dominant to *i*. The I^A and the I^B alleles are said to be *codominant*, because neither dominates the other—both alleles are expressed in the heterozygote.

Now that we have seen how the ABO genotypes determine the blood types, let us examine the manner in which ABO genotypes are inherited. To illustrate the inheritance of blood types, we will consider a specific example: Charlie Chaplin's blood type. Charlie Chaplin was a well-known motion-picture star who appeared in films from 1914 to 1952. In 1941, at the height of his career, Chaplin met an aspiring young actress from Brooklyn named Joan Barry. Apparently infatuated with Barry, Chaplin signed her to a movie contract and arranged for her to study acting at The Max Reinhart School. He planned to produce a motion picture starring Barry and even coached her himself. Their work together led to an affair, which Chaplin claimed ended in February of 1942. Subsequently, Barry became pregnant and gave birth to a baby girl on October 2, 1943, some 20 months after Chaplin said the affair ended. Barry, however, insisted that Chaplin was the father and sued Chaplin for child support.

To help determine the paternity of the child, blood tests were carried out on the baby, Barry, and Chaplin. The child's blood type turned out to be type B. As we have seen, two different genotypes—$I^B I^B$ and $I^B i$—produce the B blood type, so the child's genotype was one of these. Barry was shown to have blood type A. Once again, two genotypes are capable of producing this blood type: $I^A I^A$ and $I^A i$. However, the baby's blood type tells us that the mother must have been heterozygous, possessing the genotype $I^A i$. Recall that one of the alleles in the genotype is always inherited from the mother and the other from the father. Because Barry's blood type was A, the only alleles she could have possessed were I^A or *i*. Because the only genotypes possible for the baby were either $I^B I^B$ or $I^B i$, the baby clearly inherited the *i* allele from Barry; Barry could not give her child its I^B allele. Therefore, the mother's genotype was $I^A i$, and she passed her *i* allele to the child, who then possessed the genotype $I^B i$. If the mother donated the *i* allele to the baby, then the father must have given the child its other allele—the I^B allele. Chaplin's blood type, however, was O, which means that his genotype must have been *ii*. Because he was type O, it was impossible for Chaplin to transmit an I^B

allele to Barry's baby. Therefore he could not be the father. The genotypes of Chaplin, Barry, and her baby are outlined in Figure 2.4. During the trial, three pathologists gave expert testimony on the blood types and explained how Chaplin could not be responsible for the pregnancy. In spite of the genetic evidence to the contrary, the jury declared that Chaplin was indeed the father and ordered him to pay $75 per week for child support and $5,000 in attorney fees.

Three Girls and Pregnant Again; Will It Be a Boy This Time?

Chance plays an extremely important role in heredity, and, yet, the concept of chance is frequently misunderstood. As we have discussed, a genotype consists of two alleles but only one of those alleles will be passed on to each child. Which of the two alleles the child receives is random and determined by chance. Because of this element of chance, it is frequently impossible to say with certainty whether a child will actually inherit a trait. The best we can do is state the *probability* that the trait will be inherited. Probability is simply chance expressed as a mathematical ratio; it represents the fraction or percentage of the time that an event will occur. For example, when both parents are heterozygous for albinism, the probability that each of their children will be an albino is $\frac{1}{4}$. This means that on the average, one out of four children whose parents are heterozygous will express the trait. If 1,000 children are produced by a large number of heterozygous parents, about $\frac{1}{4}$ or 250 of these will be albinos. Although $\frac{1}{4}$ is the probability of having the trait, the number of albino children in any one family may deviate from this ratio as a result of chance. For simplicity, let's consider only families with four children. If both parents are heterozygous, on the average we expect one child out of the four to be an albino. However, not all families will have exactly one albino. Just by chance, some of the families will have no affected children. Other families will have one albino child, and still others two or

Figure 2.4.   Blood types and corresponding genotypes of Joan Barry, Barry's baby, and Charlie Chaplin. The baby must have inherited a gene for the B antigen from the father. Because Chaplin was blood type O, he could not be the father.

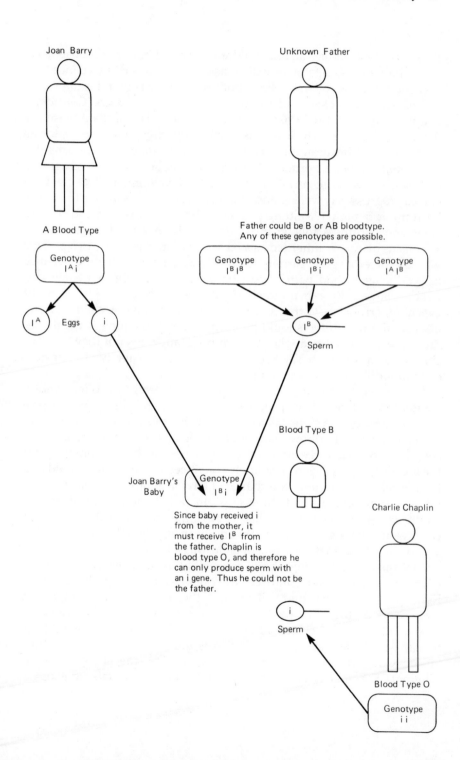

Joan Barry

Unknown Father

A Blood Type

Father could be B or AB bloodtype.
Any of these genotypes are possible.

Genotype
$I^A i$

Genotype
$I^B I^B$

Genotype
$I^B i$

Genotype
$I^A I^B$

I^A Eggs i

I^B

Sperm

Blood Type B

Joan Barry's
Baby

Genotype
$I^B i$

Since baby received i
from the mother, it
must receive I^B from
the father. Chaplin is
blood type O, and therefore he
can only produce sperm with
an i gene. Thus he could not be
the father.

Charlie Chaplin

i

Sperm

Blood Type O

Genotype
i i

three. In a few families all four children will be albinos; the probability of this is low, but such families will occasionally occur just by chance.

A common misunderstanding about probability is that it is altered by the presence or absence of the trait in previous children. Consider a couple with a child who has Tay-Sachs disease. Tay-Sachs disease is a devastating illness, which results from a defective gene coding for an enzyme called hexosaminidase. The child who inherits Tay-Sachs disease usually appears normal at birth, but after about six months begins to experience a delay in physical and mental development. The child becomes progressively weaker and after several months is unable to hold its head up or remain in a sitting position. The head enlarges, and convulsions and blindness follow; the child usually dies by the age of four. Tay-Sachs disease is inherited as a recessive trait. Therefore, two parents who are heterozygous carriers for the Tay-Sachs gene have a $\frac{1}{4}$ chance of producing a child with Tay-Sachs disease. Suppose that Allen and Rebecca have a three-year-old child with Tay-Sachs disease; they might conclude, erroneously, that since they have just had one child with the disease, the next three should be normal. This reasoning is wrong because the $\frac{1}{4}$ probability applies to each pregnancy. Even if they had five children in a row with Tay-Sach's disease, the probability of their next child inheriting the disease remains $\frac{1}{4}$.

This principle also applies to the sex of offspring. Everyone understands that the chance of producing a boy is $\frac{1}{2}$ and the chance of producing a girl is $\frac{1}{2}$, but many fail to recognize that this probability applies to each child, no matter how many brothers or sisters have come before. A couple I know had three girls in a row. When Susan became pregnant for the fourth time, they were absolutely convinced that this baby would be a boy. Surely, they argued, the chance of having another girl was remote, because they already had three girls. In fact, their chance of having another girl was $\frac{1}{2}$; even if they had 11 girls, the probability that their next child would be a girl is still $\frac{1}{2}$. When Susan finally delivered, I wasn't surprised to hear that their fourth child was a baby girl.

This misunderstanding about probability arises from two different questions that are often confused. If we ask, what is the probability that Ken and Susan's next child will be a girl, the answer is $\frac{1}{2}$, no matter how many boys or girls they have previously conceived. This is because at each conception, the chance of being male is $\frac{1}{2}$ and the chance of being female is $\frac{1}{2}$. If, however, we ask what is the probability that Ken and Susan will have four children, all of them girls, the answer is very different. The answer is different because now we are talking about a group of children, not a single conception. If the probability of being a girl at conception is $\frac{1}{2}$, the chance of four such conceptions in a row is $\frac{1}{2} \times \frac{1}{2} \times \frac{1}{2} \times \frac{1}{2} = \frac{1}{16}$. However, at the next conception, the chance of being a girl is still $\frac{1}{2}$. The probability at conception is not altered by previous events, but the probability is changed if we consider the likelihood of seeing the same trait in a group of people.

One final caution about probability. The probability of having three girls is $\frac{1}{2} \times \frac{1}{2} \times \frac{1}{2} = \frac{1}{8}$, and the chance of having three boys is $\frac{1}{2} \times \frac{1}{2} \times \frac{1}{2} = \frac{1}{8}$. But the chance of having one boy and two girls is not, as you might first assume, $\frac{1}{2} \times \frac{1}{2} \times \frac{1}{2} = \frac{1}{8}$. The reason for the difference is that there is only one birth order that will produce three girls (a girl, a second girl, and a third girl), but there are three ways to have one boy and two girls: you might have a boy, followed by two girls (boy, girl, girl); a girl followed by a boy and then another girl (girl, boy, girl); or two girls and then a boy (girl, girl, boy). Because the chance of having a boy is $\frac{1}{2}$ and the chance of having a girl is $\frac{1}{2}$, the probability of each birth order listed above is $\frac{1}{2} \times \frac{1}{2} \times \frac{1}{2} = \frac{1}{8}$. To get the total probability of having one boy and two girls in a family of three children, we add the probabilities of each birth order that will produce this result; since there are three different combinations of one boy and two girls, each with a probability of $\frac{1}{8}$, the total probability is $\frac{1}{8} + \frac{1}{8} + \frac{1}{8} = \frac{3}{8}$. Figuring probabilities of multiple events like this can become quite complex, but these calculations are not necessary for understanding what follows in this book.

DNA: The Blueprints of Life

Now that we have discussed the manner in which genes are inherited, let us turn to the physical nature of the genes themselves. I have portrayed the genes as hereditary blueprints, coding instructions for the development of our anatomical, biochemical, and behavioral characteristics. How are these blueprints written? What is the genetic code?

The information contained within a gene is encoded in the structure of a particular chemical called *deoxyribonucleic acid*, or DNA for short. A simple molecule, DNA consists of two chains twisted around one another in an elegant spiral, as shown in Figure 2.5. Each of these two chains is composed of repeating units called *nucleotides*, which are linked

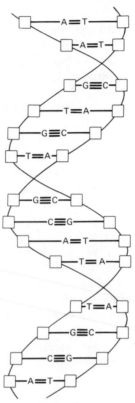

Figure 2.5.   DNA (deoxyribonucleic acid) is composed of two chains of nucleotides, twisted together in an elegant spiral.

end to end. Four types of nucleotides are found in the DNA; these are
termed *deoxyadenosine 5-phosphate, deoxythymidine 5-phosphate, deoxygua-
nosine 5-phosphate,* and *deoxycytidine 5-phosphate.* Fortunately, scientists
abbreviate these unpronounceable words with the letters A, T, G, and C,
and we shall employ this convention in our discussion of genes. The four
types of nucleotides make up the letters of the genetic code, and the
genetic instructions consist of a string of such nucleotides along the DNA
molecule.

Each DNA molecule then consists of two nucleotide chains twisted
together in a spiral, but the DNA sequences on the two chains are not
identical. Rather, they are complementary. Complementary means that

the sequences on the two chains are not independent of one another; given a sequence on one chain, there is only one sequence that can pair with it. This is because the nucleotides on the two chains are physically joined, and they join together in a very specific manner. An A nucleotide on one chain always pairs with a T nucleotide on the opposite chain; in a similar way G always pairs with C (Figure 2.5). This pairing between the bases of the two chains plays an important role in how the DNA copies itself, and it provides stability to the molecule. However, only one of the complementary sequences is important for heredity, because normally only one of the strands actually carries genetic information.

Sequencing the Human Genome

Each human cell contains approximately three billion pairs of DNA nucleotides, what is commonly called the *human genome*. This enormous amount of genetic information carries the coding instructions for all of our traits, from the color of our hair to the chemicals in our brain that allow us to think. Although the total amount of DNA is quite large, the size of each nucleotide is incredibly small. A single nucleotide is only about one one-hundred-millionth of an inch long. Thus, it is impossible to see an individual nucleotide, even with science's most powerful microscope.

For 20 years scientists knew that genes were composed of the nucleotides in the DNA, but because the nucleotides are so small, they had no way to read nucleotide sequence. Then in 1977, methods were developed for determining the nucleotide sequence of the DNA. These methods do not observe the nucleotides directly; rather they read the nucleotide sequence indirectly through the use of chemical reactions. This procedure is called *DNA sequencing*. The details of DNA sequencing are beyond the scope of our discussion here, but in general terms, chemical reactions are used to generate many fragments of DNA that differ in length. The fragments are separated according to size, and the length of each fragment indicates the position of a particular nucleotide (A, T, G, or C) along the DNA molecule.

The ability to sequence the DNA has provided us with a detailed look at the structure and functioning of our genes. Once a gene that causes a particular trait has been located, sequencing the gene may indicate how the gene produces the trait. For example, comparing the DNA of an individual who has a genetic disease with the DNA of a healthy person may lead to a better understanding of the underlying nature of the disorder, as illustrated by recent research on the Duchenne muscular dystrophy gene (see Chapter 1). This information may suggest better treatments for those suffering from the disorder. It also increases our general understanding of how genes work. Also, knowledge of the DNA sequences responsible for a disease allows genetic tests to be developed, tests that can identify the carriers of the defective gene and diagnose the disease in unborn babies.

The realization that DNA sequences are of immense importance to medicine and basic biology has lead to the start of a project to sequence the entire human DNA. This project has been called the *Human Genome Project*. Efforts to sequence the human genome are currently underway in the United States, Europe, and Japan. Recently, a Human Genome Organization (HUGO) was set up to increase international collaboration of the sequencing effort. Already, several million nucleotides of the human genome have been sequenced.

The enormous time and effort required to sequence the remainder of the human DNA is seldom appreciated. Recall that the human genome contains approximately 3 billion nucleotides of DNA. Just to print out this DNA sequence as a series of continuous letters, each letter representing one nucleotide (such as ATGCTTA . . .) would require 1 million pages of print, the equivalent of over 600 volumes, each the size of a large dictionary. The actual sequencing will require years. With present techniques, a skilled scientist is capable of sequencing 50,000 to 100,000 nucleotides of DNA in a single year. At this rate, 1,000 skilled scientists working nonstop would require 30 years to sequence the entire human DNA. Sequencing the human genome in a reasonable time frame and at a reasonable cost will require new, yet to be developed sequencing technologies. Several new approaches are already being studied. One experimental technique employs lasers to read DNA fragments tagged with special chemicals that glow under the laser light; each of the four different nucleotides glows a different color. Another approach utilizes robotics to handle many of the time-consuming steps now done by hand. Undoubtedly, new techniques will be developed in the future. Even with advances in technology, the National Research Council estimates that sequencing the total human DNA will require $200,000,000 per year for 15 years.

Genes and Proteins

A question of central importance is how does the string of nucleotides, the sequence of A's, T's, G's, and C's, produce traits like blue eyes, hemophilia, or high intelligence. The answer to this question turns out to be quite complicated, and scientists don't yet have all the details. We do have a critical part of the answer, however: We know the first step in the transfer of information from genotype to phenotype. Genes code for traits by first specifying the construction of molecules called *proteins.* Proteins are known to almost everyone as an important component of the foods we eat; they occur in abundance in meats, eggs, and beans. However, proteins are much more. The red substance that carries oxygen in our blood is a protein. Many of our hormones are proteins. Each and every cell in our body is held together by proteins, and certain proteins, called *enzymes,* control the synthesis of other substances in our body. At the chemical level, our traits are derived directly or indirectly from proteins, and genes function by coding for proteins.

To illustrate the relationship between genes, proteins, and phenotypes, let's examine the gene that causes PKU. PKU is an abbreviation for phenylketonuria, a recessive genetic disease that leads to severe mental retardation in newborns. In children with PKU, retardation results from the excess accumulation of a chemical called phenylalanine in the blood. Phenylalanine is ingested in the foods we eat, and some phenylalanine is essential for proper development. Normally the amount of phenylalanine in our body is kept low, because it is broken down by an enzyme (a protein) called phenylalanine hydroxylase. PKU arises because of a defect in the gene that codes for this enzyme. In a normal individual the gene produces plenty of phenylalanine hydroxylase, which then breaks down phenylalanine, keeping the chemical at a low level. In the child with PKU, however, this gene is defective, and phenylalanine hydroxylase is not produced. Consequently, phenylalanine is not degraded and elevated levels of it lead to mental retardation. How excess phenylalanine causes brain damage is unknown, but PKU results from a defective gene that fails to produce an essential protein, the enzyme phenylalanine hydroxylase. Fortunately, mental retardation can be prevented in children with PKU by restricting the amount of phenylalanine in their diet (see *Phenylketonuria* in "The Catalog of Genetic Traits"). All genes ultimately work in this manner, by affecting the production of a specific protein.

Germ Line Genes and Somatic Genes

Contrary to the impression I may have given in our discussion of how genes work, the genes do not float around in our body. Indeed, we don't possess just one copy of our genes, but in fact trillions of copies of them. Each cell in our body has its own set of genes, and our body is composed of over 100 trillion cells. Think of the genes as information contained in a textbook. The individual cells are like students in a class, each with their own copy of the book. Just as a book begins as a single copy of a manuscript written by the author, a human body also begins with a single copy of the genes. At conception, the DNA from a sperm joins with the DNA of the egg cell and endows the new individual with its genes. At that moment, the individual is a single cell and possesses only a single set of genetic instructions. Soon the cell divides, giving rise to two cells, each with an exact replica of the original genetic information. These two cells then divide to four, the four divide to eight, and the eight to sixteen. Each time a cell divides, the two new cells receive an exact copy of the genetic information. Cell division occurs again and again, eventually producing a body full of cells, each cell with the same set of genes.

Although each cell in our body contains a complete set of genetic information, the vast majority of these cells are never involved in heredity. In other words, the genetic information they possess is not passed on to another individual. This is because only a few of the trillions of cells in the body are directly involved in reproduction. The cells that give rise to sperm and eggs are a select few—they are termed the *germ cells*. Only the genes in the germ cells are potentially transmitted to future generations. We can think of our body as containing two types of genetic information. One type consists of the genes in all of our nonsex cells, the so-called *somatic genes* in the technical language of genetics. The other type consists of those genes in our germ cells or sex cells; these are called the *germ line genes* or simply the *germ line*. Our somatic genes are important in the functioning of our body, but they are not inherited by future generations. Only the genes of the germ line count in heredity.

A Tangled Coil of Barbed Wire:
The Chromosome

In most cells, 46 pieces of DNA are found (if we exclude tiny loops of DNA found in special structures termed *mitochondria*). Each of the 46 pieces of DNA makes up a *chromosome*. The chromosome is actually more than DNA alone; it also consists of the proteins that are attached to the DNA. One purpose of this DNA–protein structure is to condense the tremendous amount of DNA found in a cell into a small space. Take a human cell for example. Each human cell contains approximately three billion nucleotides of DNA. If all of this DNA was stretched out straight, it would measure over three feet in length. Yet this DNA must fit inside a cell that is less than 0.0004 inch in diameter. To cram itself into the tiny confines of a cell, the DNA first wraps itself around tiny protein spheres called *histones*. This creates a string of DNA and histones, somewhat similar to a string of beads, except the string is on the outside. Then the DNA–histone string coils up on itself, like a tangled mass of barbed wire. The resulting structure is what we call a *chromosome*. A typical human chromosome is shown in Figure 2.6.

Each chromosome consists of a single piece of DNA, and because there are 46 pieces of DNA, the cell contains 46 chromosomes. (Exceptions are the sperm and egg cells, which contain only half this number.) Each chromosome has a pairing partner, called its *homologous chromosome;* thus each cell possesses 23 pairs of homologous chromosomes. The two homologous chromosomes carry information for the same traits. For example, suppose that a gene for green eye color is found on chromosome 19. The homolog of chromosome 19 will also carry a gene for eye color, although the allele on the homolog might code for blue eyes instead of green. The chromosomes are paired because each person inherits one chromosome of the pair from the mother and the other one from the father. This probably sounds familiar. When we discussed alleles, we said that each genotype consisted of two alleles, one from the mother and one from the father. This similarity between alleles and chromosomes is not coincidental—the alleles are actually DNA sequences on the chromosomes. Thus, one chromosome of each homologous pair carries alleles from the father; the other chromosome carries alleles from the mother.

The genes that determine a particular trait are sometimes called a *locus*. The word *locus* literally means a place—a place on a chromosome that

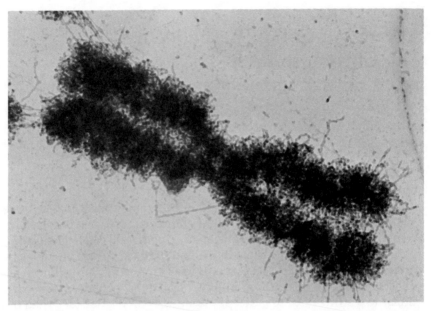

Figure 2.6.   A human chromosome, magnified approximately 28,000 times. (Gunther Bahr, Armed Forces Institute of Pathology/BPS.)

determines a trait. So we can speak of the locus that determines the presence or absence of red hair in humans. This locus holds a pair of genes, the two alleles that make up the genotype. The genotype might be *RR*, *Rr*, or *rr*. Each of these would be a genotype at a single locus.

Genetic Traits Come in Several Types

Genetic traits can arise in several ways. First, some genetic traits are determined by a pair of genes (alleles) at a single locus. The genes at that locus code for a protein that then produces a specific phenotype. The ABO blood type, PKU, and albinism are all examples of *single-locus traits*. However, not all genetic traits arise from genes at a single locus. The inheritance of many traits is more complex, involving genes at many loci. Environmental factors may also influence the trait. Traits that are influenced by a number of genes and environmental factors are called *multifactorial*. Many of the common traits in humans, such as height, weight, intelligence, and susceptibility to many types of disease are multifactorial and have complex inheritance. We will discuss these types of traits and how they are inherited in Chapter 4.

Another type of genetic trait arises from a *chromosome abnormality*. Too many or too few chromosomes may be present, or sometimes a piece of a chromosome is missing. Because many genes reside on a chromosome, a number of genes are affected by such an abnormality, and many traits are altered simultaneously. In most cases this leads to gross developmental problems and miscarriage of the fetus. The few individuals born with chromosome abnormalities usually exhibit severe mental and physical problems. We will discuss how these chromosome abnormalities arise and their phenotypic effects in Chapter 5.

A fourth and final type of genetic trait occurs as a result of a change in our somatic genes, a change that is called a *somatic mutation*. Recall from our earlier discussion that we possess two types of genetic information—the germ line genes found in our reproductive cells and the somatic genes found in all of our other cells. The germline genes are passed on to future generations; they contain the genetic information that our children will inherit. The genes contained in somatic cells will be passed on to other cells in our body, as the cells divide and give rise to new cells. However, a somatic mutation will not be passed on to our descendents, because only the genes in the sperm and the eggs contribute genetic information to our offspring. Thus, traits that result from somatic mutations are genetic, but they are not hereditary.

Somatic mutations are responsible for most if not all cancers. In this way, cancer is a genetic trait, but most cancers are not hereditary. For cancer to arise, one or more genes in a somatic cell must undergo mutations that cause the cell to divide in an uncontrollable manner. As the cancer cell divides, it passes these somatic mutations on to other cells, so that they too divide uncontrollably. However, because these mutations have occurred in somatic cells, they will not be passed on to one's children. In some cancers—breast cancer and colon cancer, for example—a predisposition to the cancer can be inherited. Here, several mutations are probably required for the cell to turn cancerous. One or more of the required mutations may occur in the germ line genes, and these can be passed on, creating a genetic predisposition to the cancer. However, additional somatic mutations would have to occur before the cancer arises. Thus some individuals—those that inherit the germ line mutations—are predisposed toward the cancer. However, most cancers show little tendency to be hereditary. (See *Cancer* in "The Catalog of Genetic Traits.")

Reproduction

From the standpoint of heredity, it is useful to think of reproduction as encompassing three connected, but distinct stages: (1) formation of the sex cells—the sperm and eggs; (2) fusion of the egg and sperm in the process of fertilization; and (3) development and birth of the individual that results from fertilization.

Genes on a Charter Bus: Meiosis and the Formation of Sex Cells

Chromosomes are the vehicles on which genes travel from one generation to the next. Each chromosome contains a number of genes, and like passengers on a charter bus, those genes riding on the same chromosome end up at the same destination—the same sex cell. This first step in the process of reproduction takes place in the germ cells of the sex organs, in the testes of a male and in the ovaries of a female. Recall that each cell of the human body contains 46 chromosomes. These are grouped in twos to form 23 pairs. If each of us passed on all 46 chromosomes, our children would be in serious trouble, for they would inherit 46 chromosomes from their mother and another 46 from their father. This would give them 92 chromosomes, which is twice too many! If they then passed on all of their chromosomes, our grandchildren would inherit 184 chromosomes. In the next generation, the chromosome number would double again to 368, and in a short time each cell would be bursting with chromosomes. Fortunately, nature has worked out a simple solution to this problem. As our sex cells are produced, they go through a special process that reduces the number of chromosomes by half. This process is called *meiosis*. Meiosis reduces the chromosome number from 46 to 23 and thus ensures that when two sex cells fuse in the act of fertilization the original chromosome number of 46 is restored (Figure 2.7).

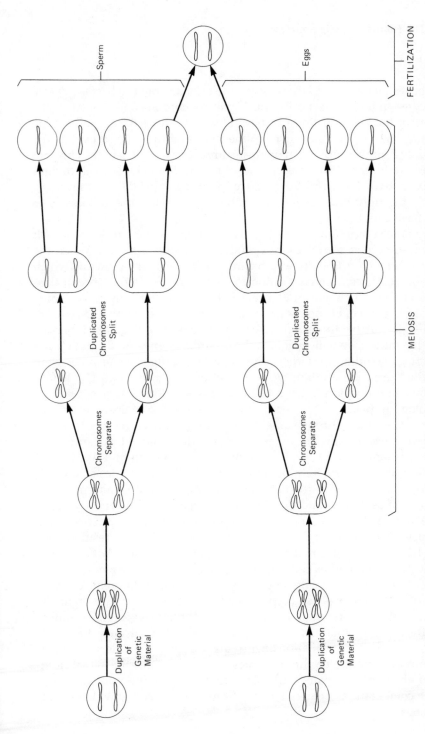

Figure 2.7. Sex cells—sperm and eggs—are produced through the process of meiosis. During meiosis, the number of chromosomes is reduced by half. The original chromosome number is restored after fertilization. For simplicity, only a single pair of chromosomes is illustrated.

Meiosis takes place in those germ line cells destined to become sperm and eggs. In these select cells, the 23 pairs of chromosomes march to the center of the cell and line up two by two. Then each pair splits. One chromosome of the pair moves to the right and the other moves to the left; they continue moving in opposite directions until half of the chromosomes are bunched up at each end of the cell. Finally, the cell divides neatly in two. Each resulting sex cell now contains 23 chromosomes, exactly the right number to ensure that the chromosome number is 46 after fertilization.

From the standpoint of heredity, a critical aspect of meiosis is that each chromosome pair separates independently of all other pairs. When the chromosome pairs line up, which chromosome is on the right and which is on the left is completely random. To illustrate the importance of this, consider the cell shown in Figure 2.8. For simplicity, this cell contains only three pairs of chromosomes; the chromosomes are labeled AA, BB, and CC. Recall that three of these chromosomes were originally inherited from the father; we will designate these chromosomes A_f, B_f, and C_f, the subscript f standing for father. The three remaining chromosomes were inherited from the mother; we will label these A_m, B_m, and C_m. Before chromosome division, such a cell contains six chromosomes, or three homologous pairs: A_fA_m, B_fB_m, and C_fC_m. During meiosis, each pair separates, and one chromosome of the pair moves to each side of the cell. However, *how* the chromosomes separate is determined by chance. As a result of chance, A_f, B_m, and C_f might move to the left, and A_m, B_f, and C_m might move to the right. After the cell divided, two types of sex cells would result: one with the chromosomes A_f, B_m, and C_f and one with chromosomes A_m, B_f, and C_m. Or, just by chance, A_f, B_f, and C_m might move to the left, and A_m, B_m, and C_f might move to the right. This would produce a different combination of chromosomes in the resulting sex cells. It is even possible that all the paternal chromosomes (A_f, B_f, and C_f) might end up in one sex cell, and all the maternal chromosomes (A_m, B_m, and C_m) in another. As illustrated in Figure 2.8, eight different combinations of chromosomes can be produced when three pairs are originally present. With more than three pairs of chromosomes, the number of different combinations is even greater. We can calculate the number of different combinations with the formula 2^n, where n equals the number of pairs of chromosomes. With 23 pairs—the actual number of chromosome pairs found in a human cell—the number of different combinations that can result from meiosis is 2^{23}, which equals 8,388,608!

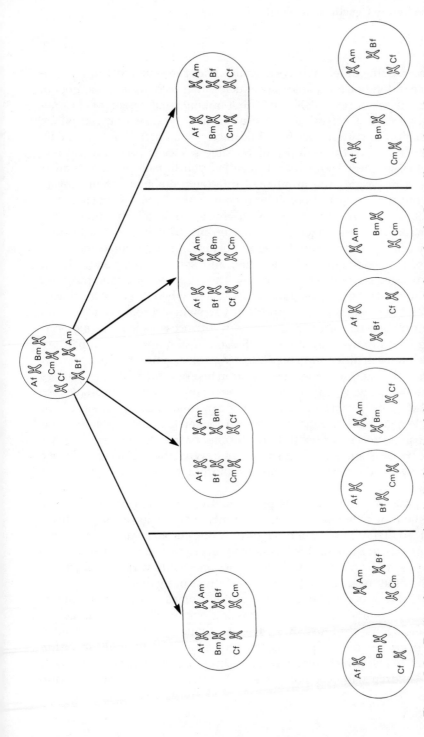

Figure 2.8. During the process of meiosis, the pairs of chromosome separate independently. In a cell with three chromosome pairs, as illustrated here, the chromosomes can divide in four different ways, yielding eight different combinations of chromosomes.

51

Because of the different ways chromosomes can separate during meiosis, each individual is capable of producing an incredibly large number of different types of sex cells, each with a unique combination of chromosomes. Of course, offspring will result from only a few of these; which combination of chromosomes a child receives is determined strictly by chance. In reality the number of possible sex cells produced by one individual is much larger than I have led you to believe. The number 8,388,608 represents the number of different combinations of *chromosomes*, but the number of possible combinations of *genes* is much larger. We said earlier that the genes on a chromosome all go to the same destination, like passengers on a charter bus. This is only partly true. Shortly after its ride through meiosis begins, each chromosome stops next to its homologous chromosome, and some of the genes switch places between the two chromosomes. The chromosomes then travel on to their destinations, to the particular sex cells where they meet up with 22 other chromosomes. The opportunity to switch chromosomes occurs in the early stages of meiosis, through a process called *crossing over*. During crossing over, the two chromosomes of a homologous pair are attracted to each other and enter into a very close pairing association. At this time, the two chromosomes are stretched out, their DNA molecules elongated and laying side by side. A piece of one chromosome may cross over the other chromosome, and they can then exchange a stretch of DNA. When this happens, we can no longer talk about whether the chromosome was inherited from the mother or from the father. Part of it may be paternal and another part maternal. What this means for heredity is that even genes on the same chromosomes may not be inherited together.

The process of meiosis thus produces two results important for our understanding of heredity. First, the number of chromosomes is reduced by half, so that each sex cell receives only one chromosome of each pair. Another way to think of this is that we possess two alleles at each of our genotypes, but only one of those alleles makes its way into each sex cell. The other result is that meiosis reshuffles our genes into new combinations. This occurs because the chromosomes can divide in many different ways and also because crossing over switches up the genes on homologous chromosomes. The consequence of this reshuffling is that every sex cell we produce is genetically different, and except for identical twins (which result from a single egg and sperm), no two of our children will ever possess exactly the same combination of our genes.

Fertilization: Egg Meets Sperm

Meiosis is initiated in the gonads, in the testes of a male and the ovaries of a female. In the ovaries, the process of chromosome division actually begins before the woman is even born. The chromosomes pair up and crossing over takes place. At this point meiosis stops, and the chromosomes remain suspended in meiosis, half divided, until after puberty. With the onset of puberty a small gland at the base of the brain, the pituitary, begins producing sex-stimulating hormones and the monthly cycle of menstruation begins. These hormones cause the eggs in the ovary to ripen and grow. They also stimulate the continuation of meiosis. After about two weeks, one egg becomes larger than all the others and is destined to develop into a mature egg cell, ready to be fertilized. This egg is encased in a special packet of cells called a *follicle*. Around Day 14 of the menstrual cycle, a surge of hormones causes the follicle to rupture, and the egg bursts out of the ovary into the abdominal cavity. The egg finds its way to the open end of the Fallopian tube, which is about 4 ½ inches long and connects to the uterus (the womb). Entering the Fallopian tube, the egg travels slowly toward the uterus, propelled by gentle rhythmic contractions of the tube. If sperm are present in the Fallopian tube at this time, fertilization takes place. Meiosis is not fully completed in the egg until after a sperm penetrates the outer layers, moments before the genes carried by the sperm and egg fuse.

The male sex cells are the sperm, which are produced in special cells found within the testes. Unlike meiosis in the female, which takes years to complete, chromosome division in males is a rapid process that occurs continually, day after day, from puberty to old age. Also unlike females who produce only one mature sex cell each month, males produce hundreds of millions of sperm daily. During ejaculation, several hundred million of the sperm are deposited in the vagina. The sperm, each only about 0.0024 inch long and propelled by a rapidly beating tail, slowly make their way up the vagina, into the uterus, and eventually up into the Fallopian tube. Attrition along the way is enormous and only a few of the hundreds of millions of sperm originally deposited in the vagina will complete the entire journey. Arriving at the egg, one sperm successfully penetrates the outer layer of the egg. This sperm then ruptures, spewing its contents of genes into the egg. The egg immediately undergoes a change in its outer layer, effectively locking out other sperm, so that fertilization occurs only once. Division of the female chromosomes finishes and the male and female genes fuse to create a new individual.

Development: Growing into a Person

The new individual is called an *embryo* or a *zygote*. Endowed with genes from its mother and father and possessing the genetic instructions for all the traits of a complete human, the embryo starts to divide. Meanwhile, it continues its downstream movement toward the uterus. The trip down the Fallopian tube requires about a week. The embryo finally arrives at the uterus, its home for the next 259 days. There it buries itself into the surrounding tissue of the mother, which nourishes the tiny embryo, providing it with food, water, oxygen, and a number of other essential elements.

The embryo develops rapidly, although at first it remains incredibly small. After about 4 weeks, it is still only about ¼ inch long. Yet, it now has a head, trunk, and tail. Tiny buds that will eventually develop into the arms and legs have formed. Its heart is beating. By the end of the fifth week, eyes and vestiges of fingers and toes are visible. During the embryo's second month of life, the limbs assume shape. Arms, legs, knees, and elbows form; fingers and toes appear. The major organs, including the liver, pancreas, gall bladder, heart, and brain have begun to develop. At the end of 8 weeks, the embryo is distinctly human and is now called a *fetus*. All the major human features have been established by this time, their development directed by the genes received from the mother and father. Amazingly, the fetus is still less than 1 inch long. During the remainder of its life in the uterus, the fetus grows rapidly, enlarging until it is almost too big to pass through the birth canal. At that point, birth occurs and a genetically unique person enters the world.

Chapter 3

SIMPLE PATTERNS OF INHERITANCE

In 1833 a child was born with a peculiar gene that would handicap his descendants for three generations. For our purposes, we will call this child "Joseph," although that was not his real name. Joseph was born into a large family, the fourth of 12 children. We have no record of Joseph's delivery, but his outward appearance was probably normal at first. As Joseph grew older, however, his parents undoubtedly saw that the boy was disproportioned—his head and trunk were of normal size, but his arms and legs were too short. When the boy began to stand, his legs bowed outward, and he began walking with a waddling stride. These traits persisted and became more pronounced as the child grew. By adolescence, it was clear to all that Joseph was a dwarf.

In spite of his considerable handicaps, Joseph worked hard throughout his life and rose to be a successful leader in his community. He practiced polygamy, supporting two wives; together they provided him with a large family of 22 children. Seven of these children, three girls and four boys, were dwarfs like their father (see Figure 3.1, which shows Joseph's complete pedigree). Although short in stature, these dwarf children were otherwise normal; all seven eventually married. They produced a total of 49 offspring (Joseph's grandchildren), 24 of whom were also dwarfs. Joseph's other 15 children were completely normal, and they gave Joseph another 80 grandchildren. To these normal parents, not a single dwarf child was born. In the fourth generation, over 250 great-grandchildren were produced, but only seven were dwarfs. The small number of dwarfs in this last generation was largely due to the fact that only seven of the grandchildren with dwarfism married; some of the affected individuals in this generation stated that they had deliberately foregone marriage because they did not want to perpetuate the trait.

Human dwarfism comes in a number of varieties, differing subtly in which bones are involved and how they are affected. Joseph and his descendants possessed a form called *Schmid-type metaphyseal chondrodysplasia*, although it was originally misdiagnosed as a more common form of dwarfism know as *achondroplasia*. Dwarfism is often inherited as a simple genetic trait, and the dwarfism that Joseph passed to his descendants was clearly a dominant trait. Let us examine Joseph's family history for clues about the manner in which a dominant trait is inherited.

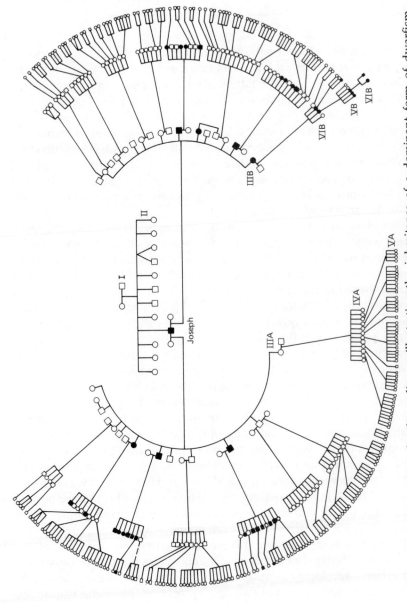

Figure 3.1. "Joseph's" family pedigree, illustrating the inheritance of a dominant form of dwarfism. (Redrawn with permission from *The Journal of Heredity* 34:232.)

Joseph's Dwarfism: A Dominant Trait

You may recall from our earlier discussion of genes and genotypes in Chapter 2 that each person inherits two sets of genes, one set from the mother and one set from the father. Thus, each gene, or allele, is paired with another gene that codes for the same trait. The pair of genes that an individual possesses is referred to as the *genotype* and it resides at a specific place on a chromosome called a *locus*. An individual who has two different genes at their genotype is said to be *heterozygous;* an individual with two identical genes is said to be *homozygous.* The particular trait that the genotype produces depends upon how the two genes interact, and the interaction between these matched genes also plays an important role in how the trait is inherited.

Some genes are *dominant.* This means that when the dominant gene is paired with a different gene, the dominant gene is stronger, and it determines the trait. Short fingers are caused by a dominant gene; if you inherit a gene for short fingers from your father and a normal gene from your mother, you will have short fingers. To put this another way, in a dominant trait the homozygous individual (possessing two copies of the gene) and the heterozygous individual (possessing only a single copy of the gene) both exhibit the features of the trait.

Dwarfism in humans is most often a dominant trait. Individuals with the disorder are usually heterozygous, possessing one copy of the dwarf gene and one copy of a normal gene; the few individuals who inherit two copies of the dwarf gene usually have severe deformities and die in infancy. The genes involved in dwarfism code for bone development. Dwarfs possess one defective copy of the gene, and this defective copy prevents proper growth of the long bones in the arms and legs.

Joseph's family provides us with an excellent illustration of the pattern of inheritance expected of a simple dominant trait. Joseph was the first individual in his family to exhibit dwarfism—neither his mother nor his father was a dwarf, and his 11 brothers and sisters were all normal. Most likely, a mutation occurred in a sex cell of one of his parents; in the testes of his father or in the ovaries of his mother a genetic accident took place. This accident changed a normal gene that provides the genetic signals for proper bone development into a defective gene that causes dwarfism. The defective gene was then passed to Joseph in either the egg or the sperm. Another possibility is that the mutation occurred shortly after fertilization, when Joseph was just a tiny embryo consisting of no more than a few cells. Either way, we can be certain that Joseph was heterozygous for the trait, possessing one defective gene and one normal gene for bone growth, because the chance of his receiving two mutations is extremely small. Also, had he been homozygous for the trait, Joseph's disabilities would have been far more severe, and it is likely he would have died in infancy.

Each of Joseph's own cells possessed the defective gene that causes dwarfism; every time Joseph produced a new sperm, the chromosome bearing the normal gene and the chromosome with the defective gene separated in the process of meiosis (see Chapter 2). Because only one of these chromosomes made its way into each sperm, the probability of a particular sperm cell acquiring the gene for dwarfism was 50 percent. Thus, half of Joseph's sperm carried a normal gene and the other half carried the defective gene. Both of Joseph's wives, however, were free of the disorder, and within their ovaries only normal genes were passed to the egg cells. When one of Joseph's sperm fertilized an egg cell at conception, that sperm had a 50/50 chance of carrying the defective gene for dwarfism. Therefore, each of Joseph's children stood a 50 percent chance of inheriting the gene for dwarfism; because only a single copy of the gene is sufficient to produce a dwarf, we would predict that approximately half of Joseph's children would be dwarfs.

We expect, then, that 50 percent of Joseph's children would exhibit the characteristics of dwarfism, providing that the trait was caused by a simple dominant gene. Joseph had 22 children, and seven were actually dwarfs. The difference between the 11 expected (50 percent of 22) and the seven actually observed could easily occur by chance. We know that 50 percent of Joseph's sperm carried a defective gene and 50 percent carried a normal gene. However, which particular sperm fertilized the eggs that produced his children was completely random, and therefore we might actually see more or less than 50 percent with the trait.

This role of chance in inheritance is analogous to flipping a coin. When we flip a coin, we expect 50 percent heads and 50 percent tails. If we flipped a coin 22 times, however, we probably would not get exactly 11 heads and 11 tails. We might obtain 10 heads and 12 tails, or 14 heads and 8 tails. Once in a long while we might even get 22 heads out of 22 flips, just by chance. In the case of Joseph's dwarfism, we expect the trait to be passed to 50 percent of his children, which would be 11, but by chance he passed it on to only 7 out of his 22 offspring.

Several other characteristics of Joseph's pedigree confirm the dominant pattern of inheritance for this trait. In an autosomal dominant trait (*autosomal* means that the genes are located on one of the nonsex chromosomes), the trait should appear with equal frequency in male and female offspring; in Joseph's own offspring, three of the dwarfs were girls and four were boys, as close to half and half as possible in seven children. Also, throughout the family each individual with the disorder had one parent who was also a dwarf. This is characteristic of an autosomal dominant trait. Because each affected individual must inherit the gene from a parent, one of the parents must also be affected. The only exception to this rule in Joseph's family is Joseph himself—neither of his parents exhibited the trait. This indicates that Joseph acquired the trait as a new mutation. Thus, Joseph's dwarfism was passed from generation to generation in a way that is entirely consistent with a simple, autosomal dominant mode of inheritance.

Let us briefly summarize the important characteristics of a simple, dominant trait.

Characteristics of Traits Determined by Simple, Autosomal Dominant Genes

1. The trait is expressed in individuals who possess one copy of the gene for the trait (heterozygotes), as well as individuals with two copies of the gene (homozygotes).
2. The trait appears equally in males and females.
3. Every individual with the trait has at least one parent with the trait, except for the first person in a family to receive the mutation.
4. When a person with the trait who is heterozygous mates with a person lacking the trait, approximately half of the children should inherit the trait (Figure 3.2).
5. The trait does not skip generations.
6. A person who is free of the trait cannot pass it to his children, unless he passes on a new mutation (an unlikely event, because new mutations are rare).

These characteristics apply to autosomal dominant traits with a simple mode of inheritance. Other factors sometimes affect dominant traits, with the result that the pattern of inheritance may be more complex than the example of dwarfism just presented. At this point, I will mention two of these complicating factors.

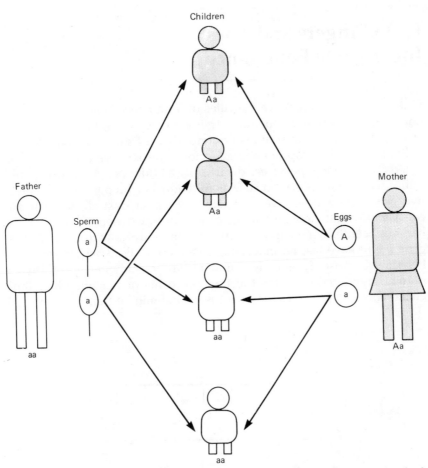

Figure 3.2.   A cross involving an autosomal dominant trait. Shaded individuals have the trait. When one parent has the trait (is heterozygous), an average of one out of two children will exhibit the trait.

Extra Fingers and Toes: Incomplete Penetrance

One factor that can change the rules of inheritance is *penetrance*. Penetrance indicates how frequently a trait is expressed in individuals possessing the genes for the trait. For example, dwarfism is dominant and all individuals with a copy of the gene for dwarfism are expected to be dwarfs. In Joseph's pedigree, dwarfism was fully penetrant (the penetrance was 100 percent), because all individuals who possessed a defective gene for dwarfism were actually dwarfs (at least all the facts are consistent with the notion that the gene was fully penetrant). If the gene had not been fully penetrant, then some individuals with the defective gene might have had normal stature. Penetrance becomes important in heredity, because if a gene is dominant but not fully penetrant, then a normal individual can pass the trait on to his or her offspring, thus violating one of our rules for an autosomal dominant trait.

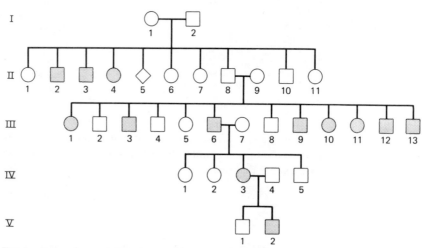

Figure 3.3. A partial pedigree illustrating incomplete penetrance of polydactyly (extra fingers and toes), a dominant trait. Polydactyly is absent in individual II-8, yet this person passes the gene for polydactyly to his children, grandchildren, and great-grandchildren. (Redrawn with permission from *The Journal of Heredity* 34:48–49.)

Incomplete penetrance is seen in *polydactyly,* the scientific name for the presence of extra fingers and toes. This trait is more common than is often recognized, and for unknown reasons, polydactyly is ten times more frequent in blacks than Caucasians. The genetic causes of polydactyly are complex (several different forms of polydactyly exist), but the trait is usually produced by a dominant gene. However, some individuals that inherit the gene for polydactyly do not develop extra digits. Although these individuals carry the gene for polydactyly, they do not express the trait; thus we say that polydactyly has incomplete penetrance. Figure 3.3 illustrates a family with polydactyly in which the trait is not fully penetrant. Notice that individual II-8 was free of the trait and yet passed the gene for polydactyly on to his children, grandchildren, and great-grandchildren. The expression of polydactyly is also quite variable; the extra digits may be on the hands, the feet, or both. Sometimes the extra digits consist of small flaps of skin, while at other times they may be fully formed fingers and toes.

Baldness, Breast Cancer, and Precocious Puberty: Sex-Influenced and Sex-Limited Traits

Another factor that sometimes alters the pattern of inheritance is a person's sex. Sex can affect genetic traits in a number of ways, and the traits involved often have nothing to do with male and female characteristics. Later, we will see that some genes are located on the X and Y chromosomes (these are called *sex-linked genes*). Because females have two X chromosomes and males have an X and a Y, the pattern of inheritance for sex-linked genes differs from that of autosomal genes. What we want to discuss here, however, is not sex-linked genes, but genes located on nonsex chromosomes, whose expression is affected by the sex of the individual. These genes, often referred to as *sex-limited* and *sex-influenced genes*, are inherited in exactly the same manner as other autosomal genes, but the expression or the penetrance of the genes differs in males and females.

A sex-influenced trait is one in which the genes are autosomal and occur equally in males and females; however, the trait is more commonly expressed in one sex than the other. Pattern baldness is an example of such a trait. In pattern baldness, which is the common form of premature baldness seen in men, hair is lost from the front and top of the head but not from the sides. This trait tends to be dominant in men, and therefore a single copy of the gene will turn a man bald. Women, however, are much less likely to become bald, because two copies of the gene are required to produce baldness. Furthermore, the trait is not as strongly expressed in the female sex, and women who do become bald frequently lose less hair than men. These differences between men and women give the appearance that the inheritance of pattern baldness differs in the two sexes; in reality, the genes for pattern baldness are the same in men and women, and they are inherited in the same manner, but they are expressed differently in males and females. This is what is meant by a sex-influenced trait.

Sometimes a trait is so strongly influenced by sex that it appears only in males or only in females; this type trait is said to be sex limited. In most cases, both sexes carry the genes for sex-limited traits, so the trait can be inherited from either the mother or the father. However, the trait will only be expressed in one sex. For example, breast cancer is a trait that is largely sex limited to women. (Breast cancer does occur occasionally in men, but it is rare.) Although breast cancer in most women arises sporadically, with little or no hereditary tendency, in a few families it is inherited as an autosomal dominant trait (see *Breast cancer* in "The Catalog of Genetic Traits"). In these breast cancer families, the gene for breast cancer may be inherited from either the mother or the father. Although the males in such families do not have breast cancer, they can pass on the gene for breast cancer to their daughters, who will then be predisposed to developing breast cancer.

Male-limited precocious puberty is an example of a trait that is sex limited to males. In this condition, young boys undergo puberty at an early age, usually at age two or three, but sometimes as early as 12 months. At this time, the child experiences a growth spurt and develops an enlarged penis; his voice deepens, and pubic hair begins to grow. Although boys with this condition initially experience rapid growth, most end up short as men, because their long bones stop growing after puberty occurs. Male-limited precocious puberty is inherited as an autosomal dominant trait. Males and females may possess the gene for precocious puberty, but the gene has no effect on females; thus the condition is sex limited to males. Although unaffected, females may transmit the gene to their children; if a son inherits the gene from either his mother or his father he will undergo precocious puberty. Several other types of precocious puberty exist that are not sex limited; these have different causes and may occur in males or females.

Rice-Bran Earwax: A Recessive Trait

As we have seen, when a single copy of a dominant gene is present, the trait determined by that gene is expressed; consequently, both heterozygous and homozygous individuals will exhibit a dominant trait. Many traits are not dominant, however, but are *recessive*. With recessive traits, two copies of the gene are required for the trait to be expressed; an individual will express the trait only if he or she inherits a recessive gene from both the mother and the father. When a recessive gene is paired with a dominant gene, the dominant gene tends to hide or suppress the recessive trait, and the trait is therefore absent in heterozygotes.

Consider a recessive gene in humans that determines the type of wax found in our ears. Earwax, technically termed *cerumen*, actually comes in two distinct types. Some individuals have wet and sticky earwax, which is usually light to dark brown in color; others possess gray-colored earwax, which is dry, granular, and brittle. Almost all Caucasians and blacks in North America have the sticky variety, but Orientals, native American Indians, and many other ethnic groups exhibit both types. In Japan, where dry earwax is most common, the sticky type is called *honey earwax* and the dry form, *rice-bran earwax*. Each person produces only one type of earwax, either sticky or dry, but never both. Individuals with earwax intermediate between sticky and dry are rare.

Genetic studies have determined that these differences in earwax are controlled by two genes at a single locus. One gene codes for sticky earwax and is dominant to another gene that produces dry earwax. To illustrate how a recessive gene is inherited, let us designate the gene for dry earwax with the small letter *w* and the gene that codes for sticky earwax with a capital *W*. Remember, each individual possesses two genes or alleles at a locus, and these two genes make up the genotype. So, an individual might have genotype *WW*, *Ww*, or *ww* at the earwax locus. Because dry earwax is recessive and requires two genes to be expressed, all individuals with dry earwax must have the genotype *ww*. In contrast, individuals with sticky earwax may be *WW* or *Ww*, because sticky is dominant to dry and requires only a single gene to be expressed.

The genotypes and their corresponding phenotypes are, therefore,

Genotype	Phenotype
WW	Sticky earwax
Ww	Sticky earwax
ww	Dry earwax

Thus far, scientists have been unable to find any differences between the earwax of WW and Ww individuals.

Recessive traits display a pattern of inheritance very different from that which characterizes dominant traits. First, some individuals are *carriers* for recessive traits. Carriers do not themselves have the trait, but they carry a gene for the trait that can be passed on to their children. For example, individuals with the genotype Ww have sticky earwax, but they also carry a recessive gene for dry earwax. When the carriers produce *gametes* (eggs or sperm), the gene for dry earwax goes into 50 percent of the gametes and the gene for sticky goes into 50 percent. If the other parent is also a carrier, some children may inherit two copies of the recessive gene and therefore produce dry earwax, even though both parents have only sticky earwax, as shown below.

Sticky (Ww) × sticky (Ww) → some children with dry earwax (ww)

In fact, when both parents are carriers for a recessive gene (both are heterozygotes), approximately $\frac{3}{4}$ of the children will have the dominant trait (in our example, sticky earwax) and $\frac{1}{4}$ will have the recessive trait (dry earwax). This is illustrated in Figure 3.4. When one parent is a carrier and the other parent has the recessive trait, about half of the offspring will have the trait and half will not. Another cross involves one parent with the recessive trait and the other parent homozygous for the dominant gene. Suppose we have a cross between a father with dry earwax (ww) and a mother homozygous for sticky earwax (WW). In this cross, each offspring will receive a dry gene, w, from the father and a sticky gene, W, from the mother; thus each child will be genotype Ww and will have sticky earwax. None of the children have dry earwax, but all of them will be carriers of the dry gene. When both parents have a recessive trait, all of the offspring will also exhibit the trait. Therefore, a cross between parents both of whom have dry earwax will produce only children with

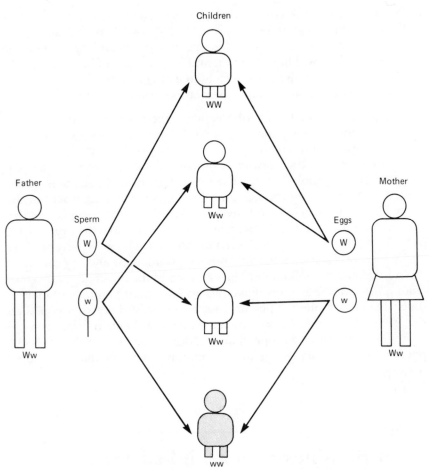

Figure 3.4. A genetic cross between two heterozygous carriers of an autosomal recessive trait. On the average, one out of four offspring will have the trait.

dry earwax ($ww \times ww \rightarrow ww$). These are the common crosses that occur with a simple recessive trait.

The essential characteristics of a recessive trait include the following:

Characteristics of Traits Determined by Simple, Autosomal Recessive Genes

1. If both the mother and the father possess the recessive trait, all their children should also exhibit the trait.

2. When one parent is a carrier (heterozygous) and the other parent has the trait, about half of the offspring should also have the trait.
3. If both parents are carriers (heterozygous), on the average 25 percent of the children will have the trait and 50 percent will be carriers. The other 25 percent will be completely free of genes for the trait.
4. Recessive traits tend to skip generations within a family.

As with dominant traits, the inheritance of recessive traits may be complicated by incomplete penetrance and differences in the expression of the trait in males and females.

The frequency of dry earwax in humans varies considerably among different ethnic groups. Only about two percent of Caucasians in the United States have dry earwax, and the frequency among blacks in the United States is even less. Yet, over 80 percent of Japanese possess dry earwax. In Taiwan, about 58 percent of the people have the dry variety, in Malaysia the frequency is 27 percent, and in Iran it is 33 percent. Why sticky earwax is common in some human populations and dry earwax is the rule in others is unknown. The variation in the incidence of this trait among human populations illustrates an important point about genetic traits: Dominant phenotypes are not necessarily more common than recessive phenotypes. Sticky earwax, which is a dominant trait, is more common in people of European and African descent, but the recessive phenotype—dry earwax—is more common among people from some parts of Asia.

Color Blindness: An X-Linked Trait

Humans have 23 pairs of chromosomes, and one of those pairs consists of the sex chromosomes. The sex chromosomes are so-called because males and females possess different chromosomes at this pair—females have two X-shaped chromosomes, whereas males have one X-shaped chromosome and a smaller chromosome called the Y chromosome. The Y chromosome appears to carry very little genetic information, but the X chromosome is filled with important genes. Those genes located on the X chromosome are referred to as *X-linked genes*, or more frequently *sex-linked genes*.

The inheritance of X-linked genes differs from that of autosomal genes because males and females have different numbers of X chromosomes.

Females possess two X chromosomes, and one X chromosome goes into each egg cell when the chromosomes divide during the process of meiosis. (See Chapter 2 for a discussion of meiosis.) In a male, however, each cell contains an X chromosome and a Y chromosome; during meiosis, half of the sperm receive the X and the other half get the Y. When one of the X-bearing sperm fertilizes an egg, the resulting offspring possesses two X chromosomes and is a girl; when the sperm has a Y chromosome, the offspring is a boy with an X and a Y chromosome. The essential fact to remember about the inheritance of X-linked genes is that males have only a single copy of an X-linked gene, which they always inherit from their mother. Males receive a Y chromosome from their father, but the Y chromosome contains essentially no genes that match up with those on the X. Females, on the other hand, have two X chromosomes, one from the mother and one from the father, so both parents contribute X-linked genes to their daughters.

Contrary to a common misconception, most genes on the X chromosome do not code for female traits. This makes sense when you recall that both males and females have X chromosomes, though males only possess a single X in each cell. The X chromosome carries a variety of genes important to both sexes, including genes that code for proper mental development, genes for muscle function, genes for normal skin development, genes for factors involved in blood clotting, and genes for a number of essential enzymes.

As was the case for autosomal genes, X-linked genes may be dominant or recessive. In *X-linked recessive genes,* the effect of a single copy of the gene is blocked or suppressed in females if a different gene lies on the other X chromosome. For example, Duchenne muscular dystrophy—a debilitating and lethal disease that we discussed in Chapter 1—is an X-linked recessive disorder. If a female inherits one X chromosome with the gene for Duchenne muscular dystrophy, she does not have the disease, because her other X carries a normal gene and one correct copy is enough to ensure normal function. Males, on the other hand, have muscular dystrophy if they possess a single copy of the gene, because there is no additional X chromosome with a normal gene to prevent the disease. In order for a female to have the disease, she would have to inherit two X chromosomes with the muscular dystrophy gene—one from the mother and one from the father. However, males with Duchenne muscular dystrophy do not live long enough to reproduce and pass on the gene to a daughter; consequently females rarely have the disease. Because females require two copies of the gene to have an X-linked recessive trait, while males need only a single copy, most X-linked recessive traits are more common in males.

A relatively common X-linked recessive trait in humans is color blindness. Color blindness occurs in about eight percent of males from western Europe but in less than one percent of the females from the same region. Actually, several distinct forms of color blindness occur. The most common type is called green weakness, or deuteranomaly; this defect arises from a deficiency in structures called *cones* found at the back of the eye. The cones contain several pigments that are sensitive to light of different wavelengths, and these pigments enable us to perceive and distinguish color. Those individuals with green weakness have a deficiency in the amount of one of the pigments; as a consequence, red colors appear reddish brown and bright greens appear tan. About 75 percent of European males with color blindness have green weakness. The remaining 25 percent mostly have red weakness, or protanomaly. This type of color blindness is similar to green weakness and also results from a deficiency in a color-vision pigment. Green weakness and red weakness are caused by different loci, but the genes for both forms of color blindness are located on the X chromosome.

The inheritance of X-linked color blindness is illustrated in Figures 3.5 and 3.6. In the first family shown (Figure 3.5), the mother is color blind and the father has normal color vision. Because the trait is recessive, the mother must be homozygous, possessing two copies of the color blind gene. The father is normal, however, and therefore his single X bears a gene for normal color vision. Any son born to this couple will be color blind, because boys always inherit their X chromosome from the mother, and the mother has color blind genes on both of her X chromosomes. Daughters receive one X from the father and one from the mother. Thus all the daughters will be heterozygous for the color blind gene and are referred to as *carriers*, since they carry a copy of the gene for color blindness without having the trait themselves. In this example, notice that the sons inherit their mother's trait and daughters inherit their father's trait. This pattern of inheritance is sometimes called *crisscross inheritance* and is a characteristic feature of X-linked traits.

The second family presented in Figure 3.6 represents a cross between a normal male and a female who is a carrier. Both the mother and the father have normal vision, but the mother carries a color blind gene that she passes on to half of her sons and half of her daughters. Since males have only a single X, those sons that receive the X with the color blind gene will be color blind. Half of the daughters also inherit the X chromosome with the defective gene, but they receive a normal X chromosome from the father, and therefore all the daughters will have normal color vision. Consequently, this couple is capable of producing four different types of

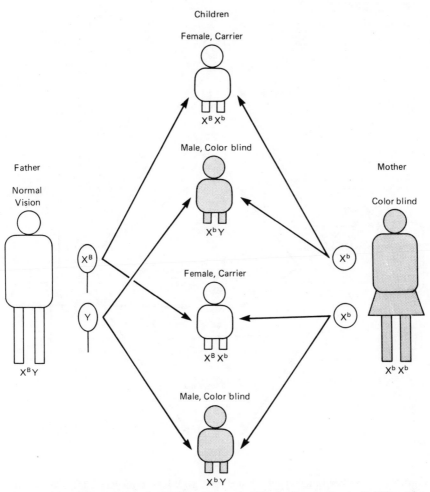

Figure 3.5.   Inheritance of color blindness, an X-linked recessive trait. When the mother is color blind and the father has normal vision, all sons will be color blind. All daughters will have normal vision, but will be carriers.

offspring with respect to color blindness: on the average 50 percent of the sons will be color blind, and the other 50 percent will be normal; approximately 50 percent of the daughters will be carriers and 50 percent will be homozygous for normal color vision.

When the father has the trait and the mother carries two normal genes, all the daughters will receive a copy of the gene for the trait, since every

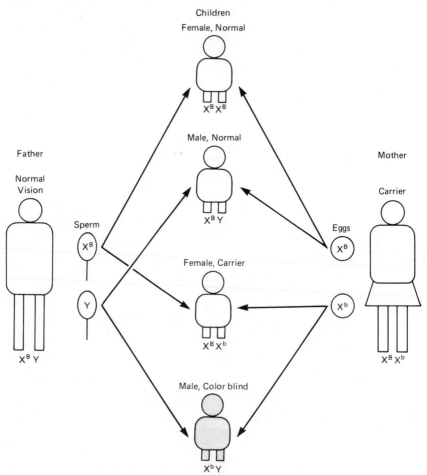

Figure 3.6.   Inheritance of color blindness, an X-linked recessive trait. When the mother is a carrier and the father has normal vision, half the sons on the average will be color blind. All daughters will have normal vision and approximately half will be carriers of the color blind gene.

daughter receives one of her X chromosomes from her father. But each daughter also receives an X from her mother. Because both X chromosomes in the mother are normal, each daughter will be a carrier. The sons will all be normal, since they receive their X chromosome from the mother, who has only normal genes on her X's.

Let us now summarize some of the key characteristics of an X-linked recessive trait.

Characteristics of Traits Determined by
X-Linked Recessive Genes

1. If a female has an X-linked recessive trait, all of her sons will also have the trait. If the father is normal, all the daughters will be normal in appearance but will carry a copy of the recessive gene (they are hetero-zygous).
2. If a father has the trait and the mother is normal (not a carrier), all the daughters will be carriers and all the sons will be normal.
3. If the mother is a carrier and the father is normal, on the average half of the sons will have the trait and half of the daughters will be carriers.
4. When both the mother and the father have an X-linked recessive trait, all of the offspring will also exhibit the trait.

Some X-linked traits are dominant, which means that any female who possesses even a single copy of the gene for the trait will be affected. Thus, females with the trait may be homozygous (two copies of the gene) or heterozygous (one copy of the gene). In practice, almost all females with X-linked dominant traits are heterozygous, because most X-linked dominant traits are uncommon, and the chance of inheriting two X chromosomes with a rare gene is small.

The pattern of inheritance for *X-linked dominant traits* is similar to that for X-linked recessive traits; males receive their X chromosome from their mother, and females inherit an X from the mother and another X from the father. A major difference between X-linked recessive and X-linked dom-inant traits is that there are no carriers with dominant traits; any female who carries a gene for the trait will also display the trait.

Hairy Ears: A Y-Linked Trait (Maybe)

A final type of simple genetic trait is a *Y-linked trait*. Y-linked traits, also called *holandric traits*, are those determined by genes located on the Y chromosome. Because all individuals with Y chromosomes are males, Y-linked traits only occur in males. As mentioned earlier, the Y chromo-some appears to carry very little genetic information. In fact, only two genes have been definitely assigned to the Y chromosome of humans. One is the so-called testis determining factor gene. All humans begin development as females, but around 8 weeks after conception, this gene on the Y chromosome—the testis determining factor gene—somehow causes the development of testes in males. Cells in the testes then begin to produce male hormones, and these hormones stimulate the development of other male characteristics. Occasionally a genetic accident occurs, in which a small part of the Y chromosome containing the testis determining factor gene breaks off and becomes attached to the X chromosome. A person who inherits this X along with a normal X will have two X chromosomes; thus chromosomally, they appear to be female. However, their appearance is basically male, because they have the male determining gene.

The only other gene known to be Y linked is the gene for the H-Y antigen, a gene that codes for one of the molecules on the surface of a cell and that is important in the body's ability to recognize its own tissue. Another gene that appears to be on the Y chromosome, but whose location has not yet been definitively established, is a gene that causes hairy ears. This trait is relatively common among males in some parts of the Middle East and India. Hairy ears, like true Y-linked traits, appear only in men. In several pedigrees that have been studied, the trait is always inherited from the father, and if the father possesses the trait, all of his sons are also affected. This is expected, because all sons receive their father's Y chromosome. Difficulties in interpreting the inheritance of hairy ears arise in some families, however, because the age at which hair appears on the ears varies and penetrance of the trait may not be complete. Characteristics expected of Y-linked traits include the following.

Characteristics of Traits Determined by Y-Linked Genes

1. Only males have the trait.
2. The trait is always passed from father to son; it is never transmitted through the mother. For example, a male should always inherit a Y-linked trait from his paternal grandfather (his father's father) and never from his maternal grandfather (his mother's father).
3. All sons of a father with the trait also possess the trait, unless the trait has incomplete penetrance (Figure 3.7).

These are the patterns of inheritance we expect to see with traits determined by a single gene. Autosomal dominant and recessive traits, X-linked traits, and Y-linked traits all exhibit characteristic patterns of inheritance, patterns that can be easily recognized when you understand how inheritance works and what clues to look for.

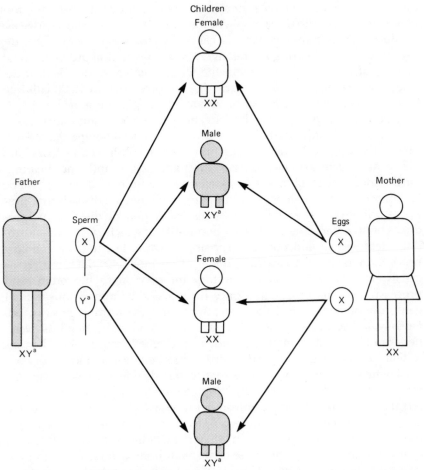

Figure 3.7. Inheritance of a Y-linked trait. Only males have the trait; all sons of an affected male will exhibit the trait.

Deafness: Genetic Heterogeneity

Many genetic traits do not have a single cause, but are produced by several—and sometimes many—different factors. Several people may superficially appear to have the same trait, but upon close inspection they often turn out to have different conditions and frequently different genes are responsible. This phenomenon—the same trait or disease produced by different genes—is called *genetic heterogeneity*. Consider deafness. Loss of hearing is a relatively common medical problem: about one out of every 1,000 infants in the United States is born deaf or develops severe deafness at an early age. Another one in 1,000 children becomes deaf before the age of 16, and many people lose some hearing as they grow older. A large number of genetic factors can cause deafness— in fact, over 100 inherited types of hearing loss are known. Deafness is caused by recessive genes, dominant genes, and X-linked genes. Complex genetic factors (to be discussed in Chapter 4) also influence hearing. Furthermore, hearing loss is associated with a number of other genetic conditions such as osteogenesis imperfecta (a genetic disease that produces brittle bones) and Tay-Sachs disease (a genetic disease that produces brain enlargement). The large number of genetic factors that produce deafness should not be surprising, because hearing is a complex process, involving the eardrum, bones of the inner ear, the semicircular canals, nerves that transmit auditory information to the brain, and processing of the information once it reaches the brain. Thousands of genes undoubtedly affect these structures and the hearing process; potentially, a defect in any one of the genes may produce hearing loss. Deafness can also result from a multitude of nongenetic causes, including infections during pregnancy, certain drugs, head injuries, and loud noise.

Genetic heterogeneity, such as that seen in deafness, causes problems for the geneticist. For example, *congenital deafness* (deafness present at birth) often results from an autosomal recessive gene. As we have discussed in this chapter, when two individuals with the same recessive trait marry and produce children, all of the children are expected to also bear the trait, because the parents are both homozygous and can only pass on genes for the trait. However, research indicates that when two parents are congenitally deaf, only about 20 to 30 percent of their children are also deaf. This unexpected result occurs because many parents are deaf for different reasons; in other words, they are not homozygous for the same genes. On the other hand, occasionally both parents *are* homozygous for the same genes, and all of their children will be deaf. Sometimes deafness results from a dominant gene; in this case each child of a deaf parent has a 50 percent chance of becoming deaf. At other times the parent's deafness is produced by environmental factors, in which case the trait will not be passed on at all. So, the probability of transmitting a heterogeneous trait like deafness depends critically upon the underlying cause. Unfortunately, it may be impossible to determine the precise cause in a given individual. In this case the geneticist cannot offer the patient any precise estimate of his or her chance of passing on the trait.

Genetic heterogeneity requires that caution be exercised about the inheritance of a trait. When a trait is heterogeneous, different individuals pass it on in different ways. Suppose that you possess a disorder that sometimes results from a dominant gene; if in fact your phenotype results from a dominant gene, your chances of passing it to your child are 50 percent. If the disease is heterogeneous, your phenotype might be caused by a recessive gene or it might be multifactorial (discussed in Chapter 4). If either of these were the cause, the probability of your children inheriting the trait would be considerably less. Or, your phenotype might be entirely the product of environmental factors, in which case the trait cannot be transmitted to your children. No layperson should ever attempt to self-diagnose a genetic disease or disorder. Distinguishing between the subtle genetic variants of a disease frequently requires a highly trained specialist in medical genetics, and even medical geneticists frequently rely on information from sophisticated diagnostic tests. If you have concerns about the hereditary nature of a disease or trait in your family, you should discuss these concerns with your family physician or get in touch with one of the genetic centers listed in Appendix I.

Chapter 4

COMPLEX INHERITANCE

In the previous chapter, we examined a number of traits that exhibit simple patterns of inheritance. We saw, for example, that the type of wax in our ears is inherited as an autosomal recessive trait. In a similar way, extra fingers and toes are caused by a dominant gene, and hemophilia is caused by an X-linked recessive gene. Each of these traits exhibits a different mode of inheritance, but they all have one feature in common: For each, the relationship between the trait and the genes is simple. The relationship is simple because only a single pair of genes—a single locus—determines the trait. As a result of this simple relationship, we can predict the probability that a given individual will inherit the trait. For example, dry earwax is a recessive trait; the only way to have dry earwax is to possess two genes for this trait. Thus, if two parents both have dry earwax, the probability that their child will have dry earwax is 100 percent. Such a prediction is possible because the relationship between the trait and the genes is simple and because we know how the genes involved are inherited.

African Pygmies and Human Height

Unlike the traits we discussed in Chapter 3, the inheritance of many human traits and diseases is far from simple. Consider human height or stature. Stature displays considerable variation among humans. As a group, the shortest people in the world are Africans of the Mbuti tribe, a primitive people who live deep in the forest of equatorial Africa. Numbering perhaps only 40,000 individuals, small bands of Mbuti tribespeople live together in hunting parties, moving their villages frequently. Although they possess no domestic animals except the dog and do not farm for themselves, the Mbuti nevertheless practice a successful existence based on hunting wild animals and gathering edible plants in the forest. Some cultural exchange does occur between the Mbuti people and neighboring tribes, but the Mbuti remain largely isolated from the outside world.

The Mbuti are true Pygmies. The average height of a Mbuti male is only 144 centimeters—a mere 4 feet 9 inches tall. Mbuti females are likewise short, averaging only 137 centimeters or 4 feet 6 inches in height. Other Pygmy tribes are found scattered across central Africa; all possess short stature and a primitive forest life-style.

The short stature of African Pygmies is hereditary, but exactly how and why these people are short is not completely understood. Pygmy children grow at near normal rates, and they are only slightly shorter than other African children. The extreme shortness of adult Pygmies is caused primarily by what takes place at puberty. Other humans undergo a period of rapid growth—a growth spurt—during adolescence; this growth spurt is stimulated by heightened secretion of a substance called *growth hormone.* Growth hormone acts by stimulating the secretion of other factors, one of which is called *insulinlike growth factor I* (IGF-I). IGF-I

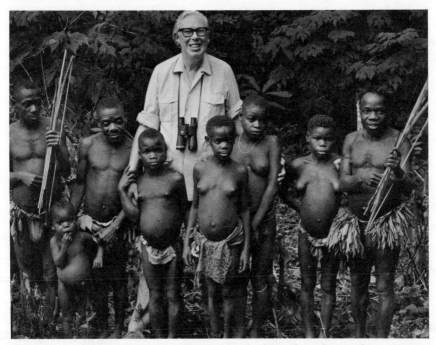

Figure 4.1. African Pygmies. These people have hereditary short stature. (George Holton, Photo Researchers, Inc.)

appears to play a key role in growing taller. Normally, levels of growth hormone and IGF-I rise during puberty and produce the usual growth spurt observed in adolescents at this time. Pygmy adolescents produce normal levels of growth hormone, but their levels of IGF-I never increase as they do in other ethnic groups. In brief, Pygmies are short because they fail to grow rapidly at puberty as other people do. Levels of IGF-I continue to remain low throughout the adult life of a Pygmy, and a deficiency of IGF-I appears to be the primary cause of short stature in these people. Exactly how genes cause the failure of IGF-I secretion in Pygmies is not yet clear.

The tallest people in the world are the Dinka, another group of Africans who reside some 500 miles to the north of the Mbuti along the Nile River. Adult Dinka average 6 feet in height. These are a tall and slender people, with extremely long legs and little fat anywhere on the body. Like short stature in the Pygmies, the precise cause of tallness in the Dinka is unknown, but heredity is almost certainly involved.

The Mbuti and the Dinka illustrate the extreme range of height found among different groups of humans. We don't have to travel across the globe, however, to observe variation in human height. Pick five adults from anywhere—it is unlikely that any two of them will have exactly the same height. In fact, height is one of the most variable of all human traits. Many studies have demonstrated that this variation in human stature has a genetic basis. However, height is also influenced by nonhereditary factors, and the inheritance of height turns out to be far more complex than any of the human traits we have discussed thus far.

Height Is a Complex Trait

Height follows none of the simple patterns of inheritance we discussed in Chapter 3; the complexity of its inheritance arises from several factors. First, the nature of the trait itself is complex. Unlike hemophilia, where the blood either clots or it doesn't and earwax, which is either sticky or dry, people don't sort out into only a few heights. If we asked 1,000 adults to line up in order of their height from shortest to tallest, we would find that no two people have exactly the same height. Thus, height is a continuous trait with an almost unlimited number of different phenotypes possible. As a result, it is impossible to observe the ratios—such as

$\frac{3}{4}$ of one type and $\frac{1}{4}$ of another—that we observed in traits with simple patterns of inheritance.

How Numerous Genes May Determine a Trait

A second complicating factor for the inheritance of height is that individual differences in the trait are determined by many pairs of genes. In the traits with simple inheritance that we examined earlier, a single pair of genes—a single locus—determined an individual's phenotype. In height, however, dozens or even hundreds of gene pairs are involved. A trait such as this, which is determined by many genes, is termed *polygenic*. Because many loci are involved, a large number of different combinations of genes are possible, and these many combinations code for many different phenotypes.

To illustrate the complexity of polygenic inheritance, let us assume for the moment that height is determined by three pairs of genes—by three loci. Certainly more than three loci are involved in this trait, but my objective here is simply to demonstrate how inheritance is complicated by the presence of multiple loci; three loci will be instructive without getting too complicated. Let us assume that at the first locus two different genes are possible: *A*, which codes for tall, and *a*, which codes for short. At a second locus, two genes also determine height: *B* for tall and *b* for short. Similarly, at the third pair, *C* codes for tall, and *c* codes for short. Now, assume that the genes at all three loci work together to determine an individual's height. Recall from our discussions in Chapters 2 and 3 that each person possesses two genes at each locus; these two genes constitute the individual's genotype. Thus, at the first locus an individual might be genotype *AA*, *Aa*, or *aa*; similarly, the individual's genotype at the second locus might be either *BB*, *Bb*, or *bb*, and at the third locus it might be *CC*, *Cc*, *cc*. Because three loci are involved and two genes are found at each locus, a total of six genes contribute to height. We will refer to this set of six genes as the individual's *multilocus genotype*. To keep things simple, we will assume that an individual's height corresponds to the added effect of all six genes . By *added effect*, I mean that the effects of all the genes are added together. For example, a person with the genotypes *AABBCC* has six genes coding for tall and thus would be quite tall—perhaps 6 feet 4 inches in height. An individual with five tall genes (say, AABBCc) would be a little shorter, perhaps 6 feet 2 inches in height. We will suppose that each tall gene contributes 2 inches in height. The different combinations of genotypes and the heights they would produce are indicated in Table 4.1. Genes that determine a trait in this manner are said to be *additive*, because the effects of all the genes can be added together to determine the trait.

Let me point out several important aspects of this polygenic system coding for height. First, a large number of combinations of genotypes are possible; in this relatively simple example involving only three pairs of genes, a total of 27 different combinations of the six genes occurred. With four pairs of genes, 81 different combinations would result, and with five pairs of genes, the number jumps to 243. If dozens of pairs of genes code for a trait, which is not an unreasonable assumption in a complex trait like height, the number of different combinations of genotypes becomes astronomical. This makes studying the individual genes involved almost impossible.

A second important feature of the polygenic system is that several different multilocus genotypes may produce the same phenotype. For example, six different combinations of genes (*AaBbcc, AabbCc, aaBbCc,*

Table 4.1 Theoretical Example of How Three Additive Loci with Two Genes Each Might Determine Stature

Multilocus Genotypes	Number of Genes Coding for Tall	Height
AABBCC	Six genes for tall	6 ft 4 in
AaBBCC,AABbCC,AABBCc	Five genes for tall	6 ft 2 in
aaBBCC,AAbbCC,AABBcc,AaBbCC AaBBCc,AABbCc	Four genes for tall	6 ft
AaBbCc,aaBbCC,AAbbCc,AabbCC AABbcc,aaBBCc,AaBBcc	Three genes for tall	5 ft 10 in
AaBbcc,AabbCc,aaBbCc,AAbbcc aaBBcc,aabbCC	Two genes for tall	5 ft 8 in
Aabbcc,aaBbcc,aabbCc	One gene for tall	5 ft 6 in
aabbcc	Zero genes for tall	5 ft 4 in

AAbbcc, aaBBcc, and *aabbCC*) produce an individual that is 5 feet 8 inches tall. Thus, the relationship between the genotype and the phenotype is not a simple one. As a result of this complexity, we cannot identify an individual's genotype by looking at his or her phenotype as we could with traits determined by a single locus.

I have purposely kept this example simple so that we could observe the features of polygenic inheritance. For most polygenic traits, more than three loci are involved; thus many combinations of genes are possible and many of these combinations produce the same phenotype. Furthermore, genes are often not uniformly additive as they were in our example with height. Frequently, one or a few genes will have a major influence on the trait, and many other genes have slight effects. Dominance on the part of some genes will further complicate the inheritance.

How Genes and the Environment Interact in Determining a Trait

There is yet a third factor that complicates the inheritance of many traits: in addition to the influence of genes on the trait, environmental factors also shape the phenotype. Unfortunately, we often have a tendency to think of human traits as the product of either heredity alone or environment alone. This line of thinking has frequently led to the so-called nature–nurture controversies, arguments about whether human traits (particularly behavioral traits such as intelligence) are genetically programmed (nature) or culturally determined (nurture). Many human traits cannot be adequately explained by either genetics alone or environment alone—both are important in determining the phenotype.

To illustrate how genes and environment interact in determining a trait, let's return to our example of human height. As we have seen, height is affected by our genes. However, genes alone do not completely explain all the differences in height we see among humans. For example, it is a well-documented fact that height has increased among Europeans and North Americans during the past 100 years. My father and I are close to the same height: between 5 feet 7 inches and 5 feet 8 inches. In his generation, my father was average in height. But today when I stop after class to speak to a male college student, I'm usually looking up. In fact, over the past 100 years average height has increased by about 1 inch per generation. While genes can change over time—this is the basis of evolution—the rise in height we have witnessed in western societies over the past 100 years has occurred much too rapidly to have a genetic basis. The real reason for this increase in height is probably better diet and health care, both of which affect growth and stature.

The genes you inherited and your environment—in the form of diet and health care—interact to determine your height. For most complex traits such as stature, we know very little about this interaction or even what specific genes and environmental factors are involved. A person might have short stature for any of a number of reasons: a particular combination of genes at many loci inherited from the parents; a single mutation at a particularly important gene like the one that produced dwarfism in Joseph's family (see Chapter 3), a chromosomal abnormality that affects many genes simultaneously, or serious illness during childhood. Traits that are influenced by multiple genes (polygenic traits) and by environmental factors are frequently called *multifactorial traits*. For multifactorial traits such as height, we recognize that genes and environmental factors are both important, but we cannot say what proportion of an individual's height is genetically determined and what proportion is the result of environmental influences.

At this point, it is critical that we discuss exactly what is meant by the term *environment*. To most of us an environmental factor means something specific in our surroundings—like temperature, income, where we live, or a virus that attacks our body. For height, diet is one of these specific factors in our environment. However, to a geneticist, *environment* refers to anything that is not genetic—anything that is not inherited. That includes temperature, income, place of residence, and viruses. It also includes less tangible, random events that take place during the development of a human body—events like which cell bumps into which cell and the precise time at which a group of cells change or move. These developmental variations are frequently random, but they may be quite important in determining our features; for example, many birth defects are thought to arise from such random developmental events. These variations are sometimes called *developmental noise*. They are part of the environmental influence of a trait because they show no tendency to be inherited, but they are not caused by diet or a chemical or some other specific factor encountered in our immediate surroundings—at least as far as we know.

The Concept of Heritability

Multifactorial traits are those features that are produced by a complex interaction of genes and environmental influences. A concept that is useful in understanding the nature of multifactorial traits is that of *heritability*. We said earlier that with a multifactorial trait we cannot determine what proportion of an individual's phenotype is genetic and what proportion is environmental. What we can sometimes do, however, is to calculate the proportion of the variation in phenotype among a group of people that is genetic. This proportion is called the *heritability*. Suppose, for example, that we examine stature among the male members of the Hopi Indian tribe living on Black Mesa in Arizona. We find that adult male height varies among the members of the tribe: the tallest male is 6 feet 2 inches, the shortest male is 5 feet 2 inches, and all the other males are in between. We might want to know how much of these differences in height is due to differences in genes and how much is due to differences in environmental factors. By comparing the heights of Hopi parents with the heights of their children and by using some complicated statistical methods (methods that are beyond the scope of this book), we could estimate the heritability for stature in this group. Suppose that the heritability was calculated to be 0.62. We would conclude from this heritability value that 62 percent of the variation in height among the male members of the tribe results from differences in their genes. Some estimated heritabilities for traits in humans are given in Table 4.2.

Heritability is usually determined by comparing the phenotypes of related and unrelated individuals or by comparing individuals with different degrees of relatedness, like identical and nonidentical twins. We must recognize that the calculation of heritability rests on a number of assumptions, assumptions that are frequently difficult to fully meet in humans. Thus, we should always view heritability values calculated for human traits with some caution. Nonetheless, they can give us a rough idea of the extent to which differences in a trait are genetically based in a particular group of people.

It is equally important that we recognize the limitations of the concept of heritability, because heritability values are frequently misinterpreted. An important limitation is that heritability should be restricted to the particular group of people and the specific environment for which it was

**Table 4.2 Heritability Values for
Representative Human Traits**

Trait	Heritability
Number of fingerprint ridges	0.7
Height	0.7
Intelligence	0.5–0.8
Muscular strength	0.3
Total cholesterol	0.7
Sitting blood pressure	0.6
Menstrual pain	0.4
IgE antibody level	0.3
Length of the eye	0.8

calculated. For example, if we calculated heritability of adult male height among the Hopi Indians to be 0.62, we would conclude that 62 percent of the differences in adult male height are due to genetic differences; however, this heritability would apply only to the Hopi Indians living on Black Mesa. If we calculated heritability for Caucasians living in Houston, Texas, we might obtain a different value. This is because the magnitude of the genetic and environmental differences among Caucasians in Houston differs from that which occurs in the Hopi, and therefore the proportion of the variation in height that is genetic—the heritability—would probably also be different. The important point to remember is that heritability is not a universal property of the trait; it is a property of the group of people and their environment. If either the group changes or the environment changes, the heritability may also change.

The Concept of Empiric Risk

Another useful concept in the study of multifactorial traits is the notion of *empiric risk*. When a trait has a simple genetic basis, we can use our knowledge of the trait's mode of inheritance to make predictions about the likelihood that relatives will inherit it. For example, webbing between the fingers and toes, a trait called *syndactyly*, is inherited as an autosomal dominant trait. If your father had webbed fingers and your mother did not, then you have a 50 percent chance of also developing webbed fingers (assuming that your father is heterozygous). The 50 percent probability of inheriting this trait is based on our knowledge that webbed fingers is caused by a single dominant gene. However, with multifactorial traits predictions based on the pattern of inheritance is impossible, because we don't know how many genes are involved, whether they are dominant or recessive, or to what degree an individual's trait is caused by environmental effects. The best we can do in the way of prediction is to look at the families of those affected with the trait and see how many of their relatives are also affected. The proportion of the relatives affected is called the *empiric risk*. The term *empiric* is used because the risk is based, not on any knowledge of how the trait is inherited, but on empirical data gathered from affected families.

To illustrate the use of empiric risk, let us examine the risks of schizophrenia in the relatives of patients with this disorder. One of the most common mental illnesses, schizophrenia occurs with a frequency of close to one percent in the United States; it is also one of the most debilitating psychiatric diseases. Typically schizophrenia has an early onset (in late adolescence or early adult life) and is characterized by delusion, hallucinations (particularly auditory), association of unrelated ideas, and an inability to function socially. The exact cause of schizophrenia is unknown, but a hereditary influence has been demonstrated repeatedly. Schizophrenia does not, however, exhibit a simple pattern of inheritance. Genetic and environmental factors both appear to play a role in the disease. Because of its multifactorial nature, geneticists use empiric risk figures to predict the probability of inheriting schizophrenia. For example, the probability of developing schizophrenia in the general population is about one percent. In contrast, the empirically calculated risk to a person who has one parent with schizophrenia is 10 to 15 percent. What this means is that 10 to 15 percent of those with one affected parent will also develop schizophrenia. If both parents have schizophrenia, the empiric risk jumps to about 40 percent. The empiric risk for a brother of a schizophrenic patient, when neither parent is affected, is seven to eight percent, but the risk for a first cousin of the patient is only two to three percent. In general, when a trait has a hereditary basis, the empiric risk is greater for close relatives than for distant ones. This is because close relatives share more genes in common, and a close relative has a greater probability of inheriting some of the genes responsible for the trait. Also, the empiric risk is greater if more than one member of a family is affected.

Estimates of empiric risk should always be used with caution. Keep in mind that they are based on the average incidence observed in those with a family history of the trait. The affected individuals in this group may have the trait for different reasons. For example, breast cancer has a hereditary influence. Suppose that Joan's mother had breast cancer; Joan's empiric risk of developing breast cancer is 14 to 20 percent, which is some two to three times greater than the risk in a woman without a family history of the disease. However, in some families breast cancer appears to be caused by a dominant gene; when a dominant gene is involved, the actual risk to a woman with an affected mother approaches 50 percent. In other patients, breast cancer apparently results from non-hereditary causes; here, the daughters of an affected woman are at no greater risk than those without a family history of the disease. Frequently, we have no means to differentiate between those cases with a strong hereditary basis and those without a hereditary basis, and so the empiric risk is just an average for all types. This obviously leads to poor estimates of true risk. Geneticists are constantly striving to improve their estimates of empiric risk by distinguishing between different forms of a disease and by including additional information about the patient that may allow better prediction of those at high risk.

Establishing a Genetic Basis for Complex Traits

Because multifactorial traits do not exhibit simple patterns of inheritance, establishing the fact that heredity is involved at all is frequently a difficult task. This difficulty arises because family members usually share more than just genes; they frequently share the same house, the same economic status, the same diet, and many other factors as well. Many traits tend to "run in families," which means that family members tend to be alike for the trait; such traits are said to be *familial*. For example, multiple members of the same family often suffer from depression. So depression is familial and runs in the family. However, we would be wrong to conclude on the basis of this observation alone that depression has a genetic basis. Perhaps depression is caused strictly by environmental factors—loss of a loved one, poverty, family violence, or an unstimulating home environment. If one member of a family develops depression as a result of these factors, other members are also likely to have depression, because they are exposed to these same precipitating environmental causes. So familial traits are not necessarily genetic, although they may be. Depression, in fact, is both familial and genetic (see *Depression* in "The Catalog of Genetic Traits").

Because observing a trait in related individuals does not definitely prove a genetic influence, other methods must be used to establish a hereditary basis. Two techniques are frequently used to separate the genetic and environmental causes of human traits: twin studies and studies of adopted children. Scientists have exploited these natural genetic experiments for years, and they have been used to establish a genetic connection for dozens of human traits.

Twins in Genetic Research

In the early years of the Depression, a young woman in Salt Lake City gave birth to two identical twin boys. Because of family difficulties (the nature of which was unrecorded), the mother and her young husband were unable to care for the twins; thus, the infants were separated and put up for adoption immediately after birth. One of the twins was adopted by a young couple in Salt Lake City, who named the boy Millan. Millan completed 4 years of high school and grew up in Salt Lake City. The other twin was adopted by a childless couple in Salt Lake City, and they named him George. When George was 3 years old, his family moved to Colorado, then to Chicago, and finally to New York City, where George grew up unaware that he was adopted. He had little high school education and went into the commercial art business.

When George was 18 years old, his parents informed him that he was adopted and that his relatives lived in Salt Lake City; at about the same time, Millan also learned of his twin brother. The following summer, George traveled to Salt Lake City to meet his relatives. The two twins met and spent a few weeks together for the first time since their birth.

Geneticists studied George and Millan during those few weeks they were together in Salt Lake City. Although separated for 19 years and reared in very different environments, George and Millan were so similar in appearance that Millan's neighbors mistook George for his brother. Their hair color and texture were identical; their hair lines were the same. Their eye colors matched perfectly. George was 5 feet 5 $\frac{1}{4}$ inches tall, whereas Millan was 5 feet 6 $\frac{1}{2}$ inches tall, but they differed in weight by less than 3 pounds. Their teeth were remarkably similar in appearance; both twins had cavities in the same teeth. Mental and personality tests administered by the geneticists indicated that the boys' mental abilities and temperament were similar. Millan scored somewhat higher than George on IQ and other mental tests (perhaps due to his increased schooling), but the scores were close and both boys displayed weakness in mathematics and word meanings. They differed some in social adjustment, but overall, their personality characteristics were quite similar. On one test of personality that included 180 different questions, the two twins answered only 20 questions differently.

Following their brief time together that summer in Salt Lake City, George and Millan parted and did not see each other again. Both entered the armed forces: Millan joined the Coast Guard and was stationed in northern California; George became a glider pilot and was stationed in the Midwest. In 1943, both twins experienced acute pain in their joints. Millan began to suffer from persistent back pain; George awoke one morning with a severe pain in his left leg that progressed to his back, hips, and other joints. The two young men were both hospitalized several times. Eventually both were diagnosed with spondylitis, a potentially crippling disease that produces inflammation of the bones in the back. Although George was treated for the illness in New York and Millan was treated in Utah, physical examinations, X-rays, and laboratory tests showed that the twins were almost identical in the onset, symptoms, and progress of the disease.

The story of George and Millan is not unique. A number of identical twins who were reared apart have made contact after years of separation and have discovered that they are remarkably similar in numerous ways. In some cases, popular accounts have overemphasized the similarities between twins reared apart. George and Millan were not identical in all respects: They differed somewhat in height, IQ, and temperament. Nevertheless, their similarities were great enough to confuse the neighbors and awe the geneticists. The often incredible similarities between identical twins reared apart are perhaps the most convincing evidence that genes influence a large number of our traits.

Twins are of two types: *nonidentical twins* (also called *fraternal twins*) and *identical twins*. As we discussed in Chapter 2, normally a woman's ovary expels a single egg each month. Occasionally, however, two eggs are released at the same time, and each may be fertilized by a different sperm. The two embryos, or zygotes, that result from this event develop into nonidentical twins. Another name for nonidentical twins is *dizygotic twins*, which literally means "from two zygotes." Nonidentical twins are therefore derived from two different eggs fertilized by two different sperm. Because each parent's genotype consists of two genes, each with a 50 percent probability of being passed on, nonidentical twins will share, on the average, 50 percent of the same genes. This is the same proportion of genes shared by all brothers and sisters; in fact, from a genetic standpoint nonidentical twins are simply siblings that happen to be the same age. As in other siblings, nonidentical twins may be the same sex or they can be different sexes.

How often nonidentical twins are born varies widely among human ethnic groups. For example, among North American Caucasians, the number of nonidentical twins is about seven twin pairs per 1,000 pregnancies. In contrast, the rate is about three per 1,000 in Japanese, and about 40 per 1,000 among Nigerians. The rate of twining also changes with age of the mother—the rate of twining increases from age 18 up to about age 37 and then declines. Producing nonidentical twins also tends to run in families. If a woman produces one set of nonidentical twins, she is more likely to produce another set. Her female relatives are also more likely to produce nonidentical twins.

Identical twins, frequently called *monozygotic twins* (from a single zygote), arise in a different way. Identical twins occur when one egg is fertilized by one sperm, initially producing a single embryo. Later, this embryo divides into two separate groups of cells, which then develop into two separate individuals. Because they originated from a single egg and sperm, these twins are genetically identical—100 percent of their genes are the same. One consequence of their identical genetic makeup is that identical twins are always the same sex. Why one embryo splits into two and gives rise to identical twins is not known, but in most ethnic groups this event occurs with a frequency of about four twin pairs per 1,000 pregnancies. Recent research indicates that the production of identical twins displays a slight tendency to run in families.

Twins can be used to estimate the importance of genes in determining the variation of a trait by comparing the similarity of identical and nonidentical twins. As an example, consider schizophrenia, a severe mental disorder that we discussed earlier in the context of empiric risk. We might begin our twin study by examining a number of twins for the presence of schizophrenia. If one member of the pair has schizophrenia, but the other does not, we say that the twins are *discordant*; if both of the twins have schizophrenia, then they are *concordant*. We calculate the percentage of identical twins that are concordant for schizophrenia and then calculate the percentage of nonidentical twins that are concordant. Now, remember that identical twins are genetically identical, whereas nonidentical twins share only 50 percent of the same genes; therefore, when genes are important in determining the trait, we expect greater similarity—higher concordance—in the identical twins. This is exactly

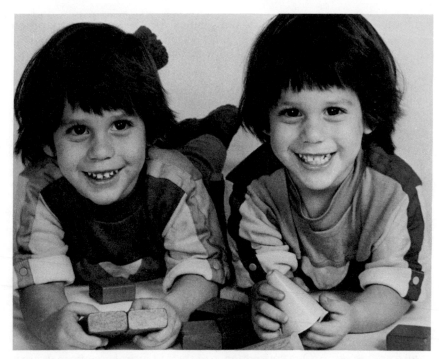

Figure 4.2.   Identical twins, who develop from a single egg fertilized by a single sperm. They are genetically identical. (Erika Stone, Photo Researchers, Inc.)

what researchers have observed with schizophrenia—higher concordance in identical twins than in nonidentical twins. In general, higher concordance in identical twins is indicative of a genetic influence to the trait. Table 4.3 lists some concordance figures for human traits.

The important thing to keep in mind about concordance is that it is the *difference* in the concordance of identical and nonidentical twins that indicates a genetic component to the trait. Many people misinterpret concordance studies, erroneously concluding that high concordance in identical twins alone signals the importance of genes. This is incorrect because identical twins usually share the same environment—the same home, the same parents, the same friends, and so on—as well as the same genes. Therefore, high concordance in identical twins might be due to their identical genes or it might result from their similarity in environment. So, by itself, high concordance in identical twins tells us nothing.

Like identical twins, nonidentical twins share the same environment, but they share only 50 percent of the same genes. If similar environments

Table 4.3 Concordance Values for Identical and Nonidentical Twins

Trait	Concordance in Identical Twins	Concordance in Nonidentical Twins
Stuttering (males)	0.75	0.45
Asthma	0.48	0.19
Hay fever	0.21	0.14
Club foot	0.33	0.03
Depression	0.65	0.14
Refractive errors requiring eyeglasses	0.63	0.03
Peptic ulcer	0.53	0.36

produce the high concordance observed in identical twins, we would also expect to observe high concordance in nonidentical twins, because they too share the same environment. However, if genes produce the high concordance in identical twins, then nonidentical twins should exhibit less concordance, because they are genetically less similar.

In summary, lower concordance in nonidentical twins signals a genetic component to the trait, although it does not exclude the possibility that environmental factors also play a role. Comparison of identical and nonidentical twins also can be used to calculate heritability values, although the mathematics involved are too complex to present here.

There are some potential problems with the use of concordance for determining the heritable basis of a trait. The method assumes that identical twins do not share a more common environment than nonidentical twins. In other words, we assume that the greater similarity in the phenotypes of the identical twins is the result of their being genetically identical and not because their environments are more similar than the environments of nonidentical twins. However, this assumption may be incorrect. Because they look alike, identical twins may be treated more similar by their peers and parents than nonidentical twins, making the environments experienced by identical twins more similar than the environments experienced by nonidentical twins.

In spite of these potential problems, studies of twins have contributed much to our understanding of human heredity. To facilitate genetic investigations of twins, a number of twin registries have been created. These are listings of identical and nonidentical twins that are available for genetic study. For example, the National Academy of Science maintains a huge twin registry containing detailed information on nearly 16,000 pairs of male twins who were born between 1917 and 1927 and who served in the U.S. armed services during World War II and the Korean War. This registry has been utilized to study the genetic basis of a number of human traits and diseases.

Adopted Children in Genetic Research

Every year, thousands of children are put up for adoption; frequently these children are separated from their mothers soon after birth and are reared by foster parents with whom they have no genetic relationship. These children, called *adoptees*, carry none of their foster parents' genes, but they do share a common environment with them. Conversely, the adoptees carry 50 percent of their biological parents' genes, but they have no common environment with them. (Actually, every child shares some common environment with its biological mother—the nine months of life in the womb.) If adoptees display similarity to their foster parents, then that resemblance must result from the influence of the environment, because foster parents and adoptees share no genes in common. On the other hand, if adoptees resemble their biological parents in some trait, then the trait must have a genetic basis, because only genes are shared with their biological parents (except for the in utero environment). So comparing adoptees with their foster parents and with their biological parents provides a powerful means of determining the extent to which genes affect a trait.

To illustrate the adoption approach, consider the inheritance of obesity. There is little doubt that obesity tends to run in families; multiple members of the same families are frequently overweight. We cannot, however, conclude from this observation that obesity is genetic, for family members frequently eat at the same table, and eating habits and activity patterns may be learned. Recent studies of twins have suggested that genes do play an important role in obesity; the studies found that identical twins were more concordant for obesity than nonidentical twins. Nevertheless, many people remained skeptical that genes significantly influence obesity. In 1986, however, *The New England Journal of Medicine* published a large adoption study that firmly established the hereditary influence on obesity. This study was carried out on 540 Danish adults, who were adopted by unrelated foster parents between 1924 and 1947. These adoptees are now adults and the relationship between their weight and the weights of their biological and foster parents was examined. Weights and heights of the adoptees, their biological parents, and their foster parents were obtained and analyzed. Because weight is correlated with height and height is inherited, the weight and height values were converted to a body-mass index, which provided an estimate of weight that was independent of height. The adoptees were then placed into one of four weight classes—thin, median, overweight, or obese—on the basis of their body-mass index, sex, and age. When the weight class of the adoptees was compared to the body-mass index of their biological parents, a strong relationship was observed, as is shown in Figure 4.3. Obese adoptees tended to have heavy parents, whereas thin adoptees tended to have thin parents. When the adoptees were compared to their foster parents, no such relationship was found. After rigorous analysis of the data to exclude the possibility that nonhereditary factors could produce the observed relationship, the investigators in the study concluded that genes play an important role in determining fatness in adult humans.

The results of this study demonstrated that adult body weight is influenced by heredity, but this does not mean that fatness is totally deter-

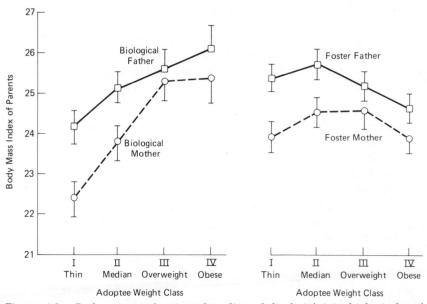

Figure 4.3.   Body mass index (weight adjusted for height) in biological and foster parents of adoptees. Heavier adoptees have heavier biological parents, but no consistent relationship exists between the weight of the adoptees and body mass index of the foster parents. (Redrawn with permission of the *New England Journal of Medicine*, vol. 314: 195.)

mined by genes—obesity is not a trait that is set for life at conception. Environmental factors certainly influence fatness, as evidenced by the fact that, regardless of one's genes, starvation produces weight loss and overeating produces weight gain. Nevertheless, the results do show that genes predispose some individuals to obesity; other things being equal, some individuals are more likely to become fat than others. How the genes involved cause obesity is not clear; they might influence the amount of food consumed, perhaps affecting appetite or eating habits. Alternatively, they might control the rate at which calories are burned. Whatever the physiological basis of obesity, this example illustrates how adoption studies can be used to study the genetic basis of complex traits.

Characteristics of Multifactorial Inheritance

We have now discussed why some traits display complex inheritance and how multifactorial traits are studied. At this point, we should review some of the characteristics of multifactorial traits—some of their distinguishing features.

1. Multifactorial traits tend to run in families. What I mean by this is that the trait is not randomly distributed among families, but tends to cluster within certain families. If one member of the family has the trait, another member is more likely to have it than is a person without a family history of the trait.
2. Although multifactorial traits tend to run in families, they do not exhibit any regular pattern of inheritance, such as the patterns we observed with recessive inheritance, dominant inheritance, X-linked inheritance, and so on.
3. If one family member has a multifactorial trait, the probability that a relative will also be affected depends on how many genes the two share in common. Suppose you have a relative with high blood pressure. Because high blood pressure is multifactorial, you are more likely to have high blood pressure than an individual without a family history of hypertension. If your relative with high blood pressure is your father, with whom you share 50 percent of your genes, you are much more likely to have trouble with high blood pressure than if the

affected relative is a cousin, with whom you share only 12.5 percent of your genes.
4. The probability of inheriting the trait is higher when more than one member of the family is affected.
5. Identical twins are more likely to be the same (concordant) for the trait than are nonidentical twins.

In summary, many human traits display complex inheritance and are said to be multifactorial. This complexity arises because many genes are involved and because environmental factors also influence the trait. The concept of heritability provides information about the relative importance of genetic and environmental factors in phenotypic variation; more precisely, heritability is the proportion of the variation in phenotype that results from differences in genotype. Although we cannot make precise predictions about the probability of inheriting a multifactorial trait, as we did for simple genetic traits, estimates of empiric risk provide some information about the likelihood of having the trait when one or more family members are affected.

Chapter 5

CHROMOSOMES AND CHROMOSOME ABNORMALITIES

Dr. Turner and Seven
Short Women

In the summer of 1938, Dr. Henry Turner spoke to a small group of hormone specialists at a medical meeting in San Francisco. Turner described seven female patients he had recently examined. All seven exhibited a common set of peculiar traits, traits that appeared to result from some type of hormone deficiency. The seven women ranged in age from 15 to 23, but all were short and sexually immature. Furthermore, the women were distinguished by folds of skin on the neck, a low hairline on the back of the head, and deformed elbows. Although Turner didn't know the underlying cause of the condition, he believed that these traits represented a previously undescribed syndrome. Later, Turner encountered several additional cases of this strange disorder. Other physicians and hormone specialists observed similar characteristics in some of their patients, and they began to refer to the disorder as *Turner syndrome.*

For many years, the cause of Turner syndrome remained obscure. Then, in 1954 Dr. P. E. Polani and his colleagues at Guy's Hospital in London made a startling discovery. When they examined the cells of women with Turner syndrome, they could not find a structure that is normally present in female cells. This structure was the sex chromatin or Barr body. All cells from normal females possess sex chromatin, whereas cells from normal males lack sex chromatin. The finding that Turner women lacked the sex chromatin suggested that this syndrome might result from an abnormal set of sex chromosomes.

The idea that Turner women might suffer from an abnormality of the sex chromosomes was confirmed in 1959. Using newly developed techniques for preparing cells and viewing chromosomes, a team of researchers lead by C. E. Ford demonstrated that a 14-year-old girl with Turner syndrome possessed only a single X chromosome, instead of the two Xs found in normal females. In that same year, two other syndromes were associated with chromosome abnormalities: Down syndrome was shown to result from three copies of chromosome 21, and Klinefelter syndrome was shown to result from the presence of two X chromosomes and a Y chromosome. These discoveries forced geneticists to recognize that chromosome abnormalities cause a number of disorders in humans.

Chromosomes: Number and Structure

Chromosomes are the vehicles of inheritance, carrying the genes that encode our traits. In each of our cells we possess 46 chromosomes arranged in 23 pairs. It is the movement of these chromosomes before and after reproduction that really creates heredity. As our gonads produce sex cells—either sperm or eggs—the chromosome pairs divide, one chromosome of each pair entering into an individual sex cell. Consequently, each sex cell contains only half the number of chromosomes, and because the genes are carried on the chromosomes, each sex cell also contains only half of the genes. When an egg and a sperm later meet in the process of fertilization, the two sets of chromosomes carried by the sex cells unite, endowing the new embryo with a full complement of genes for all of its traits.

Unfortunately, occasional accidents occur in this process; the chromosomes may not divide properly, or part of a chromosome may duplicate, break off, or become rearranged. These accidents, termed *chromosome mutations*, may lead to an individual with an abnormal set of chromosomes, such as those with Turner syndrome. These accidents occur rarely, but their effects are often catastrophic.

Let us consider the structure of a normal chromosome. Imagine that a sperm and egg have just fused, creating an entirely new person. This one-cell individual now has a complete set of genetic information, consisting of 46 chromosomes grouped in 23 pairs. For simplicity, we will consider only one of the 46 chromosomes. Let us look at chromosome 4, which is illustrated in Figure 5.1.

As we discussed in Chapter 2, all the genetic information on a chromosome actually exists in the molecular structure of DNA. Each chromosome contains a single DNA molecule (at least initially), but the DNA is not stretched out straight. Instead, the DNA coils around beads of histone proteins, wrapping up on itself to form the compact structure we call a chromosome.

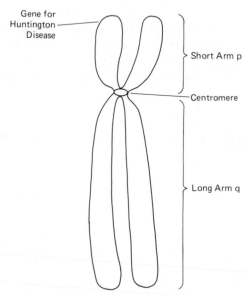

Figure 5.1.   Human chromosome 4.

On each chromosome is a special region called the *centromere*; under the microscope the centromere appears as a constricted region on the chromosome. Although the precise nature of the centromere is still poorly understood, the centromere serves as a useful reference point on the chromosome, like a prominent landmark along a highway. The centromere divides a chromosome into two parts, which are called *chromosome arms*; for the chromosome illustrated in Figure 5.1, one of these chromosome arms is considerably longer than the other. Geneticists label the shorter arm of a chromosome with the symbol *p* and the long arm with *q*. For example, the gene that causes Huntington disease—an inherited neurological disease—occurs on chromosome 4. The specific location of the Huntington's gene is *p16.3*, which indicates that this gene resides on the short arm (*p*) of the chromosome in a region designated 16.3.

Initially, the chromosome consists of a single copy of the DNA and appears as illustrated in Figure 5.2. When the cell divides and gives rise to two new cells, each new cell must receive a complete copy of the DNA to function properly. So, prior to cell division, the chromosome doubles itself in a process called *replication*. Following replication, the two copies

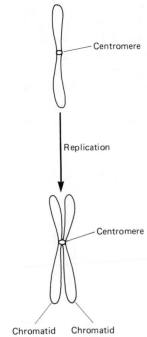

Figure 5.2.   Before replication, each chromosome consists of one chromatid. After replication, two chromatids are present, held together by the centromere. Each chromatid consists of one DNA molecule.

of the chromosome are held together at the centromere, as shown in Figure 5.2. Each of these chromosome copies is called a *chromatid*. Geneticists usually examine chromosomes when each consists of two chromatids, and we will illustrate our chromosomes in this way.

Types of Chromosomes

Geneticists classify chromosomes on the basis of the position of the centromere. In *metacentric chromosomes*, we find the centromere at or near the center of the chromosome; here, the centromere divides a metacentric chromosome into two approximately equal halves, so p and q are more or less equal. In other chromosomes, the centromere is displaced toward one end, producing a long and a short arm; these are termed *submetacentric chromosomes*. Finally, in *acrocentric chromosomes*, the centromere is located near one end, creating a chromosome with a long arm and a very short arm. These three types of chromosomes are illustrated in Figure 5.3. Now that we are equipped with some basic terms to describe chromosomes, we can examine a complete set of human chromosomes.

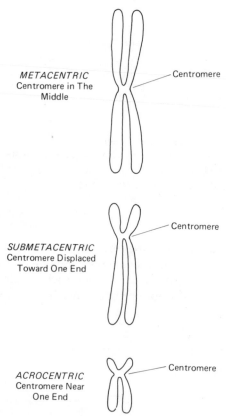

Figure 5.3.   Three types of chromosomes, based on the location of the centromere.

The Human Karyotype

At the age of 37, Sandy married for the second time. Her first marriage produced three healthy children but after 15 years ended in divorce. Following two years as a single parent, Sandy met Kenneth; they dated for 9 months and then decided to marry. Kenneth loved Sandy's children, but felt a strong desire to father a child himself. Sandy was also eager to have a baby with Kenneth.

Soon after their wedding, Sandy visited her obstetrician and explained her desire to have another child. Because of her age and the fact that she had given birth to her last child over 13 years before, she feared that there might be complications. She wanted her obstetrician's opinion.

Sandy's obstetrician pointed out that she was in excellent health and in good physical condition; there was no reason to assume that the pregnancy would be particularly difficult or the labor threatening. He explained, however, that there was one potential problem: The risk of having a child with a chromosomal abnormality is greater in older mothers.

"Let's consider Down syndrome as an example," he said. "This disorder results from an extra copy of chromosome 21, and older women are more likely to conceive a child with the extra chromosome. At age 20, your chance of giving birth to a child with Down syndrome is about 1 in 2,000. At age 30, the frequency remains quite low: a probability of only 1 in 800. By age 38, however, the risk climbs to 1 in 175. If you decided to have a child at age 45, your chances of producing a Down's child would be about 1 in 30. Other chromosomal abnormalities are similar—the older the mother, the more likely she is to conceive a child with an abnormality. The age of the father appears to have little or no effect on the incidence of chromosome mutations.

"Let's suppose you get pregnant in the next six months; you will be 38 years old when the baby is born" he pointed out. "At that age, the probability of having a child with some type of chromosome mutation is about 1 in 100. That's still fairly low," he added. "Another way to look at this probability is to consider that 99 percent of the children born to women your age have perfectly normal chromosomes. Nevertheless, many women are still concerned about that 1 chance in 100."

Her obstetrician then suggested that if Sandy wanted to get pregnant, she might consider having *amniocentesis* performed during the pregnancy and a chromosome check done on the fetus. He explained that amniocentesis is a relatively simple outpatient procedure. A needle is inserted through the mother's abdominal wall into the amniotic sac that surrounds the growing fetus. A small volume of the amniotic fluid is removed. This fluid contains a few of the baby's cells, and the baby's chromosomes can be examined in these cells.

"The discomfort involved in this procedure is brief," he reassured her, adding "It's a safe procedure, with only minimal risk of complications for you and your child." He went on to discuss what these possible complications might be. He also cautioned that occasionally amniocentesis does not provide an adequate sample for a chromosome analysis and must be repeated.

Sandy and Kenneth discussed the possibility of amniocentesis and decided to have the procedure done if Sandy was successful in getting pregnant. Eight months later, Sandy missed her menstrual period, and a trip to the doctor confirmed that she was pregnant.

In the sixteenth week of her pregnancy, Sandy underwent amniocentesis. A sample of the amniotic fluid taken from her womb was sent to a special genetics laboratory. There, a lab technician put the fluid in a tube and spun it in a machine called a centrifuge. The centrifuge forced the cells in the fluid down to the bottom of the tube, concentrating them. The technician then removed the cells, placed them on a special culture plate, and added a liquid containing nutrients needed for the cells to grow. Within a few days the cells began to divide and proliferate, each new cell containing a complete set of the baby's chromosomes. After a week of growth, enough cells had accumulated for a chromosome check to be done.

To prepare the chromosomes for analysis, the technician added a chemical to the cell culture that stopped the cells from dividing. An hour later, he placed the cells in a solution that caused the cells to swell. He then added chemicals that fixed (preserved) the cells and dropped the solution containing the cells onto a glass slide. As the solution dried on the glass, the cells spread out and burst, spewing forth the chromosomes onto the slide. Finally, he stained the chromosomes with special dyes and chemicals that made the chromosomes visible.

Once the chromosomes were prepared, a cytogeneticist (a person trained in the study of chromosomes) examined them under a microscope. After looking at a number of different cells, she picked out several cells in which the chromosomes had separated and spread nicely; these cells she photographed. Later the photographs were developed and enlarged. From one of the photos, the chromosomes were carefully cut out and arranged in groups according to their shape and size, as shown in Figure 5.4. This picture, representing the baby's complete set of chromosomes, is called a *karyotype*. The cytogeneticist then carefully studied the karyotype for any evidence of chromosome abnormalities.

Two weeks after undergoing amniocentesis, Sandy had an appointment scheduled with her obstetrician to discuss the results of the karyotype. "The chromosomes all look normal." he said. "Do you want to know the sex of your baby?" Sandy and Kenneth had already discussed this option, and, though tempted, she declined, preferring the traditional surprise at delivery.

Chromosome Abnormalities

A normal karyotype does not guarantee a normal baby. Only relatively large chromosomal defects can be observed with the microscope, and

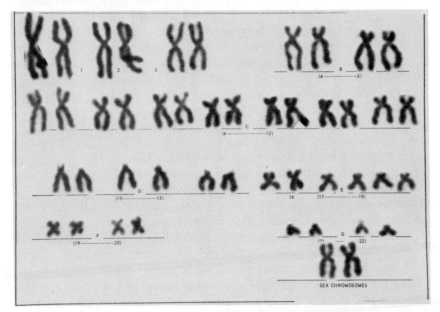

Figure 5.4.   A karyotype or set of chromosomes from a normal female. (Courtesy of the Armed Forces Institute of Pathology.)

recall that each chromosome contains millions of bits of genetic information. Consequently, the types of genetic disorders we discussed earlier—those involving only a single gene like hemophilia or dwarfism—cannot be observed on a karyotype. Other methods of prenatal diagnosis exist for some of these single gene defects; we will discuss these tests in Chapter 6. The karyotype is, however, useful for diagnosing large defects in the number or the structure of the chromosomes.

Most Chromosome Abnormalities Are Rare

Most chromosome abnormalities are rare in newborn infants. For example, Down syndrome is the most common chromosomal defect observed in humans, and yet the incidence in the general population is only about 1 in 800 births (although, as we have seen, the incidence in older mothers is considerably higher). Turner syndrome, a condition that arises when an X chromosome is missing, occurs with a frequency of only 1 in 10,000 female births. And Patau syndrome, caused by an extra copy of chromosome 13, is seen in only 1 out of every 20,000 newborns.

Two reasons exist for the relative rarity of chromosome abnormalities. First, the process of cell division is precise, and the majority of cells get the correct complement of chromosomes. Even when an accident does occur and a human is conceived with a major chromosome mutation, an abnormal baby is rarely born. Instead, the mother's body usually rejects the embryo early in pregnancy, resulting in a miscarriage.

A surprising number of human conceptions result in miscarriage. Because many miscarriages are never reported and some occur before a woman is even aware of her pregnancy, precise numbers are difficult to come by. However, recent studies that measured changes in hormone levels to detect early pregnancies indicate that almost one third of all conceptions result in a miscarriage; the majority of these take place before the woman is aware of her pregnancy. Miscarriage may occur for a variety of reasons. In a few cases the developing embryo is healthy, but the mother's body is unable to carry it. However, most miscarriages result from a genetic, chromosomal, or developmental problem in the embryo. For example, some studies indicate chromosome defects occur in 50 percent of all recognized miscarriages.

Let's consider what happens in a typical group of 1,000 conceptions. Among our 1,000 conceptions, 22 percent will spontaneously abort before the pregnancy is recognized by the woman or her doctor, usually in the first 30 days following conception. Thus, only 780 of the original conceptions will result in a recognized pregnancy. Of these 780 recognized pregnancies, 11 percent will result in a miscarriage after the first 30 days. Therefore 690 of the original conceptions will end in a live birth; of these, perhaps two children will have a chromosome abnormality of some type. If 50 percent of the miscarriages involved a chromosome problem, then 155 of the original conceptions possessed chromosome defects, but less than two percent of these survived to birth. The important point is that very few of the chromosome abnormalities that arise at conception result in the birth of a chromosomally abnormal child.

Types of Chromosome Abnormalities

What are some of the types of chromosome abnormalities that can be observed in a karyotype? Two basic kinds of chromosomal defects are seen: abnormalities of chromosome number, where too few or too many chromosomes are present; and abnormalities of chromosome structure, where the correct number of chromosomes is present, but something is wrong with the structure of one or more individual chromosomes.

Errors in Chromosome Number: Down Syndrome

Down syndrome, which we have already mentioned several times, is the most common and the best known of the chromosomal abnormalities; it is an example of a defect in the number of chromosomes. In the past, many people called this disorder Mongolism because of the somewhat Oriental appearance of the eyes in affected individuals. However, the name is really inappropriate, because people with the disorder do not possess Oriental traits, and the disease occurs in all ethnic groups, not just in Mongolians. The disorder is more properly referred to as *Down syndrome* or *trisomy 21*. *Trisomy* is a technical term that means three copies of one chromosome are present, instead of the usual two copies found in cells of normal individuals. Trisomy 21 signifies that individuals with Down syndrome have three copies of chromosome 21.

The presence of an extra chromosome in Down syndrome produces a set of traits that are the hallmark of this disorder (Figure 5.5). First, people with Down syndrome generally have poor muscle tone, which gives them a somewhat limp and floppy appearance. They typically possess slanting eyes and a relatively large tongue that often protrudes from the mouth. The bridge of the nose is flattened, the feet are short and broad, and frequently a wide gap occurs between the first and second

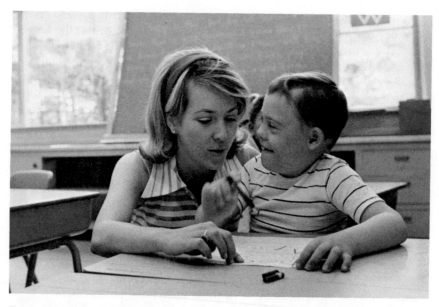

Figure 5.5. This child has Down syndrome, a genetic disorder that results from the presence of an extra copy of chromosome 21. (Courtesy of Rapho/Photo Researchers, Inc. © Bruce Roberts.)

toes. Their hands exhibit unusual palm and fingerprints; often the little finger curves inward, a condition called *clinodactyly*. All individuals with Down syndrome are mentally retarded, with an average IQ of around 50. (For comparison, the IQ of normal individuals averages 100.) Physical growth is also retarded, and most individuals with Down syndrome are short. Walking is delayed, and speech development is slow, although most children with Down syndrome do eventually learn to walk and talk. About 40 percent of the affected individuals have defects of the heart, and they have an increased risk of leukemia, as well as other medical problems. In spite of their considerable physical and mental problems, most Down's children are lively, cheerful, and affectionate.

About 92 percent of the cases of Down syndrome arise largely from random accidents that occur during the formation of a sperm cell or an egg cell: The two copies of chromosome 21 fail to divide and thus a sex cell (egg or sperm) is produced with two copies of this chromosome. When this sex cell fuses with a normal sex cell (containing a single chromosome 21) at fertilization, the resulting embryo receives three of chromosome 21 instead of the usual two. Down syndrome arising in this way—from the failure of chromosome division, producing a child with three of chromosome 21—is termed *primary Down syndrome*.

The failure of the chromosomes to divide properly appears to be a random event, there is little hereditary tendency to produce a child with primary Down syndrome. In other words, relatives of a person who has a primary Down syndrome child are not usually themselves likely to have children with the disorder. However, approximately four percent of the children with Down syndrome possess 46 chromosomes, yet they have all the typical features of Down syndrome. Initially this observation was puzzling to geneticists: How can these children have Down syndrome if they possess the correct number of chromosomes. Further study revealed that these individuals do indeed have three copies of chromosome 21, but one copy is attached to another chromosome, usually chromosome 14. Geneticists call this type of chromosomal abnormality a *translocation*. A translocation is a rearrangement of the chromosomal material, occurring when a piece of one chromosome breaks off and sticks to another chromosome or when segments are exchanged between two chromosomes. Down syndrome occurring from a translocation is appropriately called *translocation Down syndrome.*

Whereas the tendency to produce children with primary Down syndrome is not usually inherited, producing a child with translocation Down syndrome may be passed on. This occurs when one of the parents is a *translocation carrier*. The translocation carrier has only 45 chromosomes; one copy of chromosome 21 is attached to another chromosome. Because the translocation carrier possesses two functional copies of chromosome 21—the translocated copy and the normal copy—this individual does not have Down syndrome. When the translocation carrier produces sex cells, however, problems frequently arise: The two copies of chromosome 21 do not pair up properly (remember that one copy is now attached to another chromosome and travels with it), and they may not separate. Consequently, sex cells are produced that fail to have the correct number of chromosomes, and a child with Down syndrome is more likely to be conceived, as shown in Figure 5.6. Furthermore, about 50 percent of the normal children of a translocation carrier will be carriers like the parent; thus, the tendency of a translocation carrier to produce Down syndrome children is passed on to future generations.

In a few cases of Down syndrome, the affected individuals are *mosaics*, which means that some cells in their body possess two copies of chromosome 21, while other cells have three copies. Mosaics arise from accidents occurring in cell division of the embryo (after fertilization) or from a

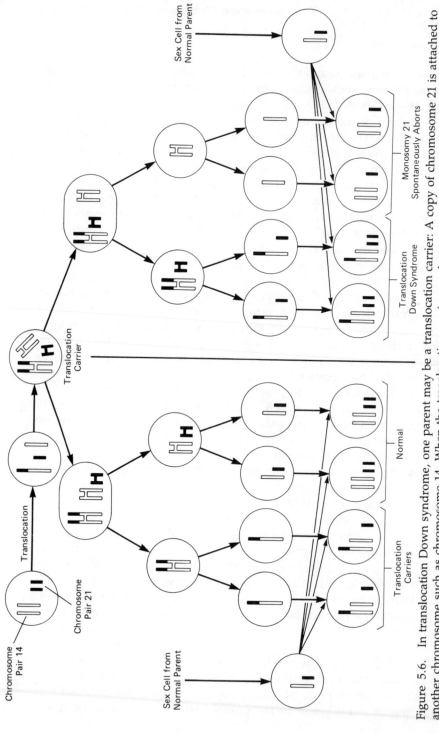

Figure 5.6. In translocation Down syndrome, one parent may be a translocation carrier: A copy of chromosome 21 is attached to another chromosome such as chromosome 14. When the translocation carrier produces sex cells, some sex cells may contain two copies of chromosome 21. Fusion with a normal sex cell will then produce a child with translocation Down syndrome.

combination of accidents in the formation of sex cells and cell division of the embryo. Frequently these individuals are less retarded than those with typical Down syndrome.

There are other ways in which abnormal chromosomes can produce Down syndrome, but these are rare, and we will not delve into the mechanics of how these mutations occur. What I want to emphasize is the fact that Down syndrome can arise in several different ways, and all these causes involve, in some manner, an extra copy of the genetic information on chromosome 21. How the extra copy arises becomes important for predicting the probability of having another child with Down syndrome. For example, if a young mother has a child with primary Down syndrome, her chance of having another Down's child is only about one percent (1 in 100). But if her child has translocation Down syndrome and she is a translocation carrier (chromosome 21 is translocated to chromosome 13, 14, or 15), the chance of conceiving another Down's child is about 10 percent. If, on the other hand, the father is a translocation carrier, the risk of another affected child is around 5 percent. These risk figures are only approximate; calculating the precise risk for a given individual is quite complicated and should be done by someone trained in medical genetics only after a thorough review of the individual's family history.

Other Errors of Chromosome Number

A few additional chromosome abnormalities involving defects in chromosome number also occur, but these are generally rare. For example, Patau syndrome results from an extra copy of chromosome 13. Children with this disorder are grossly deformed and usually die within a few months. The condition is rare, occurring in only 1 in 20,000 live births. Edward syndrome, involving three copies of chromosome 18, also produces numerous deformities and results in early death; its incidence is only 1 in 8,000 live births.

Abnormal numbers of sex chromosomes also occur and frequently produce sterility. Klinefelter syndrome arises when two X chromosomes and one Y chromosome are present. (Recall that normal females have two X chromosomes and males have one X and one Y.) Individuals with Klinefelter syndrome are male in appearance, but they possess poorly developed sexual characteristics, are frequently tall, and are almost always sterile. This condition occurs with a frequency of about 1 in 1,000 male births. Turner syndrome, which we discussed at the beginning of the chapter, is another abnormality of sex chromosome number, occurring when only a single X chromosome is present. It occurs with a frequency of only about 1 in 10,000 female births. These conditions are discussed more fully in "The Catalog of Genetic Traits."

Defects in Chromosome Structure

Some chromosome abnormalities arise, not from abnormal numbers of chromosomes, but from defects in chromosome structure. For example, an individual may possess the correct number of chromosomes, but a piece of one chromosome may be missing. This type of chromosome mutation is termed a *deletion*. Chromosome deletions typically include a number of genes and thus many traits are affected. For example, when a large part of chromosome 5 is deleted, the Cri-du-Chat (which means cat-cry) syndrome results. In infancy, a child with this disorder frequently has a round face, a small head, low-set ears, and wide-spaced eyes. Furthermore, the child is severely retarded. The name of this syndrome derives from the peculiar cry that these infants have—a high-pitched wail that resembles the cry of a kitten.

About 1 infant in 10,000 to 25,000 is born with a small segment of chromosome 15 missing. The deleted part of this chromosome is so small that it was not even recognized until just a few years ago. Nevertheless, missing this small piece of chromosome 15 results in abnormalities in a number of traits, known collectively as Prader-Willi syndrome. Infants with this condition have poor muscle tone, are undernourished, and have difficulty feeding. After about one year of age, however, they develop voracious appetites, becoming obese and frequently diabetic. Prader-Willi children have small hands and feet, short stature, and poor sexual development. Most Prader-Willi syndrome children are also retarded. Langdon Down, the first person to study Down syndrome, described a young girl with Prader-Willi syndrome in 1887, calling it *polysacria*. At the age of 13, this girl was only 4 feet 4 inches tall, but weighed 196 pounds. Actually, only about half of the children with Prader-Willi syndrome possess a recognizable chromosome abnormality; the cause of the disorder in the other 50 percent is not known.

Some additional types of defects in chromosome structure include *duplications*, where a portion of the chromosome is duplicated, and *translocations*, which involve the exchange of genetic material between chromosomes. *Inversions* are chromosome mutations in which a chromosome segment has become inverted; the chromosome breaks in two places, the segment flips over, and then reattaches. Some of these chromosome abnormalities and the traits they affect are listed in Table 5.1 and are discussed in "The Catalog of Genetic Traits."

Table 5.1 Chromosome Abnormalities

Name	Chromosome Abnormality	Symptoms
Cri-du-chat syndrome	Missing part of short arm of chromosome 5	Small head, widely spaced eyes, a round face, shrill cry, mental retardation
Down syndrome	Three of chromosome 21	Mental retardation, short stature, numerous medical problems
Edward syndrome	Three of chromosome 18	Severe mental retardation, low set ears, short neck, deformed feet, clenched fingers, heart defects, and numerous other deformities; less then 10% live more than 1 year
Fragile X syndrome	X chromosome has fragile site	Mental retardation, large ears, large testicles
Klinefelter syndrome	XXY or XXXY	Scant facial hair, small testes, and sterile; a few show mild to moderate retardation
Patau syndrome	Three of chromosome 13	Severe mental retardation, small head, sloping forehead, small eyes, extra fingers and toes, numerous other problems; most die within first year

Table 5.1 (*continued*)

Name	Chromosome Abnormality	Symptoms
Prader-Willi syndrome	About 50% are missing a part of chromosome 15	Poor muscle tone, light color, and small hands and feet; become obese after 2 to 3 years of age
Turner syndrome	A single X chromosome	Webbing of the neck, low hairline, deformed elbow; do not mature
Wolf-Hirschhorn syndrome (4p−)	Missing part of chromosome 4	Severe mental and growth retardation; small head with a high forehead and seizures; cleft lip and/or cleft palate are common; many die at an early age
XYY male	XYY	Tall; may have severe facial acne in adolescence; intelligence may be reduced in some; higher rate of criminality
3q+	An extra piece of chromosome 3	Severe mental and growth retardation; small head, seizures, a square-shaped head, deformed chest, and many other deformities; many die before the age of 1

In summary, we have seen that chromosomal defects typically affect many traits and have devastating consequences. Fortunately, few children are born with these disorders, primarily because the mother's body rejects embryos with chromosome mutations soon after conception. It is important to keep in mind that although chromosomal abnormalities are genetic traits, they are rarely inherited. Most occur as random accidents in the process of chromosome division, and the chance of another accident happening in the same family is usually low. There are exceptions, however, such as in translocation Down syndrome, where one parent carries a chromosome mutation, but is unaffected him or herself. Because of these exceptions and the severe physical and mental problems produced by chromosome abnormalities, anyone with a close relative who possesses a chromosome mutation would be well advised to seek genetic counseling.

Chapter 6

LEARNING ABOUT YOUR GENETIC RISKS THROUGH GENETIC COUNSELING

All of us are intrigued by our heredity. We speculate about which of our ancestors gave us our features or whether we will pass a particular trait on to our children. We argue over which side of the family is responsible for our good looks and which side gave us our bad habits. This book can help to answer some of the questions you may have about how heredity works, whether a particular trait is genetic, and how that trait might be inherited. In the preceding chapters, I have attempted to give you an appreciation for the importance of genetics and a basic understanding of the principles of heredity. In "The Catalog of Genetic Traits" that follows Chapter 7, I briefly summarize what we know about the hereditary basis of some human traits and diseases.

My hope is that the information contained in this book will help you to begin to understand your own genetic traits and their transmission. Some readers, however, may require more specific information about a particular genetic problem in their family. Perhaps a genetic disorder runs in your family, and you are concerned about your chances of inheriting it. Or you might be worried about the possibility of passing a disease on to your children. These concerns should always be discussed with a trained specialist, one who has the opportunity to study your family history and examine family members affected with the disorder. Earlier we discussed some of the factors that complicate the inheritance of a trait: genetic heterogeneity, incomplete penetrance, the interaction of genetic and environmental influences. These processes may confuse the diagnosis of a genetic disease and make predictions about its inheritance difficult. Because of these difficulties and the many variants of genetic diseases that cannot be discussed in this book, anyone with a serious concern about a genetic disease or disorder in their family should seek genetic counseling.

What Is Genetic Counseling?

The term *genetic counseling* refers to counseling about heredity. Providing information about how heredity works is at the heart of genetic counseling, but good genetic counseling involves much more. Genetic counseling is an educational process—a process that strives to help the patient and family members deal with all aspects of a genetic disease or disorder. Ideally, this includes an accurate diagnosis of the disorder, information about the medical consequences of the problem, help with understanding of the mode of inheritance, and information about the probability that the disorder will recur in other family members. Genetic counseling also provides facts about the reproductive options that might be available to those at risk for the disease. Furthermore, it seeks to help those involved—patient and relatives—come to grips with the reality of the problem and to make the best possible adjustment to the circumstances. Obviously, no single person can do all of these things; medical specialists, geneticists, laboratory personnel, counselors, and family physicians are all required. Consequently, most genetics clinics utilize a team approach, with many different individuals contributing to the counseling process.

Who Should Seek Genetic Counseling?

In general, genetic counseling is appropriate for anyone who has questions about their chances of inheriting or passing on a serious genetic disease or disorder. However, because of the high cost of diagnostic procedures, certain risks, and the limited availability of genetic specialists, prenatal diagnosis and genetic counseling are rarely available on demand. These services are usually reserved for those individuals or couples deemed to be at risk for a genetic disorder. The criteria for determining who is at risk vary from center to center, but here are ten common situations where genetic counseling is appropriate.

1. A person has a family history of a known genetic disease.
2. A couple has given birth to a previous child with a birth defect, or a close relative of the prospective parents possesses a birth defect.

3. An older woman becomes pregnant or wants to become pregnant. Although experts disagree about the age at which genetic counseling is appropriate for women without any other risk factor, many suggest that any pregnant woman age 35 or older should be counseled.
4. A couple has had problems with infertility, sterility, or multiple miscarriages.
5. A couple has given birth to a child with a chromosome defect.
6. One of the parents is, or may be, a carrier of a chromosome rearrangement.
7. A couple has given birth to a previous child with a neural tube defect (a birth defect in which the spinal column or brain is not completely enclosed), or there are other indications of increased risk of a neural tube defect.
8. One of the parents has a major growth disorder, or a previous child has a major growth disorder.
9. Mental retardation has occurred in a previous child or in a close relative.
10. Husband and wife are genetically related. For example, they might be first cousins.

Who Does Genetic Counseling?

The answer depends, in part, on the nature of the disorder you are concerned about. You might begin by consulting your personal physician. Much genetic counseling is provided by primary care physicians, including family practitioners, obstetricians, pediatricians, and internists. Your own doctor can probably tell you something about the nature of the disease and whether it is likely to be hereditary. If the disease is hereditary, your physician may be able to give you some estimate of the probability that you or your children will inherit it. For complex cases, he or she may refer you to a special genetics center, which will probably be associated with a major hospital or a medical school. A list of genetics centers offering comprehensive genetic counseling services is provided in Appendix I.

Private genetics clinics are available in some larger cities. Another source of information is state and federal agencies and private organizations that specialize in genetic disorders. For example, many states have special genetic services coordinators, who can provide information about genetics educational programs, genetics clinics, and genetics support services; addresses for these are listed in Appendix II. You might call your state health department and inquire about genetic services available in your region.

The National Center for Education in Maternal and Child Health publishes a number of books, pamphlets, and other resources on genetic diseases and birth defects. The March of Dimes also provides information, pamphlets, and films on a variety of genetic disorders. Addresses for these organizations are provided in Appendix III. There are a number of nonprofit organizations that assist patients with selected genetic diseases and their parents, such as the Cystic Fibrosis Foundation and the National Hemophilia Foundation. A list of these organizations may be obtained from the National Center for Education in Maternal and Child Health.

Prenatal Diagnosis

Within the past few years, our ability to accurately diagnose genetic diseases in an unborn baby has increased tremendously. Today, geneticists and physicians employ a wide array of sophisticated technology to examine the fetus; these diagnostic tools provide prospective parents with information about the risks of bearing a child with a genetic disorder. Although many genetic diseases are not yet amenable to prenatal diagnosis, the list of those that can be detected is growing at an impressive rate. Most of these tests are highly specific for a particular condition; that is, each test determines the presence of only one or a few related disorders. Unfortunately, no test can guarantee that a baby is free of all possible disorders, nor is such a test likely in the foreseeable future. Some prenatal diagnostic tests are routinely available to most physicians, but others are limited to a few genetics centers.

One of the primary goals of prenatal testing is to offer parents who are at risk the opportunity of having a healthy child. Consider a couple who has a previous child with Hurler syndrome, a metabolic disorder that results in short stature, mental retardation, and death usually before the age of 15. Because this disorder is a recessive condition and the couple has already produced one affected child, both parents must be heterozygotes. Thus, their chance of producing another child with the disease is 1 in 4 for each subsequent pregnancy. In the past, most parents faced with this prospect simply chose not to have any more children. Now, with the aid of prenatal diagnosis and the option of abortion if the fetus has the disease, many couples in this situation choose to risk another pregnancy. Seventy-five percent of these pregnancies result in a normal child, enabling the majority of such couples to experience the joy of children.

When a prenatal test is positive (the fetus is found to have the disorder), the parents have several options. Only in a few diseases is prenatal treatment available. The primary decision to be faced is whether the pregnancy should be terminated with an abortion. Even when the parents elect not to abort, the prenatal diagnosis provides an early warning that is frequently useful: Specialists can be consulted about treatment, special diets can be prepared in advance, and special surgical or other treatment facilities can be readied for the critical period that follows birth. Also, the parents have time to adjust psychologically to the birth of a sick or deformed child.

A number of different techniques are available for prenatal diagnosis. We will discuss only some of the more widely used methods here.

Ultrasonography

Ultrasonography—commonly called *ultrasound*—works much like the sonar that allows submarines to see underwater. In ultrasonography, high-frequency sound waves are beamed into the uterus. When these waves encounter dense tissues in the fetus, they bounce back; a special instrument detects the reflected sound waves and transforms them into a picture. In this way we can visualize the fetus without invading the womb.

Although the picture produced by ultrasound is often unintelligible to the average person, an experienced radiologist can measure the size of the baby's head, detect major deformities, and sex the baby from the utrasound picture, although sexing with ultrasound is not always accurate. Genetic disorders that produce major physical defects, such as dwarfism, hydrocephalus, or osteogenesis imperfecta, can sometimes be diagnosed directly with ultrasound. More commonly, however, ultrasound is utilized in conjunction with other diagnostic procedures. For example, ultrasound is routinely employed in amniocentesis to guide the needle that collects the sample of amniotic fluid. (Amniocentesis is discussed in the next section.) Ultrasound is also utilized to estimate the age of the fetus and to check for twins.

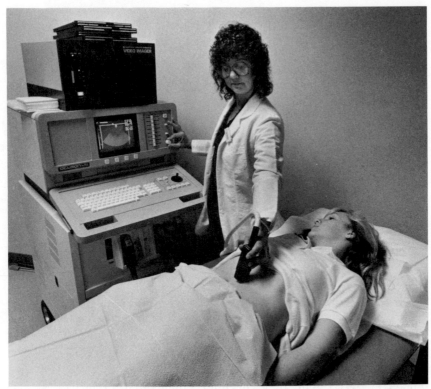

Figure 6.1. A pregnant women undergoing ultrasound examination. (Spencer Grant, Photo Researchers, Inc.)

Amniocentesis

Amniocentesis is the most commonly used method for collecting a sample of fetal tissue for chromosome and biochemical analysis. This procedure is usually performed during the sixteenth week of pregnancy. At that time, the amount of fluid in the amniotic sac is usually sufficient for withdrawal. Also, this is early enough for laboratory tests to be completed in time for the fetus to be safely aborted, if the diagnosis is positive and the parents choose this option.

Amniocentesis is routinely performed as an outpatient procedure, usually by an obstetrician. First, an ultrasound scan is done to determine the position of the fetus. A long sterile needle is then inserted through the mother's abdominal wall into the amniotic sac, and a small amount of

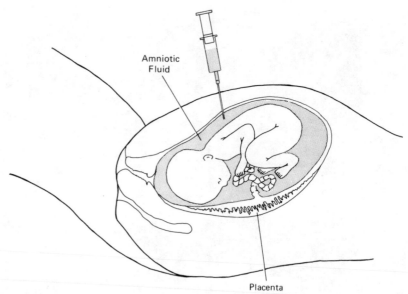

Figure 6.2.   Amniocentesis. A sterile needle is inserted through the abdomen into the amniotic sac, and a sample of amniotic fluid containing fetal cells is removed.

fluid is removed (Figure 6.2). This fluid contains some of the baby's cells, which can usually be coaxed to grow under laboratory conditions. Once the cells have multiplied, the baby's chromosomes can be examined from them. In addition, biochemical tests can be carried out on the amniotic fluid and on the growing cells. Amniocentesis carries only a small risk— about 1 in 200—of medical complications for the mother and fetus; the primary complication is a miscarriage.

Chorionic Villus Sampling

The major disadvantage of amniocentesis is that it is not usually carried out before the sixteenth week of pregnancy. Only a small number of cells are present in the amniotic fluid, and therefore the cells must be grown in the laboratory for a week or more before sufficient material is available for testing. This means that in some cases a diagnosis is not available until around the eighteenth to twentieth week of pregnancy. An abortion carried out at this relatively late date carries a higher risk of complications and is more emotionally traumatic for the parents. The need for a method of prenatal diagnosis that can be performed earlier in pregnancy has led to a new technique called *chorionic villus sampling* (CVS).

In CVS, a soft plastic tube called a *catheter* is inserted through the vagina and cervix into the uterus. Under the guidance of ultrasound, the tip of the tube is placed in contact with the placenta. Suction is then applied to the tube and a small piece of tissue is collected in a syringe at the end of the tube (Figure 6.3). The tissue removed is part of the chorion, one of the outer layers of the placenta. While the chorion is produced by the fetus, it does not develop into any body structures—it is expelled as afterbirth at delivery—so removing a bit of it with CVS does not endanger the baby. Chorion tissue contains millions of cells that are actively dividing. Whereas cells obtained from amniocentesis require days before diagnostic tests can be completed, chromosome analysis and many biochemical tests can be carried out immediately on the chorion cells. This means that results of genetic tests can be obtained in a matter of hours or days instead of the 1 to 3 weeks usually required with amniocentesis. Furthermore, CVS can be carried out between the ninth and eleventh weeks of pregnancy, some 3 to 5 weeks earlier than amniocentesis. If an abortion is elected, it can be completed by the twelfth week of pregnancy, at a time when complications are less likely to occur and the abortion will be less psychologically stressful to the parents.

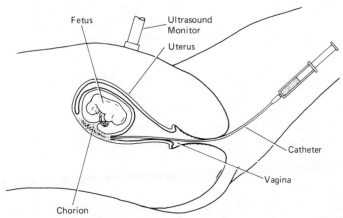

Figure 6.3.   Chorionic villus sampling. Under the guidance of ultrasound, a plastic tube is inserted through the vagina into the uterus. A small part of the placental tissue is removed by suction.

At the time I am writing this, CVS is still in the testing stages and is available only at selected centers in the United States. Recent studies indicate that the procedure is relatively safe for both the mother and the fetus, with a risk of complications only slightly greater than that associated with amniocentesis. As more physicians become experienced with CVS, this technique will likely replace amniocentesis as the preferred method for prenatal diagnosis.

Fetoscopy

Fetoscopy is a more specialized technique for sampling fetal tissue and observing the fetus. The fetoscope is a fiber-optic instrument—somewhat like a miniature periscope—which is placed into the uterus and allows direct observation of the fetus. This procedure requires great skill and must be done in an operating room. A small incision is made in the abdomen and the fetoscope is inserted into the amniotic sac. Looking through the fetoscope, the operator can examine arms, legs, the face, and other body parts of the baby, although the field of vision is very small and the illumination is poor. One of the most common uses of fetoscopy is for obtaining a sample of blood; in this case, a needle is inserted through the abdominal wall as in amniocentesis, and the operator then guides the needle to a blood vessel in the umbilical cord by looking through the fetoscope. Sometimes fetoscopy is used in the same manner to obtain skin samples for diagnosing genetic skin diseases. The risk associated with fetoscopy is much higher than that for amniocentesis and CVS. It is usually done only when other tests cannot provide the necessary information and is carried out only at specialized centers.

Fetal Blood Sampling with Ultrasound Guidance

Until recently, blood samples from a fetus could only be obtained by fetoscopy. Because fetoscopy requires making an incision in the mother's abdomen and because the risk to the fetus is relatively high, this procedure was used infrequently. Within the past few years, however, a less intrusive, safer technique for sampling fetal blood has been developed. This technique is called *percutaneous umbilical blood sampling, cordocentesis,* or simply *fetal blood sampling.* In fetal blood sampling, a needle is inserted through the abdomen of the mother into the womb; this is similar to amniocentesis except that a longer needle is used. While inserting the needle through the abdomen, the physician watches the needle and the baby with ultrasound. The ultrasound picture allows the physician to carefully guide the needle to the umbilical cord. A blood vessel in the umbilical cord is then punctured with the needle and a small volume of the baby's blood is removed.

At the present time, fetal blood sampling is still an experimental procedure and is only conducted at a few hospitals. When carried out by a physician experienced with this technique, fetal blood sampling is a safe and simple procedure. In most cases, it requires only a few minutes and is usually done as an outpatient procedure. The mother is awake during the entire operation, although a local anesthetic may be used at the site of needle insertion on the abdomen.

Fetal blood sampling has a number of potential uses. It can provide a sample of blood cells, which can be used to rapidly prepare a karyotype. In amniocentesis, so few cells are present in the sample of amniotic fluid that the cells must be grown in culture before a karyotype can be prepared. However, the blood obtained in fetal blood sampling contains sufficient cells that the chromosomes can usually be observed immediately. Many of the biochemical tests done on samples obtained through amniocentesis can also be run on blood samples obtained through fetal blood sampling. Some genetic disorders of the blood can only be detected with a blood sample, and fetal blood sampling is the safest means of detecting these disorders before birth. Furthermore, infections and some immune problems in the fetus can be assessed through fetal blood sampling. Finally, this procedure can also be used to administer drugs directly to the fetus and to provide blood transfusions to the unborn baby. Thus, fetal blood sampling provides the potential for actually treating diseases and disorders before the baby is born. Because of its low risk and many potential uses, fetal blood sampling will undoubtedly become more widely used in the future.

Diagnostic Tests for Genetic Diseases

Amniocentesis, CVS, fetoscopy, and fetal blood sampling are usually employed to obtain a tissue sample; by themselves, the techniques do not usually provide a diagnosis. The diagnosis comes from chromosomal analysis and biochemical tests that are carried out on the tissue obtained by these procedures.

Chromosomal Analysis

In Chapter 5, we discussed the procedure used to analyze chromosomes for genetic studies. You may recall that a karyotype—a picture of the chromosomes—is prepared from fetal cells obtained by amniocentesis or CVS. Karyotypes of parents and other children can be done on blood cells. The cells obtained are treated with chemicals and placed on a glass microscope slide. The cells break open, releasing the chromosomes onto the surface of the slide. They are then stained with various chemicals to make the chromosomes visible and to highlight certain features that aid in the identification of individual chromosomes.

One of the most important advances in the study of chromosomes has been the recent development of new staining techniques. In the past, the stains utilized made the entire chromosome appear dark under the microscope. Because many chromosomes are similar in shape and size, differentiating between individual chromosomes was difficult with these older stains. Also, recognizing small structural abnormalities in the chromosomes, such as small deletions or small rearrangements, was frequently impossible. The new staining techniques make individual parts of the chromosomes stand out and create banding patterns that are unique for each of the chromosomes. Q banding is one of these new staining methods. In this technique, the chromosomes are stained with a quinacrine dye and are viewed under ultraviolet light; the chromosomes glow green-yellow when viewed in this way. Most importantly, each chromosome has a specific pattern of light and dark bands, which allows it to be identified. Other staining techniques illuminate additional bands; some of these are called G bands, C bands, R bands, T bands, and prophase banding. Several different stains may be employed to thoroughly analyze an individual's chromosomes.

Once the chromosomes are stained, they are observed under the microscope. To construct a karyotype, a technician takes a picture of the chromosomes, enlarges it, and cuts each individual chromosome from the picture. The chromosomes are then identified and arranged into groups. A cytogeneticist then carefully examines the final arrangement of the chromosomes—called the karyotype—for evidence of any chromosome abnormalities. In the past few years, computer-driven systems have been developed to help analyze karyotypes. These machines employ a television camera attached to a microscope, both of which are controlled by a sophisticated computer. The microscope image recorded by the camera is transmitted electronically to the computer, which reads and analyzes the picture. First, the computer views the microscope slide,

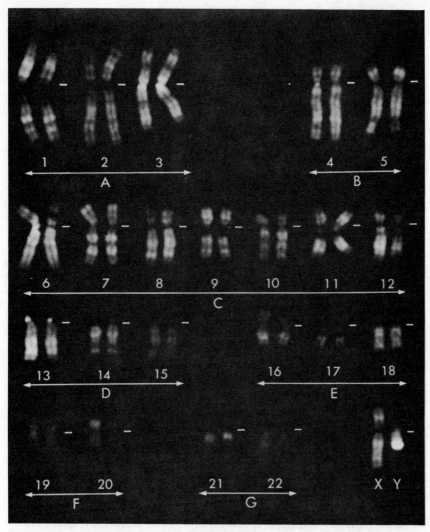

Figure 6.4.   Human chromosomes stained for Q bands. Compare this karyotype with that in Figure 5.4, in which Q bands have not been stained. (C. C. Lin, University of Calgary/BPS.)

passing back and forth, looking for spreads of chromosomes. (Each chromosome spread is a set of chromosomes from a single cell; each slide will have hundreds of chromosome spreads, but not all spreads are suitable for making a karyotype.) In its memory the computer records the location of each chromosome spread. Once it has located all the chromosome spreads, the computer assesses the suitability of each and picks out the best spread for preparation of a karyotype. The computer then finds individual chromosomes within the spread. It identifies each chromosome, straightens it electronically if necessary, rotates it and places it in its proper place in the karyotype. The computer then counts the number of chromosomes and prints out a picture of the karyotype. Not yet completely automated, these karyotype-analysis systems usually require a technician to assess the chromosomes and make a diagnosis, but the automation does shorten considerably the time required to generate a karyotype.

α-Fetoprotein Determination

α-Fetoprotein is a substance normally produced by the fetus during its development. Although its function is poorly understood, the amount of α-fetoprotein present can provide clues about the development of the fetus. The concentration of this substance is high in the blood of the fetus, moderate in the amniotic fluid, and normally low in the mother's blood during pregnancy. However, certain deformities of the nervous system—such as *spina bifida* (the spinal column is partially open) or *anencephaly* (complete or partial absence of the skull bones)—elevate the levels of α-fetoprotein in the amniotic fluid. Thus, α-fetoprotein in the amniotic fluid is usually measured any time amniocentesis is carried out. Spina bifida, anencephaly, and certain other abnormalities may also elevate the level of α-fetoprotein in the mother's blood during pregnancy, which can be detected by a blood test. Today, many physicians routinely test the mother's α-fetoprotein levels during pregnancy as a means of screening for potential problems in the fetus. It is important to point out that many other factors—for example, a miscalculated due date or twins—can also produce elevated α-fetoprotein levels in the mother's blood during pregnancy, and only a small percentage of women with elevated α-fetoprotein actually carry a malformed child. If the levels are high, the status of the fetus is then checked with follow-up tests, such as additional α-fetoprotein determinations, ultrasound, and/or amniocentesis.

Sometimes the concentration of α-fetoprotein in the mother's blood is lower than expected. This may occur for a variety of reasons, one of which is a chromosomal defect such as Down syndrome in the fetus. Although the vast majority of women with low α-fetoprotein carry a normal baby, many physicians recommend that any pregnant woman with a low level have amniocentesis or CVS performed to check for chromosome abnormalities.

Biochemical Tests

Many genetic diseases are caused by specific biochemical defects; these are frequently called *inborn errors of metabolism*. For example, *galactosemia* is a genetic disease in which a sugar called galactose is not broken down by the body. Galactose, one of the sugars found in milk, is normally metabolized by an enzyme called galactose-1-phosphate uridyl transferase, but individuals with galactosemia lack this enzyme. Although infants with galactosemia appear normal at birth, they develop digestive problems as soon as they begin to drink milk. If untreated, galactosemia can lead to cataracts, mental retardation, liver and kidney failure, and ultimately death.

Galactosemia and many other inherited biochemical disorders can be detected before birth. For most of the disorders that are amenable to genetic testing, fetal cells are obtained through amniocentesis or CVS. After growth of the cells in the laboratory, biochemical tests are performed to detect the absence of a particular enzyme or other vital substance. Some of these tests are routinely performed in many medical laboratories, but others are available only at specialized genetics centers.

DNA Studies

Fifteen years ago, geneticists had no means of directly reading the DNA. We knew that DNA carried genetic instructions and that this information consisted of a sequence of nucleotides that made up the DNA molecule. Recall from Chapter 2 that the nucleotides come in four types, abbreviated A, G, C, and T; each gene is a particular sequence of these four nucleotides on a long stretch of DNA. Although we knew that genetic information consisted of nucleotides in the DNA, each human cell contains approximately 6 billion pairs of DNA nucleotides, and many human genes are only several thousands of nucleotide pairs long. We had no technique for determining where in all of this mass of DNA a particular gene resided nor any means of viewing the sequence of a particular gene, even if we could find it. But all this has changed in the past ten years. New molecular techniques now make it possible to locate, isolate, and determine the sequence of an individual gene, although this is still a very difficult and laborious process.

As we discussed in Chapter 1, determining the location and sequence of a gene is often of immense benefit, for this information frequently gives us a better understanding of the genetic disease and may suggest ways to treat it. This information may also open the door for prenatal diagnosis of the disorder and detection of those who may be carriers of the defective gene.

Prenatal genetic tests based on analysis of DNA are of two types. First, in a few diseases we know the DNA sequence of the gene involved, and we can look directly for a defective copy of the gene. For example, sickle cell disease is an autosomal recessive trait that involves a defect in hemo-globin—an important protein that carries oxygen in the blood. Occurring in about 1 out of every 600 births among American blacks, the disease is debilitating and severely painful. The gene that causes sickle cell disease has been located, and the defect in the DNA that produces the disease has been identified. With this information, molecular geneticists have now designed highly specific "probes" that recognize the genetic defect in the DNA. DNA from fetal cells obtained through amniocentesis or CVS can be isolated and probed for the defective sickle cell gene, provid-ing parents with information about whether they will have a child with sickle cell disease.

Although geneticists have made rapid progress in finding disease-causing genes during the past five years (Table 6.1), methods for directly probing genetic defects exist for only a few genes. This is because for most genetic diseases, we don't yet know exactly where the offending gene is located or what is the specific defect in the DNA. However, for some diseases we do know of genetic markers that lie close to the gene on the same chromosome; these genetic markers are other DNA sequences that can be detected with laboratory tests. The association between a disease-causing gene and a genetic marker is similar to that of my friend and his blue '57 Chevy. I may not see my friend, but whenever I see that blue '57 Chevy, I know he is probably close by. Similarly, although we may not be able to see the gene that causes a genetic disorder, the genetic marker tells us that the gene is probably also present. The genetic mark-ers commonly used in these tests are called *restriction fragment length polymorphisms*—RFLPs. The RFLP is not directly related to the disease, but it can be used to identify whether a fetus has inherited a defective gene from one of the parents.

Table 6.1 Selected Inherited Disorders for Which the Disease-Causing Gene Has Been Found[a]

Disorder	Chromosome Location
Adenosine deaminase deficiency	20
α-1-Antitrypsin deficiency	14
Becker muscular dystrophy	X
Chronic granulomatous disease	X
Congenital adrenal hyperplasia	6
Cystic fibrosis	7
Duchenne muscular dystrophy	X
Familial hypercholesterolemia	19
Glucose-6-phosphate deficiency	X
Hemophilia A	X
Hemophilia B	X
Lesch-Nyhan disease	X
Phenylketonuria (PKU)	12
Retinoblastoma	13
Sandhoff disease	5
Sickle cell disease	11
Tay-Sachs disease	15
α-Thalassemia	16
β-Thalassemia	11
von Willebrand disease	12

[a] This list includes some disorders for which the disease locus has been identified; not all such disorders are included. This list does not include those disorders for which only linked genetic markers have been found.

To illustrate the concept of using genetic markers for prenatal diagnosis, consider *retinitis pigmentosa*. The first symptoms of this genetic disease are defective night vision and a decreasing field of vision, which progressively lead to blindness. Retinitis pigmentosa can be caused by several different genes, one of which is located on the X chromosome. Although its precise location on the X chromosome has not been determined (at least as of this writing; it may be by the time you read this), RFLPs close to the retinitis pigmentosa gene have been found. RFLPs are genetic markers that vary. For simplicity, we will consider a single RFLP with two variants, forms A and B. Some X chromosomes will have the A type and others will have the B type. Also, some X chromosomes will have a defective gene that causes retinitis pigmentosa; we will designate the defective gene r. Other X chromosomes will have a gene for normal vision, which we will designate R. So an X chromosome has one of the two types of RFLPs, and it also possesses either the defective retinitis pigmentosa gene or a normal copy. When we consider both the retinitis pigmentosa gene and the genetic marker, four types of chromosomes are possible: —A—R—, —A—r—, —B—R—, —B—r—.

Now, suppose that Joan and Frank have a son with retinitis pigmentosa. Because the disease is X-linked recessive, the son must have inherited the defective gene from Joan, because sons always inherit their X chromosome from their mother. (See Chapter 3 for a discussion of X-linked inheritance.) So we know that Joan is a carrier for the defective gene, and each additional male offspring that Joan and Frank produce will have a 50 percent chance of inheriting the disease. Because Joan is a carrier, one of her X chromosomes carries the r gene that produces the disease, and the other carries the normal R gene. From molecular studies of her DNA, we may also find that Joan has both the RFLP markers—one chromosome carries the A marker and one carries the B marker. By looking at her son with retinitis pigmentosa, we can determine whether A or B is on the same chromosome with the defective retinitis pigmentosa gene r. Remember that he has only a single copy of the X chromosome. If the son has the A marker, we know he inherited the chromosome —A—r—, because he has both the A marker and the r disease-causing gene. This means that Joan must have the following two chromosomes: —A—r— and —B—R—. In genetic terminology, we would say that the retinitis pigmentosa gene r is *linked* to the A marker.

---→

Figure 6.5.   Prenatal diagnosis using RFLP genetic markers. The gene causing retinitis pigmentosa (r) can not be detected, but the closely linked RFLP markers (A, B) can. Joan possesses RFLP markers A and B. She and Frank produce one child with retinitis pigmentosa and RFLP marker A. This indicates that the A marker is on the same chromosome with the disease gene (r), and the B marker is on a chromosome with a normal gene (R). Any additional sons produced by Frank and Joan who exhibit the A marker will have retinitis pigmentosa; any sons with the B marker will be free of the disease. This assumes no crossing over takes place between the RFLP marker and the disease gene.

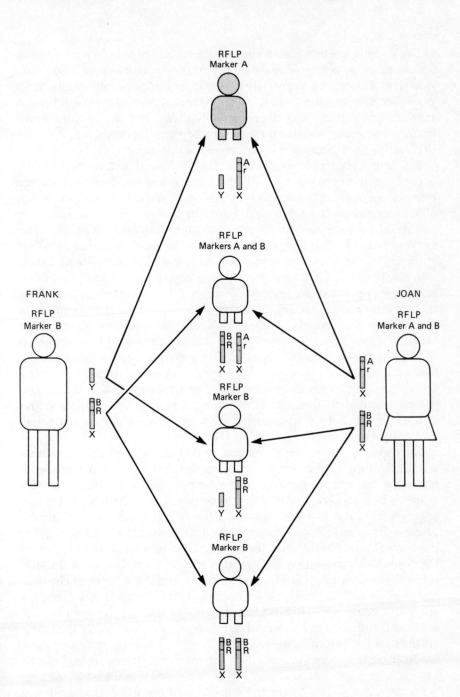

The knowledge that A and r are linked on one of Joan's chromosomes allows us to detect the disease in any future fetus that Joan and Frank conceive. Although we cannot test prenatally for the retinitis pigmentosa gene, because we don't know exactly where it is, we can test for the A marker. Any son carrying the A marker will also be carrying the retinitis pigmentosa gene, because they are on the same chromosome. Any son that carries the B marker will be free of the disease.

In practice, the RFLPs are fragments of DNA produced when the DNA is cut by special enzymes called restriction enzymes. There are a large number of different restriction enzymes; each recognizes a short stretch of nucleotides in the DNA called a restriction site. For example, one restriction enzyme recognizes the nucleotide sequence GGATCC. The enzyme not only recognizes the restriction site, but it also cuts the DNA at that spot. Some chromosomes will have the restriction site and their DNA will be cut by the enzyme; upon applying the enzyme, this DNA would end up as two fragments (we might call this pattern of fragments A, as in our example above). Other chromosomes will lack the restriction site on their DNA; consequently the DNA in these chromosomes will not be cut by the enzyme, leaving a single fragment (we might call this the B variant, as in our example above). After applying a restriction enzyme, the number and length of the fragments can be determined by sieving them through a gel with an electrical current—a method called *electrophoresis*—and visualizing the DNA with stains or other techniques. The different markers (A or B variants) are recognized as patterns of bands that appear on the gel.

The example I have just given you involving Joan and Frank is somewhat simplified; in practice several complications may occur. One problem is that the disease-causing gene must be linked to a different marker than the normal gene in the family to be tested; if the mother's chromosomes were —A—R— and —A—r—, then the chromosome bearing the disease gene could not be distinguished from the chromosome bearing the normal gene. In this case the marker is uninformative. For genes on the nonsex chromosomes, both mother and father contribute a chromosome to the offspring, and thus we must consider the types of chromosomes potentially contributed by both parents. Several family members are often required to establish which markers are on the same chromosome as the disease gene. A final difficulty is that occasionally the markers may switch chromosomes in a process called *crossing over* (see Chapter 2). If crossing over occurs, then the marker in the fetus will not be associated with the disease-causing gene as we expect, and a misdiagnosis may occur. The closer the marker is to the gene, the less likely crossing over is to occur, so close markers are preferred. Even with close markers, however, there is a small chance of a misdiagnosis. Prenatal diagnosis involving RFLPs is becoming more widespread, and it offers the possibility of genetic testing for many new diseases.

Testing for Genetic Diseases in Newborns

Up to this point, our discussion of genetic testing has been confined to the prenatal or unborn infant. Genetic testing can also be conducted after birth. Screening for genetic diseases in children and adults is done for two reasons. First, some genetic diseases are treatable if the disease is detected early; in these cases, early knowledge of the disease is clearly beneficial. Second, individuals with a family history of the genetic disease are frequently concerned about whether they might have the disease, with the potential of passing the disease on to their offspring. If shown to be free of the disease, they can have children without apprehension. If, on the other hand, they do carry a defective gene that will eventually produce the disease, this knowledge may be important in planning their future.

Many genetic diseases can be recognized by specific features that are present in the newborn. For example, infants with Down syndrome have characteristic facial features that can usually be spotted at birth. Many genetic diseases and disorders are detected when the infant is examined immediately after birth or later in a newborn checkup.

The diagnosis of other genetic diseases may require special biochemical tests. Phenylketonuria, commonly known as PKU, is an inherited biochemical disorder that can lead to mental retardation if left untreated in the first few months of life. Because of the severe effects of this disease and because treatment is available (consisting of a special diet), most states and many foreign countries now require testing for PKU soon after birth. This disease can be detected with a relatively inexpensive test conducted on a few drops of blood taken by pricking the baby's heel. If the test results are positive, additional testing is conducted to confirm the diagnosis. Some states require tests for additional diseases, which are also conducted on a small blood sample taken soon after birth.

Screening for Carriers of Genetic Disease

Detecting carriers of a genetic disease is much more difficult than screening for the disease itself; by definition, carriers lack the symptoms of the disease. Because symptoms of the disease are absent in carriers, the presence of the defective gene in these individuals can be recognized only with special tests. Sometimes the defective gene, although not producing the symptoms of the disease, may alter some biochemical function, which can then be detected. Unfortunately, biochemical tests for carrier detection are available for only a few genetic diseases; for many genetic diseases, the biochemical basis of the disease is not even known. Another possibility for detecting carriers is by examining the DNA directly. At present, this is possible for only a handful of genes, because we have no idea where on the chromosomes most disease-causing genes are located.

One disease where carrier testing is available is Tay-Sachs disease. As we have mentioned previously in this book, Tay-Sachs disease is a severe neurological disorder. The disorder is rare among the general population, but has a frequency of 1 in every 3,600 conceptions among Ashkenazi Jews. (Ashkenazi Jews are people of Jewish descent who originated from eastern and central Europe.) Tay-Sachs disease is inherited as an autosomal recessive trait, so both parents must be carriers to produce a Tay-Sachs' child. An effective program for screening genetic carriers of the disorder has been developed within the Ashkenazi community, and this has led to recent reductions in the number of children born with Tay-Sachs disease. Carriers exhibit no symptoms of the disease, but the defective gene they carry can be detected with a biochemical test conducted on a blood sample. If two carriers conceive a child, the child has a 1 in 4 chance of developing Tay-Sachs disease; a prenatal test is available to determine whether the fetus from such a couple actually has the disease.

Carrier screening is also possible with a few other diseases such as sickle cell disease, hemophilia, and β-thalassemia. With the future development of DNA diagnostic tests, screening for genetic carriers will be possible for an increasing number of genetic diseases.

Reproductive Options and Genetic Counseling

When a couple has the potential to produce a child with a genetic disease, they are confronted with difficult choices. If a prenatal test is available for the disease, prenatal diagnosis and abortion—if the test is positive—are one option. Abortion is not acceptable to many couples, however, and prenatal tests do not exist for many genetic diseases. Confronted with these obstacles, some couples simply elect to have no further children. Adoption is the answer for some, although the shortage of available infants often necessitates a long wait for those desiring a newborn.

When the husband carries a defective gene, artificial fertilization with sperm from a carefully screened donor is another possibility. If the female carries the defective gene, *in vitro* fertilization using a donor egg followed by embryo transfer may be elected. This new procedure involves removing recently ovulated egg cells from a donor, fertilizing them in a test tube with sperm from the husband, and then implanting an embryo in the uterus of the female. The first baby conceived by *in vitro* fertilization was born in 1978; more than 3,000 babies have now been born using this technique. *In vitro* fertilization is available only at selected centers around the country. The success rate of the procedure varies, and even among the most successful centers it is quite low—usually no more than 10 to 15 percent for each attempt. *In vitro* fertilization is also expensive, costing close to $6,000 per attempt at many centers.

Unfortunately, all of these reproductive options are limited and have obvious practical drawbacks. Furthermore, use of some of these techniques raises moral, religious, and social concerns. Genetic counselors can provide information about specific options available to a couple with a genetic problem, but ultimately the individuals involved must make their own decisions. Before using any of these reproductive techniques, it is important that a couple discuss their feelings about the procedure with each other, and careful consideration should be given to the opinions of both partners. Many couples may want to discuss the moral and religious issues involved with their priest, pastor, or other religious leader.

Gene Therapy

Genetic diseases cause tremendous suffering. Some are painful, debilitating, or disfiguring. Others produce mental illness or brain damage. Many are lethal. Medical treatment for those who suffer from genetic diseases costs billions of dollars annually, and these disorders inflict enormous stress and emotional suffering on the patients and their families.

Unfortunately, most genetic diseases are untreatable. In a few cases, substances missing as a result of defective genes can be supplied, relieving the patient of some of the symptoms of the disease. For example, individuals with hemophilia lack a critical component that enables the blood to clot; this component can be prepared at great cost and injected into a hemophiliac, and it will prevent excessive bleeding. In other genetic diseases, the symptoms of a biochemical disorder can sometimes be lessened by careful control of the diet, as in PKU. In a few severe genetic disorders, liver transplantation has been used to replace missing substances. These treatments help, but they do not cure the genetic disease, nor do they prevent the disease-causing genes from being transmitted to future generations. Furthermore, treatment is available for only a few genetic diseases; the vast majority of those individuals with genetic disorders cannot be helped at all.

One form of treatment that will be available in the near future is *gene therapy* or *genetic engineering*. Gene therapy basically involves transplanting genes. If an individual has a genetic disease that arises from a defective gene, the disease may be cured, or at least the symptoms lessened, by supplying a normal, healthy copy of the gene. This technique is routinely carried out in microorganisms and has even been successfully applied to plants, mice, and some farm animals.

From both a technical and an ethical standpoint, we should distinguish between two fundamentally different types of gene therapy. The first type is called *somatic gene therapy*. Somatic gene therapy involves correcting genes that reside in somatic, or nonsex, cells. For example, someday somatic gene therapy might be used to treat patients with combined immune deficiency disease, a genetic disorder of the immune system. Many individuals with this disease have a defective gene for an enzyme called adenosine deaminase; without this enzyme, their immune system is crippled and most die of common infections at an early age. If healthy genes for adenosine deaminase can be inserted into some of the patient's somatic cells—bone marrow cells are the most likely prospect at the present time—enough of the enzyme may be produced to alleviate the disease. Conceptually, this therapy is really no different than other medical treatments now in wide use, such as drug therapy, blood transfusions, surgery, or organ transplants. The only difference between somatic gene therapy and conventional treatments is that DNA is placed into the patient's body instead of other substances. An important point to emphasize is that the genes transplanted in somatic gene therapy will not be passed on to future generations, because only the genes in somatic cells are altered. The reproductive tissues—those tissues that produce sperm and eggs—will not be affected. Thus, the gene pool of the human race will not be altered by somatic gene therapy. All gene therapy currently being studied for medical use in humans is somatic gene therapy.

The second potential type of gene therapy is *germline genetic change*. This would involve altering all the cells in the body, including the reproductive cells (called the *germline*) that carry the genetic heritage for future generations. With present genetic engineering technology, this could only be carried out on human embryos; it could not be used to correct genetic problems of those already born with a genetic disease. Germline genetic changes have been accomplished in plants, mice, cows, pigs, chickens, and some other animals, but this technique has not been attempted in humans, nor are such experiments likely to be conducted in the foreseeable future. Because germline changes cannot be used to treat individuals after birth and because ethical and moral questions surround the use of this technology, it is not currently being studied for application in humans.

A number of technical problems currently preclude the use of somatic gene therapy in humans. Four major hurdles must be overcome before somatic gene therapy is available for treatment of human diseases.

1. First, the genetic defect must be located, and a correct copy of the gene must be cloned in the laboratory.
2. Next, a technique must be developed for inserting a correct copy of the gene into the patient's cells.
3. Techniques must then be perfected for ensuring that the gene functions properly once inside the cell. The introduced gene must produce the correct substance in the proper tissue, and it must produce the substance at the correct time and in the correct amounts. Too much of a gene product or the product produced at the wrong time or in the wrong place can be just as detrimental as producing none of the substance.

Chapter 7

CHARTING YOUR FAMILY HISTORY

When Melissa was 6 months pregnant with her first child, she and her husband Jeff met with the pediatrician who would care for their baby after delivery. During that first appointment, the pediatrician explained his need for some information about their families; he was particularly interested in any birth defects, mental retardation, diseases, or disorders that had occurred in their relatives. This information, he explained, would allow them to better anticipate and prepare for any potential genetic problems that the infant might have at birth or in the future.

The pediatrician then set about drawing out a pedigree for both Jeff and Melissa's families. He asked about their siblings, parents, aunts, uncles, and grandparents. As he asked detailed questions about the history of each family, Jeff and Melissa both realized that they would be unable to provide all the information that was needed. For example, Jeff's father died when he was 13, and he did not know his father's family well. His father had come from a large family—he had four brothers and three sisters; Jeff was unsure how many of these were still alive, and he knew nothing about their past or present health. Melissa knew that her mother's first child had died a few days after birth, but her mother and father rarely talked about the child. Melissa had no knowledge of why the child died.

Fortunately, Jeff and Melissa were able to obtain the needed information by telephoning their parents. Melissa's brother, who died a few days after birth, had been born with spina bifida, a birth defect that can have a hereditary basis. Melissa learned from the pediatrician that she had a slightly greater than average risk of having a child with spina bifida, and she decided to undergo prenatal diagnosis for this disorder. Jeff's father had died of a heart attack and several of his brothers also had early coronary artery disease. The pediatrician pointed out that his family history of heart disease indicated that Jeff was predisposed to coronary artery disease.

Jeff and Melissa's experience illustrates the importance of charting a family pedigree and keeping records of your family's medical history. Jeff and Melissa were lucky—both had parents alive who could supply the information they needed. Many people are not so fortunate. Sometimes medical records exist, and facts about your relatives can be obtained from these, but many people do not even know the names or addresses of some of their relatives. Frequently, medical records are simply not available for older generations. In the past, people often grew up surrounded by grandparents, aunts, uncles, and cousins. They knew firsthand that their grandfather died of diabetes or that several cousins were born with cleft lip. Today, many of us know only a few of our relatives well. Families are often scattered across the country or even across the world; we may not have heard from some relatives in years. Because people are frequently reluctant to talk about birth defects, mental illnesses, retardation, and other diseases and disorders, we may even be unaware that these problems exist in some of our close relatives—particularly if they occurred in a child who died at an early age.

My own family has always been close. I saw my grandfather regularly until he died at the age of 88. I had always assumed he had only a single brother and a single sister. However, when I recently reviewed my family history, I was surprised to learn that my grandfather actually had five siblings. Family records show that one brother died at birth, another died at age four, and a sister only lived to the age of one. These children all died near the turn of the century, before the age of antibiotics. Most likely they died of nonhereditary causes, probably infectious diseases. However, I have no way of knowing. Once my grandfather died, my link to these kindred was lost.

Everyone should chart a family pedigree and record the presence or absence of major diseases and disorders in as many family members as possible. This information should be kept in a safe place along with other valuable documents. Ideally, the records should be updated on an annual basis and passed on to your children when they start their own families.

The information contained in your family pedigree can serve several useful purposes. First, it provides a concise record of your family history, one that may be used by your descendants to learn more about their own roots and relationships. Second, the information will assist your family physician in knowing more about your susceptibility to various diseases and disorders. Almost all physicians take a family history when conducting routine examinations. They recognize that many diseases and disorders have a tendency to run in families. Knowledge that a particular disease occurs in your relatives will alert your physician to look for early signs of the disease, making an early diagnosis possible if the same disease occurs in you or other members of the family. Finally, should you, your children, or other relatives ever require genetic counseling, the information will be particularly important. With a detailed medical history of the family, a genetic counselor will be able to provide a better diagnosis of any genetic disorders and will be able to give more accurate information concerning the potential risks to other family members.

In Figures 7.1 and 7.2, special forms are provided that make recording your family history easy. Follow these directions for charting a permanent record of your family pedigree.

1. *Make copies of the family pedigree chart (Figure 7.1) and the family member information sheet (Figure 7.2).*

Begin by photocopying the family pedigree chart and the family member information sheet, making enough copies to record information for each member of your family.

2. *Fill in one copy of the family pedigree chart with members of your original family (your parents and all of their children).*

Write in the name (or some abbreviation) of your mother and father in the two boxes at the top of the chart. Next, record the names (or abbreviations) of all their children, including yourself. The children should be written from left to right in birth order, starting with the first born (the oldest child) and ending with the last born (the youngest child). (If needed, additional boxes can be added at the bottom.) The chart now contains the names of one immediate family, what geneticists call a nuclear family. A nuclear family consists of a mother, a father, and all of their children.

3. *If you have children, fill out another family pedigree chart, placing yourself and your spouse in the top boxes and all of your children in the boxes below.*

Your own name will now be in two different family pedigree charts, the one with your parents at the top and the one with you and your spouse at the top. Be sure to use the same name or abbreviation on both charts, so that you can easily connect the two.

4. *If your children have offspring (your grandchildren), fill out additional pedigree charts for each of your children's families.*

Each chart will be headed by your child and their spouse; below will be listed all of their children (your grandchildren).

5. *Next, fill out a family pedigree chart for the nuclear families of each of your brothers and sisters.*

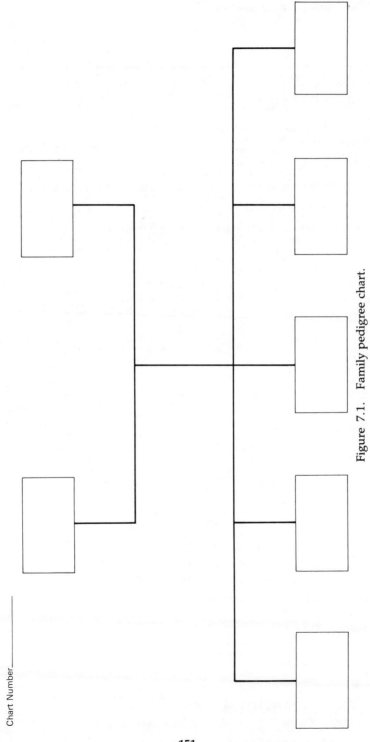

Chart Number_____

Figure 7.1. Family pedigree chart.

____ Male ____ Female

Name on Family Chart: _____

Full Name: _____

Address (if living):   _____

Birthdate: _____

Date of Death (if deceased): _____

Cause of Death (if deceased): _____

Check if this individual possessed any of the following.

Give type

Present	Absent	Unknown		
____	____	____	Birth defects	_____
____	____	____	Mental retardation	_____
____	____	____	Learning or reading disabilities	_____
____	____	____	Coronary artery disease	_____
____	____	____	Congenital heart defects	_____
____	____	____	Alcoholism	_____
____	____	____	Allergies	_____
____	____	____	Asthma	_____
____	____	____	Blindness	_____
____	____	____	Other eye problems	_____
____	____	____	Deafness	_____
____	____	____	Cancer	_____
____	____	____	Diabetes	_____
____	____	____	Fertility Problems	_____
____	____	____	High blood pressure	_____
____	____	____	High cholesterol	_____
____	____	____	Mental disorders	_____
____	____	____	Migraine headaches	_____
____	____	____	Rheumatoid arthritis	_____
____	____	____	Seizures	_____
____	____	____	Sickle cell disease	_____
____	____	____	Thyroid disease	_____

Other diseases or disorders present:

_____   _____

_____   _____

_____   _____

_____   _____

Attach any medical records or additional details.

Figure 7.2.   Family member information sheet.

6. *Fill out additional family pedigree charts for the nuclear families headed by your grandparents.*

At the top of each of these charts will be your grandfather and grandmother; below will be all of their siblings (one of your parents and aunts and uncles on their side of the family).

In this manner, you can construct a series of pedigrees, each consisting of a single nuclear family. The nuclear families will be connected by the names they have in common. You should also fill out a series of family pedigree charts for your spouse's family. Try to include all your grandparents, aunts, uncles, children, and grandchildren. These are the relatives with which you share the most genes; their medical histories will be most relevant to your own heredity. An example of a family history recorded on the family pedigree charts is given in Figure 7.3.

7. *Number the family pedigree charts.*

Once you have recorded your family history on the family pedigree charts, go back and assign a different number to each chart. For example, if you used six charts to record your family history, number the charts 1 through 6. It doesn't matter which number you assign to a particular chart; the important thing is that each chart has a unique number.

8. *Beside each name on a chart, record the number of each additional chart on which that name also appears.*

For example, your mother's name will appear at the top of one chart—perhaps chart 1—as one of your parents. Her name will also appear on another chart—perhaps chart 4—as one of the children of your grandparents. So, on chart 1, write a 4 next to your mother's name, to indicate that her name also appears on chart 4. Similarly, on chart 4, record a 1 next to her name to indicate that her name also appears on chart 1. These numbers will allow the pedigrees to be interconnected, giving one large pedigree in which the genetic relationships among all family members are depicted.

9. *Fill out a family member information sheet for each person you have recorded on the pedigree charts.*

Once you have completed the family pedigree charts, you should fill out a copy of the family member information sheet for each person on the charts. Provide the full name of each person, as well as the name or abbreviation used in the family pedigree charts. The birthdate and the

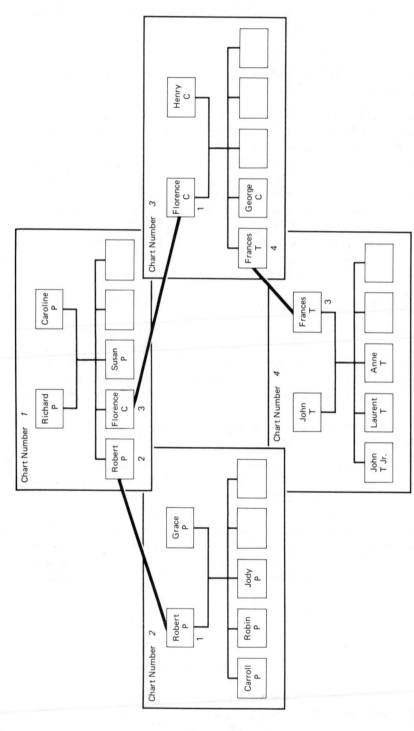

Figure 7.3. An example of a family history recorded on the family pedigree charts. Lines have been drawn between the charts to illustrate how the nuclear families are connected.

date and cause of death—if the person is deceased—should also be recorded. Finally, check off the presence or absence of any of the diseases or disorders listed on the sheet. The check list includes common diseases and disorders that have a hereditary basis. There is also space to list any additional diseases or disorders that the person presently has or has had in the past. In the space to the right, provide any additional details you know of. For example, if your father suffers from prostate cancer, check the box for cancer and list prostate cancer to the right. If your brother has high blood pressure, check the box for hypertension and give the age at which his hypertension was first diagnosed. Attach additional sheets for more details and attach any medical records you possess.

In recording family members on the family pedigree charts and medical information on the family member information sheets, keep the following points in mind. First, include only those relatives that are genetically related to the family. For example, adopted children and stepparents should not be included, because they are not "blood relatives." Second, be sure to include all births on the family pedigree charts, including stillborns and individuals that died in infancy. Stillborns and infant deaths frequently result from genetically caused problems. Therefore, information about the cause of death in these cases is particularly important. Third, the absence of a trait is almost as important for interpreting its hereditary basis as is the presence of the trait. So if you know that your Uncle Robert had excellent vision, record the fact that blindness was absent by placing a check in the appropriate space. Unfortunately, it may be impossible to know for certain that some traits are absent. For example, the presence of some birth defects are obvious, but others may be surgically corrected at an early age; thus the fact that your Uncle Robert has no obvious birth defect today does not necessarily mean that he never had a birth defect. You may be uncertain about the presence or absence of some traits in your relatives, but record as much information as you can. A final point: Try to be accurate when recording the information. Whenever possible, obtain information directly from the individual involved; if you must rely on secondhand information, try to verify it by checking with other family members.

THE CATALOG OF GENETIC TRAITS

Introduction

Several points should be kept in mind as you read the accounts of the traits listed in this catalog.

1. Read the discussion of heredity in Chapters 2, 3, and 4.

I suspect that many readers will find "The Catalog of Genetic Traits" the most interesting part of this book and will use the catalog to learn more about the heredity of those traits found in their own families. To understand the material presented in the catalog accounts and to avoid misconceptions about the traits, it is important to consult the material presented in the introductory chapters, particularly Chapters 2, 3, and 4. These chapters will help you to understand how heredity works and help in interpreting the information given in "The Catalog of Genetic Traits." You may also want to consult the glossary located at the back of the book; the glossary gives definitions for the technical terms used in the accounts.

2. There are many genetic traits that are not listed in "The Catalog of Genetic Traits."

I have included approximately 100 human traits, diseases, and disorders in the catalog that are influenced by genes. I have tried to include traits and diseases that many people have questions about or that might be interesting to the general reader. However, this is far from a complete list of all hereditary traits in humans. Indeed, Victor McKusick's latest edition of *Mendelian Inheritance in Man* lists over 4,000 human traits, diseases, and disorders that have a simple genetic basis. McKusick's catalog does not include the thousands of human traits that are influenced by multiple genes or a combination of genetic and environmental factors. Thus, only a smattering of all possible genetic traits are listed here. You should not assume that if a trait is missing from the catalog that it is not hereditary.

3. Traits listed in the catalog are not always genetic.

Traits included in the catalog are influenced by genes, but many of them may also result from nongenetic factors. For example, breast cancer is included in the catalog, and there are genes that predispose one to breast cancer. However, research indicates that hereditary breast cancer occurs in only a few families; in the majority of cases, breast cancer probably has no hereditary tendency. Do not assume that because a trait is included in the catalog, it is always genetic.

4. Many genetic traits are heterogeneous; in other words,
*   exceptions are common.*

Many genetic traits, diseases, and disorders exhibit genetic heterogeneity. This means that the same trait may be caused by different genes. In this book, I am forced to limit our discussion to the common genetic causes of a trait; the many exceptions that arise cannot be discussed in detail. Thus, the catalog may indicate that a trait has a particular pattern of inheritance, perhaps an autosomal recessive mode of inheritance. This pattern of inheritance will be the rule in most families, but there may be some families where the trait is inherited in a different manner, perhaps as an autosomal dominant trait or a multifactorial trait.

5. The probabilities given for inheriting a trait do not apply to all families.

Wherever possible, I have tried to give some idea of the probability of inheriting the traits included in the catalog. It is important to recognize that these probabilities apply to the majority of families in which the trait is present or they may be averages based on the experiences of many different families (termed *empiric risk*; see Chapter 4). However, because of genetic heterogeneity, these probabilities will not apply to all families. For some individuals, the chance of inheriting the trait may be very different.

6. If you have concerns about a genetic disease or disorder in your family,
*   consult your physician or seek genetic counseling.*

This book is intended to provide an introduction to human heredity. Frequently, people have questions about whether a trait in their own family is hereditary. For example, you might ask whether diabetes is hereditary or whether your child is likely to inherit your red hair. Hopefully, "The Catalog of Genetic Traits" will help to answer some of these questions. However, if you have concerns about a genetic disease or disorder in your family, about your chances of inheriting it or passing it on, talk to your physician or a genetic counselor. This book cannot and should not serve as a substitute for genetic counseling. Genetic diseases frequently come in a number of subtle variants; experts are often required to make a correct diagnosis and provide accurate estimates of the probability of inheritance. This information should only be provided by someone who can review the specifics of your individual family history. Your physician may be able to provide this information or refer you to someone who can. See Chapter 6 for a discussion of when and where to get genetic counseling.

ACHONDROPLASIA. See Dwarfism.

AFFECTIVE ILLNESS. See Manic depression and Depression.

ALBINISM. Albinos—people who lack pigment—have been the subject of human curiosity for centuries. Albinism is not a single disorder, but is instead a general term used to describe a variety of different genetic diseases affecting pigmentation. In one form of albinism, the eyes alone are affected; in other types the skin, hair, and eyes all lack pigment. Albinos are more likely to develop skin cancer, and most have difficulty seeing; many albinos are legally blind.

The most severe type of albinism is called *tyrosinase-negative albinism.* Individuals with this form of the disease lack an enzyme called tyrosinase, which normally helps synthesize pigment. Thus, no pigment is produced in tyrosinase-negative albinos. These individuals have pink skin and snow-white hair; the eyes are translucent gray or blue, but they shine red in a beam of direct light. Eyesight in these individuals is greatly reduced; even moderate light causes severe squinting, and nystagmus (involuntary jerky movements of the eyes) is common. A relatively rare condition, tyrosinase-negative albinism occurs in about 1 out of every 37,000 people in the United States.

A less severe form of the disease is *tyrosinase-positive albinism.* Here, the tyrosinase enzyme functions normally, but for unknown reasons little pigment is produced. In a tyrosinase-positive albino, the skin is pink and hair is white at birth, similar to the characteristics of a tyrosinase-negative albino. However, some pigment gradually accumulates over time, so that the hair may appear yellow with age and skin becomes cream colored. Visual problems are less severe in tyrosinase-positive albinism, and eyesight tends to improve with age. The prevalence of this form of albinism in North American Caucasians is similar to that for tyrosinase-negative albinism: about 1 in 37,000 individuals. However, the disorder occurs more frequently in North American blacks, with a frequency of 1 in 15,000. Some ethnic groups such as the Hopi, Zuni, and Jemez Indians of North America have much higher frequencies of this trait (see Chapter 1).

Most forms of albinism are inherited as autosomal recessive disorders. When albinism is due to an autosomal recessive gene, an individual with the disorder possesses two copies of the albino gene, one inherited from each parent. Thus, if both parents are normal and have an albino child, both parents must be carriers; each additional child they conceive will have a one in four chance of being albino. If one of the parents is albino, then he or she can only produce albino children if the other parent is a carrier for the albino gene. Because albinism is rare in the general population, the chance of marrying a carrier is low, and most albinos do not produce albino children. However, the chance that the spouse is a carrier is greater if the spouse is related or if both individuals come from an ethnic group in which albinism occurs in high frequency. When both parents have the same form of albinism, then all their children will also be albinos. However, because several different types of albinism occur, two albinos may have different forms of the disorder; in this case, none of the children are likely to be affected. It is important to keep in mind that in a few types of albinism, the inheritance is not autosomal recessive and the chance of passing on these forms will be different. Carrier testing and prenatal diagnosis are available for some forms of albinism.

ALCOHOLISM. Americans consume enough alcoholic beverages each year to provide every person over the age of 14 with more than $2\frac{1}{2}$ gallons of pure alcohol. Of course, many people drink alcohol infrequently, some not at all, and many who do drink regularly do not consume $2\frac{1}{2}$ gallons of alcohol annually. Thus, a few individuals drink very large quantities of alcohol; these heavy drinkers comprise only 11 percent of the general population, but they consume as much as 50 percent of all alcohol sold in this country. About 10 million people in the United States are problem drinkers, and 6 million are severely addicted to alcohol. The persistent problem of alcoholism costs hundreds of millions of dollars in medical care and social services each year and produces tremendous personal suffering in the lives of millions of alcoholics and their families.

In the past, society viewed alcohol abuse as a vice resulting from moral weakness; today alcoholism is more often seen as a chronic disease or a psychiatric illness. Researchers who study alcoholics frequently use different criteria for identifying those with drinking problems, but most agree that an alcoholic has severe alcohol dependence or addiction and exhibits several of the following characteristics: frequent intoxication; family problems and failure of marriage due to drinking; drinking-related arrests; inability to hold a job; hospitalization for alcohol problems; blackouts; tremors; and symptoms associated with alcohol withdrawal such as sweating, tremors, confusion, and delirium.

Several studies suggest that alcoholics consist of two distinct groups. The type 1 alcoholic usually develops alcohol-related problems after the age of 25, often not until middle age and frequently following an extended period of social drinking. These individuals lose the ability to stop drinking—once drinking begins it develops into a prolonged binge in which heavy alcohol consumption occurs. Periods of abstention typically follow these binges, during which the alcoholic expresses guilt feelings and "goes on the wagon." Fighting and arrests are uncommon in the type 1 alcoholic.

The second type of alcoholism occurs less frequently than type 1, but is usually more severe. The type 2 alcoholic typically begins drinking in adolescence and experiences problems with alcoholism before the age of 25. Drinking in type 2 alcoholics frequently is associated with fighting, arrests, and antisocial behavior.

Not all alcoholics fit into one of these two patterns, and some may exhibit characteristics of both. Nevertheless, recent research suggests that these two types of alcoholism are distinct and may have different causes. Males may be type 1 or type 2, but almost all female alcoholics are type 1.

Undoubtedly, different people develop alcohol-related problems for different reasons. Cultural practices, family upbringing, social background, and other environmental factors certainly play a role. Nevertheless, a growing body of scientific data indicates that heredity is important in alcoholism. Over 100 studies conclude that alcoholism is more common in close relatives of alcoholics, and adoption and twin studies demonstrate that this association within families is the result of a genetic influence on the disorder.

Alcoholism does not appear to be inherited as a simple genetic trait; it exhibits none of the characteristic signs of dominant, recessive, or X-linked factors. Almost certainly, alcohol dependence is influenced by complex interactions among many genes, and the genes involved also interact with environmental influences. Individuals with alcoholic relatives may inherit a predisposition to alcohol addiction; thus, they are said to be "at higher risk" for alcohol-related problems.

Several studies have utilized the cross-fostering or adoption approach to examine genetic influences on alcoholism. In this approach, geneticists study alcoholism in individuals (adoptees) who were separated from their biological parents at an early age (usually within two months of birth) and raised by foster parents. These individuals share genes in common with their biological parents, but the behavior of the parents does not directly influence the adoptee. Any association between alcoholism in the biological parents and their adopted-away children indicates that heredity affects the trait. (See Chapter 4 for a discussion of adoption studies.)

The adoption studies found that type 1 alcoholics usually have both a genetic predisposition and an environmental setting that encourages alcohol abuse. If either the genetic predisposition or the proper environment is present, but not both, individuals are no more likely to become alcoholic than the average person—apparently both the genes for alcoholism and an environment that encourages heavy drinking are required. Type 2 alcoholism displays a different pattern of heredity. Males with a type 2 alcoholic father are more likely to become alcoholic, about nine times more likely, than men without an alcoholic father. Environment seems to play less of a role in the type 2 alcoholic.

In spite of evidence for a strong hereditary component to alcoholism, anyone with an alcoholic relative should keep in mind certain facts: The majority of individuals with a genetic predisposition to alcoholism never become alcoholics, and many of those that do become alcoholic are able to overcome this problem. On the other hand, those without a genetic predisposition may be susceptible to drinking problems for environmental reasons. Finally, excessive alcohol consumption is capable of creating physical and mental problems in just about anyone.

ALLERGY. The body is constantly bombarded with foreign substances. Some of these are harmless, like small amounts of dust. Others, such as bacteria and parasites, may do considerable harm. To eliminate these harmful agents, the body possesses a complex defense network called the *immune system*. When this system detects a potentially harmful invader, it swings into action, producing a number of different responses to combat the invader: Antibodies, histamines, and special white blood cells are all brought forth to do battle with the invaders.

Normally, the immune system does not react to every foreign substance it encounters. Many common particles, like dust, pollen, and food substances, present no threat, and in most people these particles are ignored. However, some individuals have an immune reaction to substances that others tolerate; this abnormal reaction is termed an *allergy*. The substance that stimulates this abnormal immune reaction is called the *allergen*. Allergy symptoms occur when the body comes into contact with a specific allergen. If the allergen is inhaled, sneezing, coughing, and a runny nose may result. When the allergen is eaten, nausea, vomiting, and diarrhea may occur. If the allergen spreads through the body, hives may appear. In some cases, the immune reaction is so extreme that collapse, shock, and even death may take place.

Allergic reactions are complex and still poorly understood. Although precipitated by a specific allergen, the symptoms vary depending on a number of other factors. For example, infections and emotions frequently intensify the allergic reaction. Genes also play an important role in allergy. Allergies clearly run in families; for example, about 50 percent of the people who suffer from hay fever have other family members with hay fever. However, the genetics of allergy are poorly understood. Most likely, allergies are multifactorial, meaning that many genes and environmental factors interact in producing allergies. Thus, parents with allergies are more likely to produce children with allergies, but no simple pattern of inheritance is observed. Allergies are also likely to be heterogeneous—in other words, allergies may have different causes in different people. For example, asthmatics frequently have severe allergies. Asthma displays a strong tendency to run in families, and allergies are found more commonly in the relatives of asthmatics than among the relatives of those without asthma. In some people such as asthmatics, allergies may have a strong genetic influence; in others, genes may play relatively little role. We must also keep in mind that even when genes strongly influence allergic reactions, environmental factors are also important. Genes may produce a susceptibility, but the allergy is not expressed unless the proper environment—in this case, an allergen—is encountered.

One study conducted among college students in the state of Washington reported that when both parents had hay fever, 58 percent of their children were affected; when one parent had hay fever, 38 percent of the children were affected; and when neither parent had hay fever, only about 13 percent of the children had it. Other studies also suggest that when one parent has allergies, the children are two to three times more likely to develop allergies. However, the risk of developing allergies when other family members are affected depends upon a number of factors, including age and sex of the individual, the type and severity of allergic reactions, and whether asthma or eczema are also present. Thus, the risk figures given by these studies may not be applicable to all people.

ALOPECIA. See Baldness.

ALZHEIMER'S DISEASE. Alzheimer's disease is a common neurological disorder of the elderly, characterized by progressive mental deterioration. Typically, the first observable symptom of the disease is a failure to remember recent events. Speech problems frequently follow; for example, the patient may be unable to name common objects. Personality changes sometimes occur and all intellectual functions gradually worsen. In advanced stages of the disease, the patient becomes completely helpless, and, frequently, institutional care is necessary.

Specific alterations in the brain accompany these clinical symptoms. In a person with Alzheimer's disease, some brain cells are lost and the overall weight of the brain may decrease. Abnormal bundles of microscopic filaments that wind around each other—termed *neurofibrillary tangles*—fill the nerve cells remaining in the brain. Peculiar plaques loaded with protein are also deposited between the brain cells.

Because it is a leading cause of intellectual impairment in the elderly and the number of elderly people is increasing, Alzheimer's disease represents a major public health problem in the United States. Experts estimate that approximately 2 million people in the United States have Alzheimer's disease.

Alzheimer's disease occurs in two distinct groups of people. First, the disease most frequently strikes older people, typically those in their seventies and eighties; it is, in fact, the most common cause of intellectual impairment in the elderly. In these patients, Alzheimer's disease arises sporadically, without any obvious tendency to run in families. We also see Alzheimer's disease in a second group; these patients develop symptoms of the disease at an earlier age, usually in their fifties or early sixties. In its early form, the disease is more severe, and other family members are frequently affected. A few families with early Alzheimer's disease clearly exhibit an autosomal dominant mode of inheritance. Symptoms of the early and late forms are indistinguishable, as are the changes that take place within the brain tissue, but it is unclear whether the causes in these two groups are the same. Genes definitely influence the early form of Alzheimer's, but the role of heredity in the more common, late form of the disease is not certain.

Scientists recently demonstrated that in some families with early Alzheimer's disease, the gene responsible for the disorder resides on chromosome 21. In other families, however, researchers found no association between Alzheimer's disease and genes on chromosome 21. This finding raises the possibility that more than one gene may be capable of causing the disease.

ANDROGEN INSENSITIVITY SYNDROME. See Sex determinism.

ANENCEPHALY. See Neural tube defects.

ANOREXIA NERVOSA. Anorexia nervosa is a disorder characterized by obsessive fear of becoming fat. The disease occurs almost exclusively in young women between the ages of 12 and 18, and it is most prevalent among young women from middle- and upper-income families. The typical young woman with anorexia nervosa feels she is fat, even when she is actually thin or emaciated. She becomes preoccupied with her body size. By undereating, she loses an excessive amount of weight and fails to gain weight normally as she grows. Severe weight loss leads to cessation of her menstrual cycle; a number of medical complications may also occur. This is a serious psychiatric disorder. Hospitalization is frequently required, and some girls with anorexia nervosa literally starve to death.

Studies show that anorexia nervosa tends to run in families. Twin studies also indicate that two identical twins are more likely to both have anorexia than are two nonidentical twins, which is consistent with the idea that genes influence the disease. Close relatives of anorexics are more likely to experience depression; this suggests that anorexia may be related to depression, and depression has a genetic tendency (see Depression). In spite of these indications that genes may be involved in anorexia nervosa, there is no clear-cut pattern of inheritance. Genes may predispose certain women to anorexia, but environmental factors are probably also important.

ARTHRITIS. See Rheumatoid arthritis.

ASTHMA. The airways that connect the mouth and nose to the lungs are shaped much like the roots of a plant—the larger airways at the top divide successively into smaller and smaller passages, ultimately ending in the small air spaces of the lungs. Here in the lungs, exchange of gases occurs between the air and the blood. In a person with asthma, the airways to the lungs periodically constrict, blocking the flow of air. At the same time, excessive amounts of mucus are secreted into the passages, which further impedes the movement of air in and out of the lungs. Coughing ensues, breathing becomes labored, and the movement of air through the constricted channels produces the whistling sound called wheezing. This is an asthma attack.

Why the air passages of an asthmatic constrict is poorly understood. A variety of stimuli, including airborne substances, such as pollen and dust, respiratory infections, exercise, cold air, and emotional stress, may precipitate an asthma attack. Allergies and eczema frequently accompany asthma in many individuals. This suggests that asthma is a form of allergy, resulting from a general disorder of the immune system. However, some people with asthma do not have allergies or eczema, and the precise relationship between asthma and allergy is not clear.

For many years, geneticists and physicians have reported that asthma tends to run in families. A number of studies have demonstrated the hereditary nature of this disease. For example, surveys of asthmatics reveal that if a parent has asthma, on the average one quarter of the children in the family are also affected. For families in which both parents are affected, over one-third of the children have asthma.

Although the hereditary nature of asthma is widely accepted, the genetics of the disorder remain foggy. In some families, asthma appears to be inherited as an autosomal dominant trait; however, the inheritance appears to be more complicated in other families. Because asthma is often triggered by some environmental stimulus (cold air, dust, pollen, and so on), the genes involved must cause an underlying susceptibility, which is then expressed as the symptoms of asthma when the right environmental conditions are present. Most likely, asthma is multifactorial in nature, resulting from an interaction of several genes and environmental factors. Whatever the exact mode of inheritance, genes clearly exert a strong influence on the expression of this disease.

ATHEROSCLEROSIS. See Cardiovascular diseases.

ATTACHED EARLOBES. See Earlobes, attached.

BALDNESS. Baldness (*alopecia* in medical terminology) develops for a variety of different reasons: Illnesses, injuries, burns, and certain drugs may all produce hair loss. Baldness also tends to run in families, and heredity is the primary cause of baldness in most men.

The most common form of baldness is *pattern baldness,* which is recognized by premature loss of hair from the front and top of the head; pattern baldness does not affect the eyebrows, eyelashes, pubic hair, and hair on the sides of the head. Geneticists believe that pattern baldness is inherited as a sex-influenced trait, which means that the sex of the individual influences how the trait is expressed. (For more information on sex-influenced inheritance, see Chapter 3.) In the case of pattern baldness, the trait is dominant in men: Only a single gene for baldness will produce hair loss in a male. In females, however, baldness is recessive, requiring two copies of the gene to be expressed. For this reason, pattern baldness occurs more commonly in males than in females. Contrary to popular opinion, the gene for baldness does not reside on the sex chromosomes; thus a man's gene for pattern baldness may be inherited from either the mother or the father. But because the expression of pattern baldness requires two copies of the bald gene in females, a woman must inherit a bald gene from both her mother and her father to become bald.

When present in females, pattern baldness is usually only weakly expressed. Females who inherit two copies of the bald gene typically experience only thinning of the hair, whereas pattern baldness in males frequently progresses to a loss of over 50 percent of the hair on the head. This difference of expression between males and females probably results from the influence of male sex hormones, which apparently accentuate the effects of the bald genes.

Genes also produce several other types of baldness, but the characteristic hair loss and the patterns of inheritance are different in these conditions. For example, in *congenital universal alopecia,* the head is hairless at birth or hair loss occurs within a few months after birth. In this type of baldness, the eyebrows, eyelashes, and pubic hair are also scanty. Congenital universal alopecia is thought to be inherited as an autosomal recessive trait. Baldness may also occur as a side effect of some rare genetic disorders, some of which have a dominant mode of inheritance and some of which have a recessive mode of inheritance. For example, individuals with Alopecia-Mental Retardation (AMR) syndrome are bald at birth and have severe mental retardation; this rare condition appears to be inherited as an autosomal recessive trait.

BECKER MUSCULAR DYSTROPHY.   See Muscular dystrophy.

BEDWETTING (Functional Enuresis). Bedwetting, or functional enuresis, is repeated involuntary urination in children over the age of six. Many children experience bedwetting up to the age of six, and the trait should not be considered abnormal in this younger age group. After seven years of age, however, the number of bedwetting children decreases, and bedwetting is very uncommon by age 12. Nevertheless, bedwetting continues to occur in some older children, and, in most of these, physical causes such as diabetes or seizure can be excluded. Although many theories have been proposed to explain bedwetting in such children, no consensus exists regarding the underlying nature of the problem.

A number of studies indicate that bedwetting tends to run in families, and many children with the disorder have a parent or a sibling who also had problems with bedwetting. Studies of twins demonstrate that for identical twins, more twin pairs exist where both individuals of the pair show the trait than for nonidentical twins, which is the expected result if hereditary factors are important in bedwetting. In spite of these observations indicating that genes influence bedwetting, no simple pattern of inheritance has been observed for the trait, and the mode of inheritance is uncertain.

BIRTH WEIGHT.   When a new baby arrives, everyone asks two questions: "Is it a boy or a girl?" and "How much does it weigh?" Our society's preoccupation with the second question—birth weight—is not just a cultural quirk. Birth weight is strongly correlated with a baby's health and survival in the first few weeks following delivery. Thus, the answer to that simple question "How much does it weigh?" actually gives us important information about the baby's vigor. The response we hope to hear is that the baby was large, for on the average, bigger babies survive better. Actually, this is true only up to a certain point. In terms of survival, the optimum birth weight for babies is between 7.5 and 8 pounds; thus middle-size babies really thrive best. However, many postbirth complications and illnesses occur in very small babies, so with babies, bigger is generally better.

Birth weight is one of the most complex of all human traits. Numerous factors affect it, and trying to separate the genetic and nongenetic components of birth weight is a formidable task. First, we must consider the baby's own genes. At conception, an embryo inherits its genetic potential for growth from its two parents. Because half of its genes come from the mother and half come from the father, both parents contribute equally to its growth potential, at least initially. The baby's genes can be expected to influence fetal growth in the womb, just as its genes influence growth and weight after birth.

Both the mother and the father endow the baby with its genetic constitution, but the mother, unlike the father, contributes more to the fetus than a set of her genes—she also provides all of its nutrition, its immunity, its living space, and its exposure to a number of outside agents during pregnancy. Some of this contribution is a function of the mother's own genetic constitution. For example, adult height and weight are partly genetic (see Height and Weight in this catalog), and women who are tall and heavy have larger babies at birth, on the average, than small women. Furthermore, having large babies tends to run in some families, so there is probably a genetic tendency on the part of some females to have large babies, which is independent of the mother's height and weight. Thus, the mother's genes continue to influence the birth weight of her offspring even after conception. Geneticists call this type of genetic influence, where the mother's genes determine a trait in the offspring after conception, a *genetic maternal effect*. Genetic maternal effects definitely play a role in birth weight.

Environmental factors also contribute to birth weight. For example, numerous studies have documented the detrimental effects of smoking and alcohol consumption during pregnancy: Babies born to mothers who smoke or drink weigh less than babies born to those who don't. Other chemicals and many drugs also depress birth weight. Finally, certain characteristics of the baby and the pregnancy influence birth weight; these include the sex of the baby, whether it is a first pregnancy, if twins are present, and whether the baby is born full term.

In summary, birth weight is determined by complex and still poorly understood interactions among the baby's own genes, the mother's genes acting on the baby during pregnancy (genetic maternal effect), environmental agents, and several characteristics of the pregnancy. Researchers have found that all these factors contribute to birth weight. However, studies often disagree about the relative importance of these components. For example, several investigators have reported that the baby's own genes contribute relatively little to birth weight—around ten percent or less. Other geneticists, however, have estimated that the baby's genes may determine as much as 60 to 70 percent of the variation in birth weight. Additional studies reveal that the effect of the baby's own genes on birth weight may depend on the presence or absence of certain environmental factors, such as whether the mother smokes. Also, the mother's genes may affect whether certain environmental factors are present; for example, alcoholism has a hereditary component (see Alcoholism), so the mother's genes may influence whether the fetus is exposed to alcohol—an environmental agent—during development.

Thus, birth weight is determined by an exceedingly complex process that is still poorly understood. All we can say with certainty is that genetic and environmental factors are involved, but whose genes, how much they contribute, and how they act is not yet clear.

BLEEDER'S DISEASE. See Hemophilia.

BLINDNESS. Vision is one of the most precious of all human traits; tragically, over 1 million people in the United States alone have difficulty seeing, and 500,000 of these are legally blind. Eyesight commonly fails with age—over 70 percent of all blind people are 65 or older. However, many children are born blind each year, and many others lose their eyesight at an early age. Thus, blindness is not only a problem of the elderly, but is a handicap that may strike at any age.

Blindness is not a precise term. A person may be considered blind when applying for a driver's license and yet see well enough to undertake most other normal activities. Another person may be handicapped with extremely poor vision, but may be able to distinguish large objects dimly. About 20 percent of all legally blind people are totally without vision, perceiving no light at all.

Visual impairment and blindness occur for a variety of reasons. Disease and injury are responsible for many cases. Heredity also causes much blindness; researchers estimate that heredity is involved in roughly half of all cases of blindness that occur before the age of 45. A large number of different genes contribute to the development of the eye, its associated nerves, and those parts of the brain that control vision. Thus, it is not surprising that hundreds of different types of hereditary blindness exist. Some forms of blindness are inherited as autosomal recessive traits, others as autosomal dominant traits, and still others as X-linked traits. Additional eye diseases and disorders exhibit multifactorial inheritance, which means that multiple genes and environmental factors are responsible for the defect. Many genetic syndromes and genetic diseases may cause visual problems along with other deformities and medical problems. For example, galactosemia, a hereditary disorder of sugar metabolism, produces cataracts that may result in blindness, unless the disorder is treated. Also, individuals with chromosome abnormalities frequently have visual problems along with numerous other birth defects.

Because blindness exists in many genetic and nongenetic forms, the chance of developing blindness when a member of the family is blind depends upon the precise cause of the blindness. If a parent is blind and their blindness is one of those types that exhibit an autosomal dominant mode of inheritance, each child will have a 50 percent chance of inheriting the disorder. On the other hand, if the parent's blindness is due to a recessive gene, children can be affected only if the other parent is a carrier for the recessive gene, which is an unlikely event unless the two parents are related; therefore, the probability of children inheriting a recessive form of blindness from a blind parent is low. When blindness occurs as a side effect of a genetic disease or a chromosome disorder, it will exhibit the same pattern of inheritance as the disease or chromosome disorder. Once the cause of blindness has been established, genetic counselors can often provide estimates of the risk of inheriting the disorder.

See Cataracts, Glaucoma, Nearsightedness.

BLOOD PRESSURE. See Cardiovascular diseases.

BLOOD TYPE, ABO. Each day, a multitude of bacteria, viruses, parasites, and other potentially harmful substances assault the body, yet it remains healthy most of the time. Resisting these foreign invaders is the immune system. The immune system is the body's defense network—a vast array of different types of cells, each type carrying out a different function, but all communicating and interacting together in the defense of the body. A central problem that the immune system faces is distinguishing between what is foreign and what is not foreign. Although many aspects of this recognition process are still poorly understood, as long ago as 1900, geneticists learned that the immune system recognizes certain molecules on the surface of cells. These molecules are called *antigens*. An individual's own antigens are determined by his or her genes and they tell the immune system that this is part of one's self. Foreign antigens, on the other hand, are recognized by the immune system as nonself; these are attacked and destroyed. One of the weapons used against foreign antigens is the production of special substances called *antibodies*.

The ABO blood type is one of the numerous antigens that occur on the surface of our red blood cells. Most of us possess one of four common blood types: type A, type B, type AB, or type O. (Blood types are frequently designated as A *negative* or O *positive;* the positive and negative designations represent the presence or absence of another antigen called Rh, which is under separate genetic control. See Blood type, Rh.) Each person has a genotype that determines their ABO blood type. A person's genotype consists of two genes—one gene from the mother and one gene from the father. In most groups of humans, three ABO genes are common; these are designated I^A, I^B and i. An individual's ABO genotype consists of any two of these genes, so six different genotypes are possible: $I^A I^A$, $I^A i$, $I^B I^B$, $I^B i$, $I^A I^B$, and ii. The I^A gene produces the A antigen, the I^B gene produces the B antigen, and the i gene produces no detectable antigen.

The genotype $I^A I^A$ produces only A antigens, and thus a person with this genotype has blood type A. Similarly, if you have the genotype $I^B I^B$, you produce only B antigens, and your blood type is B. When a person has genotype $I^A I^B$, both A and B antigens are produced on the red blood cells, and the blood type is called AB. The i allele produces no antigen. Therefore a person with the genotype ii has no ABO antigen; their blood type is said to be O. Because i produces no antigen, a person with the genotype $I^A i$ produces only A antigen and has A blood type. Similarly, a person with the genotype $I^B i$ produces only the B antigen and has B blood type. The frequencies of the blood types vary among different ethnic groups; in North Americans, O blood type is most common.

Blood types are medically important for blood transfusions. When a person is given a transfusion, foreign cells are introduced into the body. If the immune system recognizes the transfused cells as foreign, it will attack and destroy them. This deprives the person of the needed blood. Even worse, an intense immune reaction occurs, which can lead to shock. Chemicals from the destroyed blood also upset the body chemistry, leading to numerous medical problems. Before blood types were discovered, blood transfusions frequently killed the patient. With the discovery of the ABO antigens, however, it was learned that only certain blood types are compatible. A person with A blood type can receive blood from another type A person with no ill effects. However, a person who has blood type B carries antibodies against A antigens and will destroy any A blood that enters the body. Therefore, people with blood type B cannot tolerate A blood. Normally, patients are only given blood of their own blood type. However, in an emergency, O blood can be donated to a person of any blood type, because O carries no antigens and there are no antibodies against it. Because of this ability to use O blood in any transfusion, O is said to be the universal donor. In an emergency, AB individuals can receive A blood, B blood, or AB blood, because they possess both the A and B antigens on their own red blood cells and thus recognize none of these antigens as foreign. They also tolerate O blood because O carries no antigens. Therefore, in an emergency an AB individual can be transfused with blood of any type, and the AB blood type is said to be the universal recipient. Because not all blood types are compatible and because no artificial blood has yet been developed, donations of blood from people of all types are a critical necessity.

A number of subtypes of A and B antigens have been discovered; for example the A antigen is commonly divided into two major types, A^1 and A^2. Many other variants also exist. These ABO blood types are caused by additional genes at the same locus.

BLOOD TYPE, Rh. Blood types are usually designated by a letter (A, B, AB, or O) and as either positive ($+$) or negative ($-$). The letter part of the blood type refers to the ABO antigen (see Blood type, ABO). The positive or negative designation refers to the presence or absence of the Rh antigen, which is separate from the ABO antigen.

An *antigen* is a substance that the immune system—the body's defense system—is capable of recognizing. The immune system recognizes some antigens as foreign; these antigens are attacked and destroyed. Other antigens are part of the body's own cells and are ignored by the immune system. To help the immune system differentiate between self and nonself (bacteria, viruses, and other foreign particles), the red blood cells contain dozens of different molecules on their surfaces that act as antigens; these antigens provide a unique code that tells the immune system "These cells are self."

One of the antigens that occurs on a red blood cell is the Rh antigen. Rh stands for rhesus monkeys, which were used in the first experiments leading to the discovery of this antigen. There are many different types of Rh antigens, but most of the differences are not medically important. At the simplest level, we can divide Rh blood types into two groups: those that contain the Rh antigen, called *Rh positive* (Rh+), and those that lack this antigen, called *Rh negative* (Rh−). In an Rh− person, the immune system recognizes the Rh antigen as foreign; it makes *antibodies* (proteins that help destroy foreign antigens) against the Rh antigen. Therefore, an Rh− person should not receive a blood transfusion of Rh+ blood. Usually, problems do not arise with the first transfusion of Rh+ blood in an Rh− person, because in the first exposure to a foreign antigen, the immune system is slow to produce antibodies. However, once exposed to a foreign antigen, the immune system spins off special memory cells that last one's entire life. These memory cells "remember" the foreign antigen and are capable of quickly producing antibodies against it should the antigen ever reappear in the future. (The memory cells are responsible for the lifelong immunity one acquires after having an illness like mumps or chicken pox.) If an Rh− person receives a second transfusion of Rh+ blood, antibodies against the foreign antigen are quickly manufactured, and they destroy the transfused blood; the resulting immune reaction and the breakdown products from the destroyed blood may lead to shock or even death.

The Rh antigens can also produce a disease called *hemolytic disease of the newborn*. This disorder arises when an Rh− mother carries an Rh+ fetus, which may occur if the father is Rh+. Normally, the blood of a mother and an unborn child do not mix. In the placenta, the fetal and maternal circulatory systems lie near one another, so that food, water, oxygen, and other vital substances can pass from the mother to the child. Carbon dioxide and waste products also pass from the child to the mother, but there is no direct exchange of blood between the mother and the unborn child. However, occasionally small amounts of fetal blood may pass into the mother's circulatory system. When these blood cells are Rh+ and the mother is Rh−, the mother's immune system will recognize the Rh+ cells as foreign and will make antibodies against them. The antibodies then cross into the fetal bloodstream and destroy the baby's blood.

As in transfusions of Rh+ blood, problems do not usually arise the first time the Rh− mother is exposed to Rh+ blood cells from the fetus, because the production of antibodies requires time and the baby is usually born before antibodies against its blood are made; consequently, the first Rh+ child is usually not affected. However, the mother becomes sensitized to the foreign Rh antigens in this first exposure. If she becomes pregnant with a second Rh+ child, leakage of fetal cells into her circulation quickly stimulates the production of antibodies against the fetal blood. These antibodies easily pass into the fetal circulation and destroy the baby's red blood cells. When its red blood cells are destroyed, the baby becomes anemic. After birth, destruction of large numbers of cells produces a substance called bilirubin, which causes the baby to turn yellow. The severity of hemolytic disease of the newborn varies from pregnancy to pregnancy. In some cases, if the bilirubin is not promptly removed, it settles in the brain and causes brain damage, which may lead to mental retardation or even death.

Fortunately, hemolytic disease can be prevented by giving the Rh− mother a dose of anti-Rh+ antibodies (called Rhogam) immediately after the birth of each Rh+ child. These antibodies destroy any fetal blood cells in her circulatory system and prevent her from becoming sensitized to the Rh antigen.

The genetics of the Rh blood type are complicated and not yet fully understood. For most purposes, we can consider that the Rh blood type has a simple genetic determination. Each person possesses two genes comprising their genotype for the Rh factor; one gene is inherited from the mother and one gene is inherited from the father. Two different Rh genes exist: one gene—symbolized *R*—that codes for the Rh antigen, and one gene—symbolized *r*—that codes for the absence of the Rh antigen. Thus, three genotypes are possible: *RR* and *Rr*, which produce the Rh antigen (Rh+ blood), and *rr*, which produces no Rh antigen (Rh− blood).

BRACHYDACTYLY. See Fingers, short.

BREAST CANCER. Breast cancer is the most common cancer in women. Each year, over 100,000 women in the United States discover that they have breast cancer and more than 40,000 women in the United States die from breast cancer annually.

Medical authorities recognize that breast cancer tends to run in some families. If a woman has a sister or a mother with breast cancer, she is two to three times more likely to develop breast cancer than a woman without breast cancer in her family. If a woman has a mother or a sister who develops cancer in both breasts before menopause, then she is nine times more likely to develop breast cancer. We should recognize that these figures are based on averages for all women with breast cancer. Breast cancer appears to occur in different families for different reasons. In some families, breast cancer appears to arise spontaneously or sporadically, with little or no inherited susceptibility. Because breast cancer is so common, even sporadic breast cancer may occur in two members of the same family as a result of chance. Thus, the presence of breast cancer among several members of a family does not necessarily indicate that genes are involved.

Although breast cancer has little hereditary tendency in most families, it does have a strong genetic basis in a few. In fact, in a small number of families breast cancer appears to be inherited as an autosomal dominant trait. An autosomal dominant trait is caused by the inheritance of a single copy of the gene for the trait. When a woman inherits the breast cancer gene, she has an 80 to 100 percent chance of developing breast cancer during her lifetime. Because the gene is autosomal dominant, both males and females may carry it and pass it on to their children. However, with a few rare exceptions, the gene only causes breast cancer in women; most men who inherit the gene are unaffected. This type of trait, in which both men and women carry the gene for a trait but the trait is only expressed in one sex, is called a *sex-limited trait*. Breast cancer in males is rare, but when it does occur it appears to have a strong hereditary component.

In families where a dominant gene for breast cancer occurs, the daughters of a woman with breast cancer have about a 40 to 50 percent chance of developing breast cancer. Similarly, sisters of women with breast cancer in one of these families have a 40 to 50 percent chance of developing breast cancer. However, experts estimate that women who develop breast cancer because of a dominant gene comprise less than ten percent of all women with breast cancer. In families without an inherited susceptibility to breast cancer, having a sister or mother with breast cancer increases the risk of developing the disease only slightly.

BULIMIA. Bulimia means binge eating—the rapid consumption of large amounts of food over a short period of time, usually in less than two hours. Frequently, those who engage in this behavior end their binges by gagging themselves until they vomit, or they use laxatives or rigorous dieting to control their weight. Bulimia is seen most commonly in young women, particularly university and high school students. Bulimic girls usually are aware that their eating habits are abnormal, and frequently they try to hide their binging. Many have a fear of being unable to stop eating. Depression and self-criticism frequently follow their binges, and most women with bulimia have great concern about their weight. Nevertheless, they seem unable to stop eating once they begin.

Because those with bulimia attempt to hide their binging behavior, the disorder often goes unrecognized by family and roommates. One telltale sign is the presence of scars on the back of the hand, which result from scraping the hand against the top teeth while trying to induce vomiting with the fingers. Bulimia can lead to a number of medical problems. These include destruction of the teeth from stomach acids that are regurgitated during vomiting, damage to the esophagus from repeated vomiting, stomach and intestinal problems resulting from binging, and heart problems.

Bulimia frequently occurs in association with anorexia nervosa, another eating disorder that involves obsessive dieting and self-induced starvation (see Anorexia nervosa). Bulimia also tends to run in families. People who have this eating disorder often experience depression, and a number of studies indicate that close relatives of bulimics tend to have higher than expected rates of depression. Because predisposition to depression has a genetic influence (see Depression), some experts suggest that both anorexia and bulimia are caused by some of the same genes that produce depression. However, some studies have not found more depression in the relatives of bulimics, and the relationship between bulimia and depression is controversial. These facts suggest that susceptibility to bulimia may have a hereditary component, but few genetic studies have been conducted on this disorder. The mode of inheritance (if bulimia is indeed hereditary) is unknown.

CAMPTODACTYLY. See Finger, bent little.

CANCER. Cancer is a disease that touches everyone. Everyone knows someone, a close friend or a family member, who suffers from cancer; one in five people will die of cancer. Cancer is not a single disease, but is a series of diseases that have in common the presence of cells that multiply uncontrollably. Cells throughout the body are continually dividing and multiplying. This normal process of cell division provides growth, repairs injuries, and replaces worn out cells. Under normal conditions, the cells of the body follow a carefully regulated pattern of growth and multiplication; new cells are produced only as needed. In cancerous tissue, however, the cells are out of control, multiplying and spreading relentlessly. Clusters of cancer cells—called *tumors*—crowd and compress other tissues, and frequently starve normal cells by using up all available nutrients. Cells in cancerous tumors may invade other tissue, or they may break off and travel to distant parts of the body, where they may lodge and begin to proliferate, producing new tumors.

Most, perhaps all, cancers are genetic, but few cancers are inherited. This statement might, at first, seem contradictory; how can cancers be genetic without being inherited? The answer to this question lies in the fact that every cell in the body carries a complete set of genes, but only the genes in the reproductive cells are passed on to future generations. Each person begins life as a single cell—formed by the fusion of a sperm and egg at conception. Soon after conception, this single cell divides into two cells. Each of these cells receives a complete set of genes from the first cell. The two cells then divide to four cells, and then to eight cells, and then to sixteen cells, and so forth. Eventually billions and billions of cells that make up the human body are produced, and each of these cells contains a complete set of genes. However, all of these cells do not contribute genes to the next generation. Only a few cells are destined to become sperm or eggs, the cells that will ultimately provide the genes for children. The genes in the reproductive cells, those that are passed to the next generation through sperm and eggs, are termed the *germline genes*. All the other cells of the body—the muscle cells, skin cells, brain cells, liver cells, bone cells, hair cells, and so on—contain *somatic genes*. The somatic genes are important—they provide the information necessary for our bodily functions—but they play no part in the conception of children.

Cancer arises because of defects in somatic genes. The somatic genes that cause cancer are called *oncogenes*, which literally means "cancer genes." Oncogenes begin as normal genes that are essential for proper growth and development; before they acquire the capacity to cause cancer, they are called *protooncogenes* or *cellular oncogenes*. Mutations—accidental changes in the coding instructions of the genes—may transform a protooncogene into an oncogene. Here mutation is used in a broad sense to mean any type of genetic alteration; the alteration might be a small change in the DNA sequence, it might be the deletion or addition of a large segment of DNA, or it might involve the loss or addition of a whole chromosome. Whatever the nature of the change, these genetic alterations stimulate the cell to divide rapidly, free from the normal controls on cell proliferation. The cell is now said to be *transformed*, with the capacity to cause cancer. Each time the transformed cell divides, it passes a copy of its oncogene on to the two resulting daughter cells. Because the daughter cells also contain the oncogene, they too divide in an uncontrolled manner and give rise to more transformed cells. The growing mass of cells forms a tumor. Additional genetic alterations may cause the tumor to become more aggressive, allowing it to invade other tissues and spread to distant sites.

Mutations that produce cancer arise in a variety of ways. Some mutations probably occur randomly, with no obvious cause. For example, during the process of cell division, a part of a chromosome may be lost; if the lost part of the chromosome encodes a gene that normally holds cell division in check, the absence of this genetic information may result in cell proliferation—a first step in the development of cancer. Other mutations may be caused by chemicals in the environment that alter the coding instructions of the DNA; such chemicals are called *mutagens* or *carcinogens* when the mutation leads to cancer. Many natural and unnatural substances in the environment are carcinogens. Cigarette smoke, for example, contains a number of carcinogens, with the capacity to alter the DNA and produce cancer. Sunlight and other forms of radiation such as X-rays can induce genetic alterations. Viruses can also cause cancer by inserting oncogenes into a cell. Finally, some genetic alterations that lead to cancer may be inherited. If a mutation arises in the germline genes, then a genetic susceptibility to cancer may be passed on to the future generations.

The origin of cancers is probably more complicated than that presented here. In fact, many of the details of this process are not understood. In spite of this lack of understanding, research indicates that most cancers do not arise in a single step—most are not produced by change in a single gene. More likely, several genes must be altered to transform a completely normal cell into an aggressive cancer cell. For purposes of illustration, suppose that changes in three genes—gene A, gene B, and gene C—are necessary to transform a normal cell into a cancer cell. For the cell to become cancerous, A must be altered to A', B must be altered to B', and C must be altered to C'. We will call each of these alterations a mutation, keeping in mind that the "mutation" might be a change in a single bit of DNA, a deletion or addition of a large piece of DNA, or even a loss or addition of a whole chromosome. The chance that each mutation will occur is low, but because the body contains trillions and trillions of cells, a number of cells in the body might receive one of these mutations. A much smaller number of cells might get two of the three required mutations. The chance of a cell undergoing all three mutations would be very low. However, because of the astronomically large number of cells in the body, this unlikely event becomes possible. Because a cancer cell multiplies faster than normal cells, the cell containing these mutations has an immediate advantage. It multiplies and spreads, passing on its capacity for rapid proliferation to all its descendant cells.

If one is exposed to carcinogens, mutations arise more frequently, and the risk of cancer increases. It is also possible that some people might inherit one of the mutations. Suppose that Bill inherits a copy of one of three mutations necessary to transform a normal cell into a cancerous cell: perhaps he inherits a copy of A'. Because all of his cells now contain one of the necessary mutations, only two additional mutations, B → B' and C → C', must take place for Bill to get cancer. Bill is already one third of the way toward developing cancer cells. The other two mutations might never take place, and Bill might not get cancer. However, he is clearly more likely to develop it than someone whose cell must undergo all three mutations. A geneticist would say that Bill is "predisposed" toward cancer, or he is at "higher risk" for developing cancer.

Numerous other factors undoubtedly enter into cancer susceptibility. The immune system, the defense network of the body, appears to play an important role; this is illustrated by the fact that people whose immune system is weak or faulty frequently develop certain types of cancer. For example, people who receive organ transplants are routinely given drugs to suppress the immune system, so that the immune system will not destroy the "foreign" transplanted organ. One of the side effects of this treatment is that cancers arise more frequently in immunosuppressed patients. Cancer cells may arise frequently, but the immune system destroys most of these before they proliferate and produce a tumor. Only those transformed cells that successfully evade the immune system survive and go on to cause cancer. Numerous factors may influence the ability of cancer cells to evade the immune system. Still other factors may influence the ability of cancer cells to spread and invade other tissues.

The important point to remember is that most cancers arise because of genetic defects in somatic cells. Thus, most cancers are not inherited—they are acquired through mutations that are experienced in the somatic cells during a lifetime. However, in a few types of cancer one may inherit a predisposition; in other words, certain genes that are inherited may increase the risk of developing cancer. Still, some people without a genetic predisposition may develop the cancer and some with the predisposition may never get it.

Only a few of the common cancers have a tendency to be inherited; these include breast cancer and cancer of the colon and rectum (colorectal cancer). Most other common cancers have little or no tendency to be inherited. Several rare cancers display a strong hereditary tendency; these include Wilms' tumor, a cancer that occurs in children; retinoblastoma, a rare eye cancer that also occurs in children; and certain cancers that tend to occur in hormone-producing glands.

See Breast cancer and Colon and rectal cancer.

CARDIOVASCULAR DISEASES. Cardiovascular diseases are diseases affecting the heart (cardio) and/or the blood vessels (vascular). Although many people refer to these conditions as *heart disease*, several distinct disorders produce heart problems, and these diseases frequently involve more than just the heart. Three common cardiovascular diseases influenced by heredity are coronary artery disease, hypertension (high blood pressure), and congenital heart defects.

Coronary Artery Disease. The human heart weighs about one half of a pound and is not much bigger than your clenched fist. However, its relatively small size is deceptive, for the heart does an incredible amount of work. An average person's heart beats about 70 times per minute,

4,200 times per hour, and 100,800 times in a day. This adds up to over 36 million beats per year. In one year, the heart may pump over one million gallons of blood through 100,000 miles of blood vessels. To keep up this pace, the heart must continually receive food, water, oxygen, and other essential factors. This nourishment passes to the heart through the coronary arteries, which are medium-sized blood vessels that traverse the surface of the heart.

In people with coronary artery disease, the walls of the coronary arteries become lined with plaques—deposits containing cells, fats, and other materials. These plaques narrow the space through which the blood flows. Eventually a blood clot forms in the narrowed artery, shutting off the blood supply to the cells of the heart. Without oxygen, food, and water provided by the blood, the cells of the heart stop contracting and begin to die. If not relieved, the blockage damages the heart muscle; in severe cases, a heart attack ensues.

Plaque formation occurs not only in the arteries of the heart, but in blood vessels throughout the body. This disease is technically termed *atherosclerosis*. Atherosclerosis causes stroke as well as heart disease and accounts for half of all the deaths in the United States. The process that leads to the deposit of plaques in the blood vessels is complex and still poorly understood. Many factors contribute to plaque formation. A major component of the plaque is fat, most notably cholesterol. When the blood levels of cholesterol are high, the chance of developing plaques increases; thus, transport and metabolism of cholesterol influence coronary artery disease. Diet may also play a role, but this issue is still controversial. Hypertension—high blood pressure—contributes to plaque formation, and smoking also increases the risk of coronary artery disease. Obesity and diabetes are other predisposing factors. Genes are also clearly involved; they may influence atherosclerosis by affecting cholesterol transport and metabolism, blood pressure, diabetes, obesity, or other factors.

Geneticists have long recognized that coronary artery disease tends to run in families. Indeed, having a close relative who suffered a heart attack before the age of 55 is one of the strongest indications of susceptibility to the disease. Twin studies also indicate that genes influence coronary artery disease. This genetic basis to the disease is probably heterogeneous, meaning that many genes may predispose one to early coronary artery disease in a variety of different ways.

One route by which genes influence coronary artery disease is by affecting the utilization of cholesterol and other fatty substances. Remember that cholesterol is a major component of atherosclerotic plaques responsible for coronary artery disease. Several genetic diseases prevent the normal uptake of cholesterol and other fats from the blood, leading to plaque formation and predisposition to coronary artery disease. Three such diseases are discussed below.

1. Familial Hypercholesterolemia. This is a genetic disorder involving the transport of cholesterol; individuals with the disorder have greatly elevated levels of cholesterol in their blood and are predisposed to early coronary artery disease.

Cholesterol is an essential component for the normal functioning of our bodies; it is used in all cell membranes, it is converted into several hormones that provide vital functions, and it is used to make bile salts, which aid in digestion. Cells are capable of making their own cholesterol, but much of the cholesterol used in the body comes from the diet. In the gut, the ingested cholesterol is packaged into particles that enter the bloodstream and then travel to the liver. The liver secretes the cholesterol back into the bloodstream in the form of small spherical particles called *lipoproteins*. Several different types of lipoproteins transport cholesterol, but about 70 percent of cholesterol in the blood is normally carried in the form of particles called *low-density lipoproteins* (LDL).

Because cholesterol is a fat, it cannot dissolve in the blood, just as bacon grease and water do not mix in the kitchen sink. Therefore, cholesterol is sequestered in the core of the spherical LDL, covered by an outer layer of a substance that does dissolve in blood. In this manner, cholesterol is transported to cells throughout the body. When it reaches its ultimate destination, the LDL attaches to a special hook—called a *receptor*—on the surface of the cell. The receptor latches onto the LDL and pulls it into the interior of the cell. Inside the cell, the LDL is broken apart and the cholesterol is released for use by the cell.

Individuals with familial hypercholesterolemia possess a defective copy of the gene that normally codes for the cell receptor for LDL. The disease is inherited as an autosomal dominant trait, and most affected individuals are heterozygotes, possessing one copy of the defective gene and one copy of the normal gene. These people are deficient in LDL receptors; consequently, less cholesterol is removed from their blood. Their blood levels of cholesterol become elevated and the cholesterol sticks to the walls of the blood vessels. This promotes the formation of plaques that may lead to early coronary artery disease. About 1 in 500 people is heterozygous for the defective LDL receptor gene. Because familial hypercholesterolemia is an autosomal dominant disease, a parent with the disease has a 50 percent chance of passing it on to each of his or her offspring. Similarly, a person with a brother or sister who has familial hypercholesterolemia possesses a 50 percent chance of developing the disease. About one in a million people inherit two copies of the defective LDL receptor gene, one copy from each parent. Those with two copies—homozygotes for the disease—are severely affected. Their blood cholesterol levels are more than six times normal; they may have a heart attack as early as age two and almost certainly will by age 20. When both parents have familial hypercholesterolemia, half of their children on the average will have the heterozygous form of the disease, and one out of four will have the severe, homozygous form.

2. Familial Hypertriglyceridemia. Another disorder of fat metabolism that predisposes a person to early coronary disease is familial hypertriglyceridemia, which is also inherited as an autosomal dominant disorder. This disease results in elevated levels of fatty substances called triglycerides during adult life. The cause of this disease is poorly understood. It occurs with a frequency of about 2 in 1,000 people. When a parent has this disorder, each child has a 50 percent chance of inheriting it.

3. Familial Combined Hyperlipidemia. This is yet another disease of fat metabolism, affecting 3 to 15 in every 1,000 people. The exact mechanism of the disease is unknown. About one third of the affected individuals have elevated cholesterol, about one third have elevated triglycerides, and one third have both. Affected individuals are frequently obese and are likely to develop early coronary disease. This disorder is probably inherited as an autosomal dominant disease, and affected parents would pass the disorder on to approximately 50 percent of their offspring.

Numerous other genetic diseases also affect the metabolism and transport of fats that may contribute to heart disease, but most of these are rare.

It must be emphasized that although these disorders of lipid metabolism definitely predispose affected individuals to coronary artery disease, very few people with coronary artery disease have one of these conditions. The exact cause of coronary artery disease in the vast majority of people is unknown. Heredity is clearly one factor that predisposes to coronary artery diseases, but in most families, the disease does not follow any simple pattern of inheritance. Multifactorial inheritance, involving interaction between many genes and environmental factors, is thought to be the explanation for most cases of coronary artery disease.

High Blood Pressure. Thirty-five million Americans—one in six—suffer from high blood pressure, or *hypertension*. Another 25 million exhibit borderline hypertension. Although high blood pressure alone produces no obvious symptoms, if untreated it leads to stroke, heart disease, and kidney failure. People with high blood pressure are three times more likely to have a heart attack, six times more prone to heart failure, and seven times more susceptible to stroke.

Blood pressure is the force or pressure exerted by the blood on the walls of the arteries as it flows through them. (Arteries are blood vessels that carry blood away from the heart; veins are blood vessels that carry blood toward the heart.) Blood pressure is usually expressed as two numbers, such as 120/80. The first number, which is always larger, represents the pressure in the arteries when the heart contracts and is called the *systolic blood pressure*. The second smaller number measures the pressure in the arteries when the heart is relaxing between beats; this number is called the *diastolic blood pressure*. Two physiological parameters largely determine the blood pressure in the arteries: the amount of blood pumped by the heart and the diameter of the blood vessels. As the heart pumps more blood, blood pressure rises; as the diameter of the blood vessels enlarges, blood pressure drops. This apparently simple relationship between heart activity, vessel diameter, and blood pressure is, in reality, exceedingly complex. A number of hormones and nerve impulses from the brain control heart activity and vessel diameter. Scientists do not yet fully understand how blood pressure is regulated nor what goes wrong in those with high blood pressure.

Blood pressure is not constant. Whenever the body requires more oxygen—during exercise for example—blood pressure goes up. During periods of rest, blood pressure goes down. Thus, blood pressure varies throughout the day and may differ from one day to the next. Among people in modern society, it also inches upward with age. Furthermore, blood pressure varies greatly from person to person. Therefore, blood pressure represents a continuum, ranging from those with abnormally low blood pressure to those with abnormally high blood pressure. For this reason, high blood pressure differs from many other diseases—there is no sharp distinction between those with the symptoms of the disease and those without them. Physicians generally diagnose high blood pressure when an adult patient's pressure exceeds 140/90 on several different days, but this cutoff point is somewhat arbitrary.

Physicians have recognized for many years that high blood pressure tends to run in families. The familial occurrence of high blood pressure might result from genetic factors; alternatively, common environmental predisposing factors might be shared by members of the same family. In fact, much research indicates that both environmental factors and genes are involved. One strong indication that environment plays a role is the observation that high blood pressure is primarily a disease of modern society. Among people living in primitive cultures, high blood pressure is almost nonexistent. Furthermore, in those societies that have recently undergone westernization, the incidence of high blood pressure has increased. Research points to three environmental factors—prevalent in modern societies—that appear to increase one's susceptibility to high blood pressure: high amounts of salt in the diet, obesity, and psychological stress. Although these factors influence blood pressure, they do not fully explain why some individuals suffer from high blood pressure and others do not; many overweight people consume large amounts of salt and lead stressful lives, yet they never suffer from high blood pressure.

It is clear that genes play an important role in high blood pressure. One indication that heredity is involved is the observation that different races vary in their susceptibility to hypertension. For example, black Americans are about twice as likely to suffer from high blood pressure as white Americans, and these differences do not appear to result from ethnic differences in environment. Twin studies also indicate that blood pressure is heritable. Research suggests that genes may produce a susceptibility to high blood pressure, which is then provoked by environmental factors such as stress or high dietary salt. Whether the environmental factors implicated in high blood pressure are capable of inducing high blood pressure in those without a genetic susceptibility is controversial.

The genetic susceptibility to high blood pressure does not exhibit a simple mode of inheritance. Most authorities agree that many genes are involved and the mode of inheritance is multifactorial, arising out of a complex interaction of many genes and environmental effects. Individuals with a close relative who has high blood pressure are more likely to develop high blood pressure. For example, one study found that males in Utah ages 20 to 39 were more than twice as likely to develop high blood pressure if they had a close relative with hypertension. If a male had two or more close relatives with hypertension, he was four times more likely to develop high blood pressure. Studies of heritability (the extent to which variation in a trait is genetically determined; see Chapter 4) indicate that about 50 percent of the individual variation in blood pressure is due to differences in genes, whereas the other 50 percent results from environmental differences.

Congenital Heart Defects. The human heart consists of four chambers that contract and pump blood throughout the body. At the top of the heart are two small chambers known as the right and left *atria*. The atria sit on top of two larger chambers called the *ventricles,* which are more muscular and do most of the pumping. Separating these chambers from one another and from the major vessels that fill and empty the heart are delicate valves. These valves act as one-way doors, ensuring that the blood flows in a single direction.

Congenital heart defects are birth defects in the heart; they arise because the heart fails to develop properly during fetal life. These defects are surprisingly common, appearing in about 4 out of every 1,000 newborns. Some are minor and may not produce noticeable problems until later life. Others cause severe problems; approximately 15 percent of all infant deaths result from congenital heart defects. A number of different types of heart defects may occur in the newborn. A common defect is a hole through the muscular wall that separates the two ventricles. In other defects, the blood vessels that enter and exit the heart are narrowed, or abnormal connections occur between the vessels. Another group of heart defects include faulty valves, so the blood flows backward when the heart contracts. Defects may also arise in the conduction of impulses responsible for heart contractions, so that the heart does not beat normally.

The majority of heart defects are thought to arise from genetic factors, but in most individual cases the actual cause is unknown. About 2 percent of congenital heart defects are produced by environmental causes; known environmental agents that can induce heart defects in the developing fetus include certain diseases and infections in the mother during pregnancy, maternal consumption of alcohol, and some drugs taken by the mother during pregnancy. Another 13 percent of heart defects may be caused by chromosomal disorders. For example, children with Down syndrome are more likely to be born with certain heart defects. Some heart defects exhibit simple patterns of inheritance or occur as a result of a genetic syndrome; these comprise about 3 percent of all congenital heart defects. The cause of the remaining 82 percent of heart defects is not known, but most of these are thought to be multifactorial in origin, arising from a complex interaction of genes and environmental factors. The risk of producing a child with a heart defect depends upon the type of defect and the family history of the disorder.

Some types of heart defects can be detected before birth with special ultrasound techniques that allow the structures of the heart to be visualized; these techniques are usually available only at special centers. Chromosomal abnormalities that cause congenital heart defects can be detected with amniocentesis. Prenatal testing for congenital heart defects might be desirable if a parent or a previous child has a congenital heart defect.

CATARACTS. When you look at someone's eye, the black disk you see in the center of the eye is the *pupil;* the pupil is actually an opening that permits light to enter into the eyeball. Situated just behind the pupil is a small spherical-shaped body, the *lens*. The lens serves to focus light coming through the pupil into an image on the back of the eyeball, and this allows us to see a clear image. Normally the lens is perfectly transparent and light passes through it unobstructed. In some people, however, cloudy spots develop within the lens; these spots are called cataracts. Cataracts can impair vision by blocking or distorting the light that passes through the lens. If a cataract is small, vision will be barely affected; if the cataract is large, it may produce total blindness.

Cataracts most commonly develop with age as the lens deteriorates over time. Other causes include certain eye diseases, injury to the eyeball, some drugs, radiation, and diabetes. Occasionally, cataracts are present at birth—these are known as congenital cataracts. About 1 infant in 250 is born with cataracts, and other newborns develop cataracts shortly after birth. Many congenital cataracts are caused by environmental factors, such as disease, poor nutrition, toxic substances, or inflammation. Others have a genetic basis.

A number of different types of genetically determined congenital cataracts exist; the mode of inheritance depends on the specific type. Some congenital cataracts are inherited as autosomal recessive traits, others are autosomal dominant, and still others are X-linked traits. The most common mode of inheritance for congenital cataracts is autosomal dominant. When the trait is autosomal dominant, a person with congenital cataracts usually possesses a single copy of the gene for congenital cataracts (the person is a heterozygote), and thus, he or she would have a 50 percent chance of passing this disorder to each child. In the rare circumstance that both parents have congenital cataracts, they would have a 75 percent chance of passing the trait on to each of their children. However, keep in mind that congenital cataracts do not always follow an autosomal dominant pattern of inheritance, and it may have no hereditary basis at all. Thus, the chance of a child inheriting congenital cataracts when a parent has this disorder may be considerably less than 50 percent.

Most cataracts are not congenital, but arise as part of the normal process of aging. Whether age-related cataracts are influenced by heredity is not clear.

CERUMEN. See Earwax.

CHIN CLEFT. Some people possess a distinct vertical cleft or a dimple on their chin. This feature is probably inherited as an autosomal dominant trait. When a trait is autosomal dominant, only a single copy of the

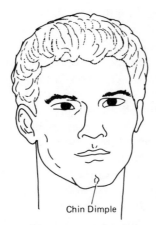

Catalog Figure 1.   Cleft chin consists of a cleft or a dimple on the chin.

gene for the trait is required for the trait to appear. The gene for chin cleft might be represented with the capital letter *C* and the gene for the absence of chin cleft with a little letter *c*. Recall from the discussion of inheritance in Chapter 2 that each person has two genes for each trait, one inherited from the mother and one inherited from the father. Thus, a person might possess two genes coding for the absence of chin cleft—*cc*. This person would lack a chin cleft. Alternatively, a person might possess one or two genes coding for chin cleft—*CC* or *Cc*; a person with these genes would normally have a cleft chin. However, the penetrance of the trait is not complete, meaning that some individuals who inherit the gene for chin cleft do not express the trait (see Chapter 3 for a discussion of penetrance). Because chin cleft has incomplete penetrance, it is impossible to give any simple predictions about its heredity. Parents with chin cleft can produce children with or without the trait, and parents without chin cleft can produce children with or without the trait. The trait will, however, tend to occur more commonly among the children of parents with chin cleft than among the children of parents without the trait.

CLEFT LIP AND CLEFT PALATE. Cleft lip, sometimes called a *hairlip*, is a notch or vertical split in the upper lip. The cleft may be only partial, or it may extend all the way to the base of the nose; in some individuals, two clefts—one on each side of the lip—are present. Frequently, cleft lip is accompanied by a cleft palate, which is a split that runs down the roof of the mouth. Although the severity of these deformities varies, cleft lip and cleft palate are distressing and disfiguring birth defects. They may make eating and swallowing difficult for the newborn, and they frequently lead to speech problems. Children with cleft lip and cleft palate also experience increased susceptibility to ear and sinus infections. Fortunately, even severe cases of cleft lip and cleft palate can usually be corrected with plastic surgery.

Cleft lip can occur by itself or in conjunction with cleft palate. Cleft lip is among the more common birth defects, occurring with a frequency of about 1 in 1,000 Caucasian births. The incidence is higher among Orientals, with a frequency of approximately 1.7 per 1,000 births, and is lower among blacks, with a frequency of about 1 in 2,500 births among American blacks. American Indians exhibit the highest frequency—about 3.6 per 1,000 births. Cleft palate by itself appears to be a different type of defect; it occurs with a frequency of approximately 1 in 2,500.

Experts consider cleft lip and cleft palate to be genetically heterogeneous, meaning that a number of different genes can produce the defects. The chance of inheriting these disorders depends upon the precise cause. Cleft lip and cleft palate most frequently exhibit multifactorial inheritance, meaning that a number of genes and environmental factors interact to produce the disorder. If one parent has cleft lip with or without cleft palate and no other family members are affected, the chance of producing a child with the same disorder is about four percent. If the parent has cleft palate alone, the risk in the children is approximately seven percent. Although most cases of cleft lip and cleft palate are isolated, occurring in only one member of the family, they are occasionally inherited as simple genetic traits, with autosomal dominant or X-linked inheritance. One recent study suggests that in some Danish families, where cleft lip and cleft palate appear to be inherited as an autosomal dominant disorder, a gene on chromosome 6 is responsible for producing the defects. Cleft lip and cleft palate also occur along with other deformities in a number of genetic syndromes (close to 200 syndromes with cleft lip and cleft palate have been identified) and in chromosomal abnormalities. In these cases, the inheritance follows that of the syndrome or chromosome abnormality. Also, both cleft lip with or without cleft palate and cleft palate alone may also be caused by environmental agents. Cleft lip and cleft palate can sometimes be detected prenatally with ultrasound.

CLUBFOOT. Clubfoot is a relatively common birth defect characterized by a foot that is twisted out of its normal position. The deformed foot may be turned inward, outward, upward, downward, or some combination of these positions. In a common type of clubfoot—called *talipes equinovarus*—the foot is turned downward and inward. Our discussion of clubfoot will deal with talipes equinovarus.

Although clubfoot occurs in about 1 out of every 1,000 births in the general population, the frequency varies among racial groups. For example, among Japanese living in Hawaii, clubfoot arises with a frequency of about 1 in every 2,000 births, and among Caucasians in Hawaii the frequency is 1 in 1,000 births. However, among native Hawaiians the frequency increases to 7 in 1,000 births. Clubfoot occurs most commonly among people of Polynesian ancestry, such as native Hawaiians. The disorder affects males more commonly than females in all groups. Clubfoot can be caused by constriction of the womb during development, but genetic factors also play an important role in the occurrence of this trait.

Recent studies of the inheritance of clubfoot suggest that the deformity results from the influence of both a major dominant gene and multifactorial effects (other minor genes and environmental factors; see Chapter 4 for a discussion of multifactorial inheritance). If two normal parents have a child with clubfoot, the risk of producing another child with the same deformity is about three percent. If one parent has clubfoot, the risk is also about three percent. When one parent has clubfoot and produces a child with clubfoot, the risk for clubfoot in additional children rises to 10 to 15 percent. Clubfoot is also a feature of other conditions and syndromes, some of which have a genetic basis. For example, certain types of heritable dwarfism produce clubfoot, and some chromosome disorders cause clubfoot along with numerous other physical deformities. In general, these conditions are rare and most clubfoot occurs as an isolated birth defect. Clubfoot can sometimes be detected prenatally with ultrasound.

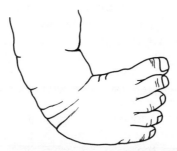

Catalog Figure 2. Talipes equinovarus, a common type of clubfoot, in which the foot is twisted downward and inward.

Once a crippling deformity, today clubfoot is almost always correctable. The treatment varies with the severity of the defect. In mild cases, the foot may be coaxed back into a correct position by repeated manipulation with the hands. In other cases, a cast or brace is applied. When the deformity is severe, surgical correction may be required.

COLON AND RECTAL CANCER. Cancers of the lower large intestine (the colon) and the rectum are termed *colorectal cancer*. Colorectal cancer is the third most common cancer in the United States, killing about 60,000 individuals in the United States each year. About 5 percent of the U.S. population will develop colorectal cancer during their lifetime.

Colorectal cancer, like all cancers, is a malignant growth of cells that multiply uncontrollably and spread to other tissues. Scientists do not yet fully understand how colorectal cancer develops. However, considerable evidence suggests that colorectal cancer is closely related to the development of polyps in the large intestine called *adenomas*. These polyps are small grapelike growths that project from the wall of the large intestine. The polyps are not themselves cancerous; hence, they are called *benign*. However, a small number of polyps may degenerate into the malignant growths that are known as cancer. Colorectal cancer probably begins as a defect that leads to the growth of polyps in the large intestine; apparently some of these polyps later develop into cancerous growths. Many people have polyps, and not all polyps will become cancerous. However, people who have large numbers of such polyps are more likely to develop cancer of the colon and rectum. Thus, a tendency to produce polyps in the large intestine predisposes one to colorectal cancer.

Although in the past most experts believed that only a few cases of colorectal cancer were inherited, evidence now suggests that the majority of colorectal cancers have a hereditary basis. Recent studies indicate that individuals with colorectal cancer inherit a gene that predisposes them to the development of polyps of the large intestine. About 60 percent of those who possess this gene will eventually develop polyps. Because the development of polyps increases the risk of developing colorectal cancer, this gene is thought to be responsible for most cases of colorectal cancer. The tendency to develop polyps is inherited as an autosomal dominant trait, which means that a single copy is enough to give the predisposition. Thus, if one parent develops polyps or has colorectal cancer, each child has a 50 percent chance of inheriting the predisposition for polyps. For people who possess the gene, the probability of developing polyps increases with age; by age 80, approximately 60 percent of those with the susceptible gene will have polyps. The presence of polyps increases the likelihood of developing colorectal cancer. However, keep in mind, that only a few of the polyps are likely to become cancerous. Thus, not all those who develop polyps get colon cancer, but the risk is great enough that those with a tendency to develop polyps should have their large intestine examined on a regular basis.

The finding that colorectal cancer is hereditary does not mean that this cancer is determined entirely by genes. On the contrary, numerous studies suggest that environmental factors—specifically diet—may also be involved. Genes and environmental factors appear to interact in the development of this cancer. Hereditary factors probably determine who is susceptible to colorectal cancer; diet and other environmental factors may then determine which of those susceptible individuals will eventually get colorectal cancer. Thus, environmental factors like diet will be most important for those who inherit the susceptibility gene. Unfortunately, there is no test at the present time that will identify those individuals who carry this gene. However, when adenomatous polyps of the large intestine or colorectal cancer are present in a parent or a sibling, the gene may be present in the family, and there is a greater likelihood of developing colorectal cancer. In such cases, regular examinations by a physician are advisable.

There are several rare genetic diseases that cause colorectal cancer. One of these diseases is *familial adenomatous polyposis,* a genetic disorder in which hundreds or thousands of polyps develop in the large intestine, often at an early age. Some of these polyps inevitably develop into cancerous growths, usually by age 40. Thus, anyone with this disorder is highly predisposed to colon cancer. Familial adenomatous polyposis is inherited as an autosomal dominant trait. If one parent has the disorder, the chance of each offspring inheriting the disorder and developing colon cancer is approximately 50 percent. Geneticists have recently discovered that the gene causing familial adenomatous polyposis is located on chromosome 5. This is a rare genetic disorder, and only about five percent of those with colorectal cancer have this particular genetic disease. Several other genetic diseases and syndromes also predispose one to colon cancer, but these are quite rare.

Also see Cancer.

COLOR BLINDNESS. Inside the human eye, light passes through the lens and shines on the back of the eyeball. As light passes through the lens, an image focuses on a layer of cells, called the *retina,* located at the back of the eye, just as a picture appears on a movie screen after passing through the lens of a projector. Cells within the retina record both intensity and color of the light and send that information to the brain, which then composes the picture that one sees.

Lining the retina are special cells that appear to be topped by upside-down ice cream cones; these cells are appropriately termed *cone cells*. A pigment that absorbs light at a particular wavelength fills each cone cell. Some cones contain a pigment that absorbs blue light, some contain a pigment that absorbs red light, and still others contain a pigment that absorbs green light. Thus, only three colors are actually seen—blue, green, and red—but the brain mixes the signals from these three pigments into the multitude of hues and shades that are perceived.

People with color blindness possess a genetic defect in one or more of the color pigments. In humans, separate genes encode each of the three pigments: the gene for blue pigment is located on chromosome 7, while the genes for the red and green pigments are found at the tip of the X chromosome. Actually, recent research indicates that most people possess at least two green pigment genes on each X chromosome; a few people even have three or four copies.

Color blindness is a relatively common trait in humans. About eight percent of western European males and about half of one percent of the females from this region are born with defective color vision. Genetic defects in the blue pigment are rare; when these occur, they are inherited as autosomal dominant traits. Most color blind people have disorders of the red and green pigments. About 75 percent of color blind individuals are deficient in green pigment and the other 25 percent are deficient in red pigment. Because the genes coding for red and green pigments lie on the X chromosome, both red weakness (termed *protanomaly*) and green weakness (termed *deuteranomaly*) are inherited as X-linked recessive traits. Color blindness occurs more frequently in males because males possess only a single X chromosome, and thus even a single copy of the color blind gene produces the trait. Females, on the other hand, possess two X chromosomes and must inherit a copy of the color blind gene on both X's to be color blind. Because a male always receives his X chromosome from his mother, he can only inherit color blindness from his mother, never from his father. Females can be carriers—having one X chromosome with the color blind gene and one normal X chromosome; carrier females possess normal color vision but they have the capacity to pass on a color blind gene. On the average, 50 percent of the sons born to a carrier female with a normal husband will be color blind. If the mother is color blind and the father is normal, then all the sons will be color blind and all the daughters will be carriers. Females are color blind only when their father is color blind and their mother carries at least one color blind gene.

CONGENITAL HEART DEFECTS. See Cardiovascular diseases.

CONVULSIONS. See Epilepsy and Febrile convulsions.

COOLEY'S ANEMIA. See Thalassemia.

CORONARY ARTERY DISEASE. See Cardiovascular diseases.

CRETINISM. See Thyroid disease.

CYSTIC FIBROSIS. Cystic fibrosis is a genetic disorder that disturbs the mucus-producing glands throughout the body, leading to respiratory problems, incomplete digestion, and abnormal sweating. For example, the air passages of a person with cystic fibrosis secrete large amounts of thick, sticky mucus. This mucus plugs up the smaller airways, preventing air from properly flowing into and out of the lungs. Respiratory infections frequently set in, and the lungs fill up with mucus and pus.

Down in the intestine, a thick, abnormal mucus is also produced. Among other effects, the mucus clogs the ducts leading from the pancreas to the intestine. Normally, these ducts carry secretions that are essential for proper digestion of food. When the pancreatic substances are prevented from reaching the intestine in the person with cystic fibrosis, food is incompletely digested; weight loss occurs in spite of a hearty appetite, and fatty, bulky, and foul-smelling stools are passed. The abdomen often protrudes, producing a "pot belly" appearance in a cystic fibrosis child. The pancreas regresses and eventually may be completely destroyed. Another complication is liver disease.

The sweat glands also malfunction and secrete too much salt in the sweat; this can lead to heat prostration during exertion. The underlying defect in cystic fibrosis involves abnormal transport of chloride ions into and out of the cell, which in turn affects fluid secretion in various glands.

Cystic fibrosis is primarily a disease of Caucasians. Among North American whites, approximately 1 in every 2,000 newborn infants has the disease, and about 1 in 20 individuals carries a gene for cystic fibrosis. In contrast, the frequency is much lower among blacks—only about 1 in 17,000.

There is no known cure for cystic fibrosis. Left untreated, a child with this condition usually dies at an early age, most frequently of severe lung infection. However, over the past several decades treatment of cystic fibrosis patients has steadily improved, and today many will live past the age of 21. Nevertheless, individuals with cystic fibrosis continue to suffer from numerous medical problems that require exhaustive and expensive therapy.

Cystic fibrosis is inherited as an autosomal recessive disease. Thus, a child with the disorder must inherit a cystic fibrosis gene from each parent. Parents who have a cystic fibrosis child must both be carriers, and each additional child they conceive has a one in four chance of having the disease. Furthermore, two thirds of their normal children will carry the gene for cystic fibrosis. If one parent has cystic fibrosis and the other parent has no known family history of the disease, the chance of producing a child with cystic fibrosis is about three percent. A few families have children with a particularly severe type of cystic fibrosis in which the child is born with an intestinal obstruction; in these families, the chance of producing another child with cystic fibrosis may be greater than one in four.

For parents with a family history of cystic fibrosis, carrier detection and prenatal diagnosis may be possible using DNA techniques (see Chapter 6). These tests are not 100 percent accurate, and they cannot be done on all families, but for many families they provide diagnosis of the condition with a high degree of certainty. Blood samples are required from family members to do the test.

Geneticists have recently isolated the gene responsible for the cystic fibrosis on the long arm of chromosome 7. Now that the precise location of the cystic fibrosis gene is known, accurate prenatal diagnostic testing and carrier testing will soon be available.

DEAFNESS AND HEARING LOSS. One out of every one thousand infants is born into a world of silence or loses their hearing during early childhood. Because normal speech does not develop without hearing, these children are also mute and only learn to speak with special training. Another 1 of every 1,000 children becomes deaf before reaching the age of 16; many more people lose significant hearing as they grow older. Experts estimate that about one in ten adults endures some degree of hearing impairment.

We can divide deafness into two major types: conductive deafness and perceptive deafness. *Conductive deafness* originates from a problem in those parts of the ear that conduct sound, including the outer ear, the eardrum, and the small bones in the middle ear that carry sound to the inner ear. In *perceptive deafness,* a problem occurs in the reception of sound within the inner ear, in the nerves that connect the ear to the brain, or in those parts of the brain that control hearing. Perceptive deafness is more likely to be present at birth, while most hearing loss that develops with age involves conductive deafness. However, either type may appear at any age, and some deaf people have both conductive and perceptive problems.

Deafness is not a single disorder, but arises in a number of different ways and has many causes. Infections, injuries, certain drugs, and continual exposure to loud noise can bring about loss of hearing. Genes are also involved in deafness; it is estimated that perhaps 50 percent of all deafness in children has a genetic origin. However, even among hereditary forms of deafness, many varieties exist. More than 100 different forms of hereditary hearing loss are known. Some types of hereditary deafness are inherited as autosomal recessive traits, while others display autosomal dominant, X-linked, or multifactorial inheritance. The mode of inheritance depends upon the specific type of hearing loss, but in many cases the cause is difficult to establish. Many genetic syndromes and some chromosomal abnormalities also produce deafness in association with other defects. In these cases, the inheritance of deafness will be the same as the syndrome or chromosome abnormality.

Deafness occurring at birth or in early childhood is more likely to be genetic in origin, although diseases, drugs, and injuries can also produce deafness in newborns and young children. Experts estimate that 20 to 30 percent of the cases of deafness that occur at birth with no obvious cause are inherited as autosomal dominant traits, about 40 to 60 percent are inherited as autosomal recessive traits, and about two percent are X-linked. The 10 to 40 percent of the cases remaining are thought to be multifactorial in origin (resulting from a complex interaction of genes and environment) or result from environmental factors alone. When there is no family history of deafness, the most likely mode of inheritance is recessive. However, if deafness occurs in several generations, dominant inheritance is more likely. The chance of a deaf person having deaf children varies greatly, depending on the type of deafness and the family history; the risks can range from minimal to 50 percent. The same applies for normal parents who have produced one deaf child and are concerned about the chances of deafness in future children. After hearing tests have been conducted and the family history reviewed, genetic counselors can often provide specific risk figures for couples concerned about the chances of producing a deaf child.

DEPRESSION. Depression is a universal human emotion—everyone experiences some sadness or depression at certain points in their lives. Disappointment, defeat, the death of a loved one, divorce, or loss of a job may induce low spirits. However, most people display an amazing ability to bounce back from tragic circumstances, and most quickly overcome stress-induced depression. On the other hand, a few people seem to be especially vulnerable to moods of depression; they experience unusually intense depression, which often arises spontaneously, without any obvious precipitating event. For these people, depression is often incapacitating and may last months. If untreated, about 15 percent attempt suicide. The periods of depression tend to recur and may be a lifelong affliction. These people are said to have depressive illness.

Depression has been recognized as a mental illness for over 2,500 years. Early Greek physicians described the disease, noting that aversion to food, despondency, sleeplessness, and irritability were typical symptoms. The Greeks attributed the disease to an excess of "black bile," one of the four humors they thought controlled the body. From the Greek word for "black bile" comes the English term *melancholy*, which is frequently used to describe the depressive symptoms.

At the broadest level, two types of depression can be differentiated. First, some people tend to have extreme mood swings, alternating between periods of euphoria or intense activity—called *mania*—and periods of depression. This condition is termed *manic depression*, or *bipolar affective disorder*. In the second type, severe depression alone is experienced; these individuals are said to have *unipolar depression*, or *unipolar affective disorder*. In this account, unipolar depression will be discussed. See Manic depression for a discussion of depression associated with mood swings.

Although there are a variety of forms of depression and individuals vary in their symptoms, many individuals who have depression exhibit a common set of characteristics. These characteristics include low spirits, a lack of interest, and feelings of worthlessness. Typically there is a loss of appetite and insomnia. The person with depression frequently has little energy and seems unable to focus his or her thoughts. Many people with depression awake early in the morning. They feel particularly low during the morning hours, but their outlook brightens as the day proceeds. Although these are typical traits of a depressed person, not all depressed people have these symptoms; for example, some people eat and sleep more, not less, when depressed.

Depressive illness is a major medical problem in the United States. Experts estimate that as many as 20 percent of the public has some depression, and approximately 2 to 3 percent of the population at any given time is hospitalized or seriously affected by depression. Depression tends to occur more frequently in women than men and is more likely to occur at certain ages—adolescence, middle age, and old age. In recent years, a number of drugs have been developed that are frequently effective in treating depression.

A large number of studies indicate that depression is hereditary. For example, studies show that in pairs of identical twins, both twins are more likely to be affected with depressive illness than are both twins of a nonidentical pair, which is the expected result if genes influence depression. Close relatives of patients with depression are also more likely to suffer from depression. If a person has unipolar depression, on the average there is an 11 percent chance that the person's children will also experience depression, as compared to a 2 percent chance among the children of a person who does not have depression. The same risk figure—11 percent—applies to siblings of a person affected with depression.

Although heredity is clearly involved in many cases of depression, nongenetic or environmental factors are also important. In people with depressive illness, an episode of depression may be precipitated by a specific environmental event, such as a death in the family or loss of a job. One does not inherit depression, but genes cause some people to be susceptible to depressive illness; depression may or may not develop in these people depending upon environmental circumstances. Susceptibility to depression does not exhibit any clear-cut pattern of inheritance; in most families it appears to be transmitted as a multifactorial trait, resulting from a complex interaction of many genes and environmental factors.

DERMATOGLYPHICS. See Fingerprints.

DIABETES MELLITUS. In the first century A.D. the Greek physician Aretaeus described a disease in which the patients possessed unquenchable thirst and passed large amounts of urine. He called this disease *diabetes* (in Greek meaning "siphon"), the name referring to the frequency of urination that characterized the affliction. Sixteen hundred years later, Thomas Willis established a simple diagnostic test for diabetes: The urine from a diabetic tasted sweet. This characteristic gave rise to the second part of the name, *mellitus,* which is Latin for "honey." These three characteristics—thirst, frequent urination, and sugar in the urine—remain the hallmark characteristics of diabetes today.

Diabetes is the fifth leading killer in this country; approximately 35,000 people in the United States will die of diabetes this year. The cost of treating diabetes is astronomical: Almost $5 billion was spent in 1984 alone. When the indirect costs associated with loss of productivity are figured in, experts estimate that the total cost of diabetes in the United States exceeds $20 billion annually.

In contrast to what the name implies, diabetes mellitus is not a single disease, but instead is a diverse assemblage of disorders characterized by problems in sugar metabolism. Under normal conditions, a hormone called *insulin* carefully regulates the amount of sugar in the blood. For example, after a candy bar is eaten, the level of sugar in the blood goes up, as the candy is digested, and its sugar is absorbed into the bloodstream. When this happens, the pancreas—where insulin is synthesized—secretes more of the hormone into the blood; insulin then stimulates the liver and cells throughout the body to take up sugar from the blood. The process is quite complicated, but basically insulin produces a drop in blood sugar. In a diabetic, the pancreas produces too little insulin, or the body is unable to use the insulin that is produced. Consequently, the blood sugar rises and excess sugar is excreted into the urine. The kidneys also excrete large amounts of water to dissolve the sugar, producing frequent urination and thirst. Other problems develop because the cells do not take up enough sugar to support their growth and day-to-day activities. The high blood sugar touches off other biochemical events, which may disrupt the entire body chemistry and lead to severe problems, some life-threatening.

In many cases diabetes occurs secondarily, as a consequence of other diseases and abnormalities. For example, an infection of the pancreas may inhibit insulin production. Also, a number of genetic syndromes produce diabetes along with other physical problems. However, in about one percent of the population the symptoms arise in the absence of other problems; this is referred to as *primary diabetes mellitus.* However, even primary diabetes mellitus is not a single disease. Physicians recognize two major forms: *juvenile-onset diabetes,* which typically first appears in childhood, and *maturity-onset diabetes,* which usually appears after the age of 40. Both types are clearly hereditary, but the genetics involved are complex and not completely understood.

Juvenile-Onset Diabetes. This form of the disease is also called *type I diabetes* and *insulin-dependent diabetes mellitus* (IDDM). It occurs less commonly than maturity-onset diabetes, but unfortunately it is also more severe. The cause of juvenile-onset diabetes remains unclear, but somehow the insulin-producing cells in the pancreas are damaged. As a result, the pancreas secretes little or no insulin. Much evidence suggests that this is an autoimmune disease, in which the body's defense network—the immune system—goes awry and attacks its own cells, specifically those cells in the pancreas that produce insulin. Other experts believe that viruses damage the pancreatic cells and precipitate the disease.

Whatever the immediate cause of juvenile-onset diabetes, genes are definitely involved. Numerous studies indicate that juvenile-onset diabetes has a hereditary basis. However, one does not inherit this disease. What is apparently inherited is a genetic susceptibility to it; some environmental factor (as yet undetermined) must then damage the insulin-producing cells in susceptible individuals. The importance of nonhereditary factors is demonstrated by studies of identical twins. Although such twins are genetically identical, when one twin has juvenile-onset diabetes, the other twin will be affected only about 50 percent of the time. How the susceptibility to diabetes is inherited is, as yet, undetermined. Most studies suggest that it is not inherited as a simple genetic trait. When one parent has juvenile-onset diabetes, each child has on the average approximately a 3 percent chance of developing the disorder.

One clue to the genetics of juvenile-onset diabetes is its association with certain genes that control the immune system, the genes of the *HLA system*. The HLA system represents a large array of genes found on human chromosome 6; these genes code for certain proteins that mark the cells and allow the immune system to distinguish between one's own cells and foreign cells that might invade the body. Many different alleles exist for the HLA genes, and individuals possessing certain HLA alleles are more likely to acquire juvenile-onset diabetes.

Maturity-Onset Diabetes. Maturity-onset diabetes typically appears after the age of 40, although it is sometimes seen earlier. This form is also called *type 2 diabetes* and *non-insulin-dependent diabetes mellitus* (NIDDM). Here the pancreas secretes some insulin, but the output is insufficient to keep blood sugar low. In most cases, the cells of the body show resistance to the action of insulin. Patients with maturity-onset diabetes are frequently obese, and obesity may contribute to the disease; however, not all patients are overweight, and the exact role of obesity is not clear.

Maturity-onset diabetes has a strong hereditary component. On the average, about 5 to 10 percent of the children of a person with this disorder will eventually develop the disease. As in juvenile-onset diabetes, no clear-cut pattern of inheritance is evident; multifactorial inheritance (inheritance involving both genes and environment) appears most likely. No association with genes of the HLA complex have been discovered.

Summary. Both juvenile-onset and maturity-onset diabetes are hereditary, but environmental factors also play a role in these disorders. Neither form follows a simple pattern of inheritance. The two types are entirely distinct diseases, each with a different genetic basis. Thus, having juvenile-onset diabetes in the family does not predispose one toward maturity-onset diabetes and vice versa. Genetic heterogeneity probably exists in both types; in other words, each form of the disease actually consists of several different genetic disorders that only appear similar. This genetic heterogeneity may account for much of the confusion surrounding the genetic basis of the disease.

Problems During Pregnancy in Diabetics. Women who are diabetics run a higher risk of producing children with birth defects. Those with juvenile-onset diabetes are at highest risk. Overall, about six percent of the children of diabetic mothers have birth defects, as opposed to two to three percent in the general population. The cause of these birth defects is not clear, but poor control of sugar metabolism in the mother during the first few weeks of pregnancy may be involved. Preliminary studies suggest that the incidence of birth defects can be lowered if strict diabetic control is begun prior to conception. Diabetic women contemplating pregnancy should consult with their physician before they become pregnant.

DOWN SYNDROME. In 1866, John Langdon Down was medical superintendent of the Earlswood Asylum for Idiots in Surrey, England. In the course of his work, Down noticed that about ten percent of his patients were so similar in appearance that he felt one might easily mistake them for children of the same parents. In a classic description, he recorded that these individuals possessed a broad flat face, a thick tongue, and a small nose. Because of their oval-shaped eyes (produced by a fold of skin called an epicanthal fold), Down thought they resembled Mongolians. Down's original description faithfully depicts the characteristics of one of the common causes of mental retardation. His reference to Mongolians stuck, and for many years these people were called *Mongolian idiots*. Unfortunately, this term is inappropriate, for the disorder occurs in all ethnic groups, and affected individuals do not really have Oriental traits. Today, the disorder is more appropriately referred to as *Down syndrome* or *trisomy 21*.

Down syndrome results from a chromosomal abnormality. Children born with this disorder have numerous medical problems and severe mental retardation. Typical features of Down syndrome include a flattened face, oval-shaped eyes, short broad hands, unusual palm creases, and poor muscle tone. Retarded growth produces short stature, and about 40 percent of the individuals with the disorder suffer from heart defects. Cataracts and other vision problems are common. Affected individuals are unusually susceptible to infections and exhibit an increased incidence of leukemia. Better health care has increased the life expectancy of individuals with Down syndrome, but the average length of life is still only about 30 years.

One of the most devastating symptoms of Down syndrome is the irreversible mental retardation it produces. IQ for these individuals typically averages about 50 (normal IQ averages 100). In spite of their low intelligence and numerous physical problems, individuals with Down syndrome are generally friendly, cheerful, and sociable. Recent research emphasizes the importance of providing affected individuals with stimulation and intensive special education; given a stimulating environment and training, today many individuals with Down syndrome are functioning at a level that was previously considered impossible. However, the moderate to severe mental retardation associated with Down syndrome cannot be prevented and these people experience a lifetime of mental and physical handicaps.

Down syndrome is the most common chromosomal abnormality seen in living humans; it results from the presence of an extra copy of the genetic material on chromosome 21. This extra chromosome material may arise in several different ways.

Primary Down Syndrome. This is the most common cause of Down syndrome, occurring in 92 to 95 percent of all liveborn children with the disorder. Affected individuals possess three copies of chromosome 21. During the production of sperm or egg cells in one of the normal parents of a child with Down syndrome, the chromosomes occasionally fail to divide properly, which then leads to the presence of two copies of chromosome 21 in an egg or a sperm. During fertilization this reproductive cell fuses with a normal sperm or egg, which contains a single copy of chromosome 21, resulting in an embryo with three copies of chromosome 21. In the majority of cases, the extra chromosome comes from the mother.

The incidence of primary Down syndrome increases dramatically in children born to women over the age of 35. For example, when the mother is age 21, the chance of producing a Down's child is only about 1 in 1,500. At age 35, the probability increases to 1 in 400. By age 40, the chance of producing a child with Down syndrome increases further to about 1 in 100, and at age 45 the probability is 1 in 30. The reason for this increase in Down syndrome with age of the mother is not clear, but the same trend is observed with most chromosomal abnormalities. One possibility is that as a woman ages, the process of chromosome division becomes more prone to errors; therefore, an older mother may produce more eggs with an extra chromosome, which then results in an increased incidence of children with Down syndrome. Apparently, the same phenomenon does not occur in men, or if it occurs the increase associated with paternal age is weak.

Translocation Down Syndrome. Occasionally a child has 46 chromosomes (the normal number), but possesses the typical symptoms of Down syndrome. Most of these individuals have an extra piece of chromosome 21 attached to another chromosome (usually chromosome 14). This type of chromosomal rearrangement is termed a *translocation*. Individuals with translocation Down syndrome have 46 chromosomes, but they possess three functional copies of the material on chromosome 21. Translocation Down syndrome accounts for about 3 to 5 percent of all individuals with Down syndrome. In this condition, one of the parents may be a translocation carrier. The translocation carrier has two functional copies of chromosome 21 and hence does not have Down syndrome. However, in a translocation carrier one copy of chromosome 21 is attached to another chromosome, and therefore the two copies of chromosome 21 may not separate properly during chromosome division; when the two chromosomes fail to separate, a sperm or egg is produced that carries two functional copies of chromosome 21 (one copy is attached to another chromosome). When this abnormal sperm or egg fuses with a normal egg or sperm carrying one copy of chromosome 21, the resulting fetus will possess three functional copies of chromosome 21 and will have Down syndrome. Thus, a translocation carrier has a tendency to produce abnormal sperm or eggs that can result in a child with Down syndrome. If a couple produces one child with translocation Down syndrome, one of the parents may be a carrier. When one parent is a translocation carrier, the couple has an increased risk of producing additional children with Down syndrome; in this way translocation Down syndrome runs in families.

Mosaic Trisomy 21. In these individuals, some cells of the body possess the normal complement of 46 chromosomes, but other cells possess 47, with an extra copy of chromosome 21. Mosaics arise from accidents occurring in cell division of the embryo (after fertilization) or from a combination of accidents in the formation of reproductive cells and in cell division of the embryo. Frequently these individuals are less retarded than those with primary Down syndrome.

There are several other ways in which abnormal chromosomes can produce Down syndrome, but these are rare. Once a couple has produced one child with Down syndrome, the risk of producing another child with the disorder depends critically on the exact type of Down syndrome and the chromosomes present in the child's parents. Therefore genetic counseling is advised for anyone who has a close relative with Down syndrome.

Down syndrome can be detected before birth by examining fetal chromosomes obtained from amniocentesis or chorionic villus sampling. Also, mothers who carry a fetus with Down syndrome frequently have abnormally low levels of a substance called α-fetoprotein in their blood (see Chapter 6). α-Fetoprotein is routinely tested in many pregnancies because abnormally high levels are associated with neural tube defects (see Neural tube defects). Low levels of α-fetoprotein can occur for reasons other than a Down syndrome fetus, so additional tests (usually amniocentesis) must be performed to confirm the presence of a Down's child. However, this test may provide a means of identifying those pregnancies that are likely to result in a Down syndrome child, especially among younger women who might not otherwise undergo amniocentesis.

DUCHENNE MUSCULAR DYSTROPHY. See Muscular dystrophy.

DWARFISM. Dwarfism refers to exceptionally short stature. There are a large number of different types of dwarfism, and many different factors may produce short stature. At the broadest level, two types of short stature can be distinguished: *proportionate short stature,* in which all body parts are shortened proportionally and *disproportionate short stature* in which only some body parts are shortened. Traditionally, people with proportionate short stature have been called *midgets*—these individuals are short all over. In contrast, those with disproportionate short stature have traditionally been termed *dwarfs;* in dwarfs, the head and trunk are frequently of normal size, but the arms and legs are short. In this account conditions that produce disproportionate short stature will be discussed; proportionate short stature will be discussed under Short stature.

Dwarfism—disproportionate short stature—results from defects in the development of the bones. A large number of types of such defects exist, differing in which bones are affected and how the developmental process is altered. In some cases these differences are obvious to an untrained observer, but in others they are subtle and a correct diagnosis frequently requires careful examination of X-rays by a specialist. Almost all forms of disproportionate dwarfism are hereditary, but the mode of inheritance differs from one type to the next. Some common types of dwarfism result from a dominant gene; others are inherited as autosomal recessive or X-linked recessive traits. There is even an X-linked dominant variety. As we discussed in Chapter 3, these patterns of inheritance differ greatly in how the trait is passed on; thus, an accurate diagnosis of the type of dwarfism is critical for predicting the probability of inheriting the disorder.

One of the most common forms of dwarfism is *achondroplasia*. In this disorder, the trunk is relatively long and the arms and legs are severely shortened; the head is relatively large, with a prominent, bulging forehead. Achondroplasia occurs with a frequency of about 1 in 40,000 births. This disorder is inherited as an autosomal dominant trait, and almost all achondroplastic dwarfs are heterozygous, possessing a single gene for dwarfism. The rare homozygote, with two copies of the achondroplasia gene, is severely deformed and usually lives for only a few months.

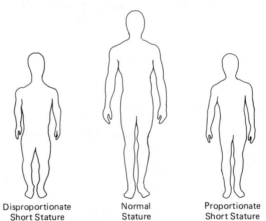

Disproportionate   Normal   Proportionate
Short Stature   Stature   Short Stature

Catalog Figure 3. In disproportionate short stature, only some parts are shortened; typically the head and the trunk are of normal size, but the arms and legs are short. In proportionate short stature, all body parts are shortened proportionally—the person is short all over.

Acondroplasia is inherited as a dominant trait, and thus a person with this form of dwarfism has a 50 percent chance of passing the disorder on to each child. However, most cases of achondroplasia are not inherited from a dwarfed parent, but arise spontaneously from new mutations. These are genetic accidents that occur in one of the reproductive cells that produced the individual with dwarfism. In this way, two normal parents may produce a dwarf child. Some forms of dwarfism can be detected prenatally with ultrasound or X-rays.

See Short stature.

DYSLEXIA. See Reading disability.

DYSMENORRHEA. See Menstrual pain.

EAR INFECTION (Otitis Media). Many young children experience infections of the middle ear, particularly during the first three years of their life. A child with an ear infection usually complains of a severe, persistent earache and frequently runs a fever. The infection occurs in the middle ear, which is found on the inner side of the eardrum. In severe cases, the middle ear fills with fluid, and the eardrum may rupture. Middle ear infection differs from *swimmer's ear,* which is an infection of the outer portion of the ear canal.

The middle ear is connected to the back of the throat by a channel called the *eustachian tube.* Normally air passes back and forth from the throat to the middle ear as the eustachian tube opens during swallowing. In young children, the eustachian tube is not well developed: it is shorter, wider, and more horizontal than in adults. The shorter and wider nature of the tube in young children may facilitate the movement of bacteria up into the inner ear, where they cause infection. Furthermore, the eustachian tube in young children becomes easily blocked, particularly during colds and upper respiratory infections. Blockage promotes the growth of bacteria in the middle ear, which then leads to infection.

Infection of the middle ear is not a genetic trait, because the infection results from a specific environmental cause—the presence of bacteria in the middle ear. However, since some children have recurring problems with ear infection and others have few if any infections, the susceptibility to infections could have a hereditary component. At least one study suggests that recurring ear infection during childhood tends to run in families. Also suggestive of a genetic basis is the fact that racial differences occur in the incidence of middle ear infections; for example, Eskimos and some native American Indians have a high incidence of infection, while low rates are typically observed among blacks. Genes may influence susceptibility to ear infections by affecting the size and functioning of the eustachian tube; consistent with this idea is the finding that the eustachian tubes of Eskimos and Native American Indians are larger than those found in blacks and Caucasians. Although these facts are suggestive of a genetic influence on ear infections, too few studies have been done to determine if the racial differences and the familial patterns of ear infection result from common environmental factors or from heredity.

EARLOBES. In most people, the earlobes hang down below the point where the ear attaches to the side of the head; this trait is termed *free earlobes*. In some individuals, however, the earlobes connect to the side of the head by skin, a condition termed *attached earlobes*. Attached earlobes is frequently said to be a recessive trait, but experts doubt that the inheritance is so simple. Earlobes cannot always be easily categorized as either completely attached or free, occasionally, the lobes are intermediate between these two extremes. Furthermore, a few people possess an attached earlobe on one side and a free earlobe on the other. Attached earlobes is most likely inherited as a polygenic trait—one controlled by a number of genes (see Chapter 4 for a discussion of polygenic inheritance).

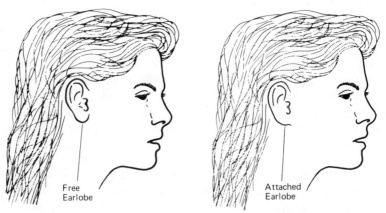

Catalog Figure 4.   Attached and free earlobes.

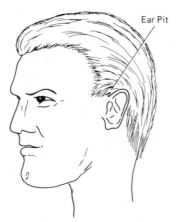

Catalog Figure 5.   An ear pit consists of a small pit at the upper junction of the ear and the head.

EAR PITS. The outer ear forms a semicircle that attaches to the side of the head. Sometimes, a small pit occurs in the skin at the upper junction of the ear and head; this trait is called an ear pit. Ear pits are present in about 1 in 500 Caucasians, and they occur more frequently in blacks. The trait is inherited in an autosomal dominant fashion. With a simple autosomal dominant trait, a parent with the trait may be heterozygous, possessing a single copy of the gene, or they may be homozygous, possessing two copies of the gene. When the parent is heterozygous, they have a 50 percent chance of passing an autosomal dominant trait on to each of their children; when the parent is homozygous, they have a 100 percent chance of passing it on to each of their children. However, with ear pits the penetrance is not complete, meaning that some individuals who inherit a gene for ear pits will not have the trait. Ear pits also exhibit variable expression: an ear pit may appear on the right ear, the left ear, or on both ears. Moreover, even within the same family, ear pits typically vary in their location on the ear and in their depth. When one parent has ear pits, on the average about 40 percent of their children will also have the trait.

EARWAX. Few people pay much attention to the texture of the wax that accumulates in their ears, but earwax, technically termed *cerumen*, comes in two distinct types. Some individuals have wet and sticky earwax; this variety of wax is usually light to dark brown in color. In others, the wax is dry, granular, and brittle, with a light gray color. Almost all Caucasians and blacks in North America have the sticky variety, but Orientals, native American Indians, and many other ethnic groups exhibit both types. In Japan, where dry earwax is more common, the sticky type is called *honey earwax* and the dry form *rice-bran earwax*. Each person produces only one type of earwax, either sticky or dry, but never both.

The type of earwax that is produced is determined by a single pair of autosomal genes—a single locus—and sticky earwax is dominant to dry. This means that two copies of the gene for dry earwax are required to produce dry earwax, but only a single gene for sticky earwax is needed to produce the sticky type. Thus, two people who both have dry earwax can only produce children with the same type. On the other hand, two people with sticky earwax may produce children with either dry or sticky earwax.

EDWARD SYNDROME (Trisomy 18). Edward syndrome is a rare chromosomal abnormality in which the affected child possesses three copies of chromosome 18. The disorder is also termed *trisomy 18*. Infants with this condition exhibit many deformities and are severely retarded; most die within the first year of life. The incidence of Edward syndrome in the general population is about 1 in 8,000 newborns. Like Down syndrome (see Down syndrome), the frequency of children born with this disorder is higher among older mothers. Edward syndrome can be detected prenatally by examining chromosomes in fetal tissue obtained through amniocentesis or chorionic villus sampling.

ENURESIS. See Bedwetting.

EPILEPSY. The word *epilepsy* comes from a Greek word that means "to lay on" or "to seize;" an epileptic is a person who has seizures or fits. In a severe epileptic seizure, the person loses consciousness and falls suddenly to the ground. The muscles contract violently in spasms, producing an uncontrollable thrashing of the body. The attack generally lasts only a few minutes, but usually seems much longer to those watching the fit. It is typically followed by a period of exhaustion and sleep. Other seizures may be less pronounced; they may produce only a short blank spell and minor muscle contractions.

Seizures are a symptom, not a disease; they may occur for a variety of reasons. For example, in some infants, high fever can induce seizures (see Febrile convulsions). İnfection, injury, brain tumors, some diseases, and certain toxic substances may also trigger convulsions. However, recurring seizures also take place in a number of people without any obvious precipitating factors; these people are said to have epilepsy.

It is important to recognize that epilepsy is not a single disease, but is a term that encompasses a large group of disorders characterized by recurring seizures. In a person with epilepsy, convulsions result from a spontaneous electrical discharge that sweeps through the brain. There are a variety of different types of epilepsy that are distinguished by the characteristics of the seizures and the parts of the brain from which they originate. The seizures may begin at any age, but in most epileptics, seizures first appear during early childhood or puberty. Exactly why people with epilepsy have seizures is unknown, but many epileptics can be successfully treated with medication.

Genes are clearly involved in epilepsy; however, the importance of heredity and the mode of inheritance depend upon the type of epilepsy. In some cases, epilepsy occurs as a part of a genetic syndrome or with a chromosome abnormality. Over 100 different genes have been described that cause epilepsy, encompassing all types of inheritance. However, most of these forms of epilepsy are rare, and all together they account for only a small proportion of people with epilepsy. Geneticists believe that multifactorial inheritance—involving the interplay of complex genetic and nongenetic factors—is responsible for most cases of epilepsy. The probability of inheriting epilepsy when a parent or another relative has this disorder depends upon the type of epilepsy, the person's sex, and the age at which seizures began in the relative. Supplied with this information, genetic counselors can frequently provide an estimate of the risk of inheriting epilepsy. Recent studies suggest that offspring of an epileptic mother are more likely to develop seizures than are the offspring of an epileptic father, but the reason for this difference is not known.

Pregnancy in an epileptic woman is associated with certain problems. Women with epilepsy are about twice as likely to have children with birth defects and mental retardation. However, in spite of this increased risk, over 90 percent of the children born to epileptic women are normal. The increased incidence of birth defects results, at least in part, from some of the anticonvulsive medicines taken by epileptic women. Unfortunately, pregnancy frequently increases the occurrence of seizures in women with epilepsy, and the seizures themselves may be harmful to the unborn baby; thus most women with epilepsy must remain on medication during pregnancy. Because some anticonvulsant medicines are more likely to produce birth defects than others, medications and doses may need to be changed during pregnancy. Thus, any woman with epilepsy who is planning to get pregnant should check with her physician.

Also see Febrile convulsions.

EYE COLOR. Eye color tends to be described as though it were a simple trait, such as someone has blue eyes, brown eyes, or green eyes. Careful observation reveals, however, that eye color is actually a complex trait, with many different shades and patterns within each basic color. The amount of pigment and its distribution in the iris largely determines the color of the eye. Individuals with brown eyes have brown pigment distributed evenly throughout the iris. Blue eye color also results from brown pigment, but the amount of pigment is less and the pigment is present only in the back layers of the iris. The structure of the iris also affects the color, and eye color may change over time, as in children whose baby-blue eyes become brown or green with age.

A popular misconception is the notion that eye color is a simple genetic trait and that blue color is recessive to brown. Although genes clearly influence eye color, blue eyes are not inherited as a recessive trait. If this were the case, then any person with blue eyes would be homozygous (would carry only genes for blue eyes), and two parents with blue eyes could bear only blue-eyed children. Yet in a number of families, parents with blue eyes have brown-eyed children. Eye color appears to be determined largely by a few major genes that interact in complex ways, and no simple pattern of inheritance is observed in all families. In general, genes for darker eye color tend to be dominant to those for lighter eyes, but because several different genes are involved, this is not always the case. One recent study of eye color among a large number of Danish families concluded that green eyes was strongly influenced by a gene located on chromosome 19.

EYELID, DROOPY. Droopy eyelid, or *ptosis*, occurs when the eyelid hangs down and cannot be completely raised. In most cases, only one eyelid is affected. Several different forms of ptosis occur. Congenital ptosis is droopy eyelid that is present at birth; this form is usually inherited as an autosomal dominant trait with incomplete penetrance, meaning that not all individuals who inherit the gene for ptosis will have a droopy eyelid.

FAMILIAL COMBINED HYPERLIPIDEMIA. See Cardiovascular diseases.

FAMILIAL HYPERCHOLESTEROLEMIA. See Cardiovascular diseases.

FAMILIAL HYPERTRIGLYCERIDEMIA. See Cardiovascular diseases.

FEBRILE CONVULSIONS. Convulsions consist of involuntary muscular contractions of the entire body, typically producing unconsciousness and lasting a few minutes. There are many different causes of convulsions. Febrile convulsions are defined as convulsions occurring in young children during high fever, without an infection of the brain or spinal column. Most febrile convulsions occur in children between the ages of three months and five years; usually they accompany fever due to respiratory infection, ear infection, or other common viral illnesses. Why a high fever produces convulsions is not known, but these seizures are surprisingly common; about 2 to 5 percent of all young children in the United States experience at least one episode of febrile convulsions. Two thirds of these children never have another seizure, and, even if they do recur, most children suffer no long-term intellectual or physical impairment. Although parents are highly alarmed by the sight of a convulsing child, the majority of the children recover quickly. However, other serious illnesses—such as epilepsy, meningitis, and kidney disorders—can also produce seizures, and a physician should always be consulted when a child has convulsions.

Febrile convulsions display a strong tendency to run in families; almost 40 percent of the children who experience febrile convulsions have a close relative who also had febrile convulsions. In fact, a child with a parent or a sibling who had febrile convulsions is 2 to 3 times more likely to have febrile convulsions. Twin studies also indicate that genetic factors are important. Febrile convulsions probably represent a heterogeneous trait, meaning that what is called febrile convulsions actually encompasses two or more distinct disorders. Children experiencing a single episode of convulsions differ genetically from at least some of those who have repeated seizures. For children with a single seizure, the inheritance appears to be multifactorial (influenced by multiple genes and environmental factors), with a heritability around 70 percent (see

Chapter 4 for a discussion of heritability and multifactorial inheritance). On the other hand, in some families with children experiencing multiple seizures, the trait may be determined by a single dominant gene.

FINGER, BENT LITTLE. A permanently bent little finger which cannot be straightened is technically termed *camptodactyly*. This trait occurs when the muscles do not attach correctly to the bones in the finger. Sometimes the little finger on only one hand is bent, whereas in other cases both hands are affected. Bent little finger is inherited as an autosomal dominant trait with incomplete penetrance, meaning that sometimes an individual with the gene for camptodactyly does not have the trait. With a simple autosomal dominant trait, 50 percent of the children born to a parent with the trait will also have it; however, because penetrance is incomplete in bent little finger, less than 50 percent of the children born to a parent with bent little finger will be affected. Bent little finger is also observed as one of several associated traits in some rare genetic syndromes. In these cases, the pattern of inheritance for bent little finger is the same as that for the genetic syndrome.

FINGERPRINTS. Our fingerprints are among the most permanent and uniquely personal traits we possess. No two individuals, not even identical twins, share the same fingerprints. Nevertheless, the fingerprints of identical twins are quite similar, and genes play an important role in determining our fingerprint patterns.

The technical name for fingerprint patterns is *dermatoglyphics*, which literally means "writing on the skin." Dermatoglyphics include not only fingerprints, but also the raised ridge patterns found on the palms and soles of the feet. These ridge patterns begin development 12 weeks after conception. They require about five weeks to fully form, and by the seventeenth week of development, an individual's fingerprints are set for life.

Several different systems exist for classifying fingerprint patterns. One simple and widely used system recognizes three basic patterns: the arch, the loop, and the whorl. Loops may open toward the thumb (termed *radial loops*) or away from the thumb (termed *ulnar loops*). Each finger possesses either an arch, a loop, or a whorl. The fingers on the same hand do not necessarily share the same patterns, and the patterns on the left and right hands frequently differ.

Geneticists began studying the inheritance of fingerprints almost 100 years ago, and yet they still don't completely understand how genes determine individual patterns. Although genes clearly influence dermatoglyphics, the patterns do not exhibit any of the simple modes of inheritance, such as recessive, dominant, or X-linked inheritance. The inheritance of fingerprints can best be described as multifactorial, meaning that multiple genes and environmental factors are involved. Heritability values for the number of fingerprint ridges on all ten digits may be as high as 0.7, indicating that 70 percent of the variation among individuals in this trait is genetic. (See Chapter 4 for a discussion of heritability.) Because fingerprints are present at birth and are permanent for life, environmental factors that influence the patterns must act during prenatal development; these environmental influences appear to be random variations in the process of development.

A strong indication that genes influence fingerprints is the observation that people with chromosome mutations frequently possess atypical fingerprint patterns, along with unusual palm and sole prints. For example, Down syndrome arises from an extra copy of chromosome 21; this chromosome abnormality produces mental retardation, delayed growth, and numerous other physical problems (see Chapter 5 and Down syndrome). Thirty-two percent of the individuals affected with Down syndrome have ten ulnar loops (one on each finger), whereas this particular pattern occurs with a frequency of only about four percent in the general population. (Don't be alarmed if you have ten ulnar loops; remember, a small percentage of normal individuals do possess this pattern.) Individuals with Down syndrome also possess distinctive palm prints, and unique dermatoglyphic patterns are frequently associated with other chromosome abnormalities.

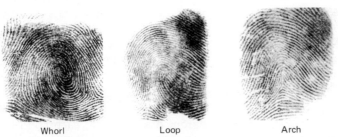

Whorl   Loop   Arch

Catalog Figure 6.   Three common fingerprint patterns. Each finger possesses either a whorl, a loop, or an arch.

FINGERS, EXTRA. Possessing extra fingers and toes is a genetic trait called *polydactyly*. For unknown reasons, this condition is about ten times more common in blacks than it is in Caucasians. In the most frequently seen polydactyly, extra digits occur on the little-finger side of the hand; this type is called *postaxial polydactyly*. Less commonly, extra digits develop on the thumb side, a condition termed *preaxial polydactyly*. Several different varieties of both postaxial and preaxial polydactyly exist, but most are inherited as autosomal dominant traits. Polydactyly frequently exhibits incomplete penetrance—not all individuals with a gene for polydactyly have extra digits. The expression of the trait also varies considerably: Some affected individuals have only a small tag of skin, whereas others may possess fully formed fingers and toes. Polydactyly is also found associated with other abnormalities in a number of genetic syndromes; in these cases the trait follows the inheritance pattern of the syndrome.

FINGERS, SHORT. Abnormally short fingers and toes is a condition called *brachydactyly*. A number of different types of brachydactyly occur in humans, affecting different bones and different digits. For example, brachydactyly type A3 involves a shortened middle bone of the little finger only, whereas brachydactyly type D is characterized by a broad short thumb and big toe. When no other abnormalities are present, brachydactyly is almost always inherited as an autosomal dominant trait, and, on the average, 50 percent of the children born to a parent with brachydactyly will also have short fingers. However, brachydactyly frequently occurs along with other skeletal abnormalities in a number of genetic syndromes; here, its inheritance follows the characteristic pattern of inheritance for the syndrome.

FINGERS, WEBBED. Webbing of the fingers, in which the fingers appear to have grown together, is a common genetic deformity of the hand. This condition, termed *syndactyly*, may also involve the toes. In some cases, the webbing consists only of soft tissue between the fingers and toes; at other times, the bones are actually fused together. Geneticists have observed at least five distinct types of syndactyly, differing in which fingers are affected, whether extra fingers are present, and whether the toes are also webbed. All five types are inherited as autosomal dominant traits; when a parent has this trait, each child has a 50 percent chance of inheriting it. This 50 percent probability assumes that the parent with the trait is heterozygous, carrying one copy of the dominant gene for webbed fingers. Homozygous individuals—those with two copies of the gene for webbed fingers—are very rare; all of their children will inherit the trait. A nonhereditary form of syndactyly also occurs; when a parent has nonhereditary webbed fingers, it is unlikely that any of their children will have the trait. Syndactyly is frequently present along with other abnormalities as part of a number of different genetic syndromes. When occurring in a genetic syndrome, syndactyly follows the inheritance of the syndrome.

FRAGILE X SYNDROME. Fragile X syndrome is a genetic disorder that has recently become recognized as the most common form of inherited mental retardation. In spite of intensive research, many of the peculiar characteristics of this disorder remain unexplained.

Fragile X syndrome affects about 1 in every 2,000 males. Males with the disorder are moderately retarded, with an IQ typically ranging from 30 to 60 (for comparison, normal IQ averages 100). Other characteristics include a large head, large or protruding ears, and enlarged testicles, although the symptoms vary a great deal. The syndrome is called fragile X because a constriction appears near the tip of the X chromosome in those with the disorder; as a result of this constriction, the X chromosome is fragile and susceptible to breakage. However, the fragile X chromosome can only be observed when cells are grown in the laboratory under special conditions, and, even then, the fragile X chromosome shows up in only some cells. What causes the constriction on the X chromosome and how it produces the features of the disorder are not known.

The inheritance of fragile X syndrome is peculiar and is still poorly understood. The disorder is clearly due to a genetic defect on the X chromosome, and thus it exhibits an X-linked pattern of inheritance. However, its transmission differs in several important respects from that of a typical X-linked recessive trait. In most X-linked recessive traits, females must possess two copies of the gene to exhibit the trait, but because males have only a single X chromosome, one copy of the gene produces the trait in a male. Also, in X-linked recessive traits, affected males pass their gene for the trait to all of their daughters; these daughters will then be carriers for the gene, but will not have the trait since they carry a normal gene on their other X chromosome (which they inherited from their mother).

Fragile X syndrome violates these basic rules of X-linked recessive inheritance. First, about 20 percent of the males who carry the gene for fragile X syndrome appear normal; such males are called *transmitting males*, since they pass the fragile X gene on to their daughters, whose sons—the grandsons of the transmitting male—may have fragile X syndrome. This pattern of inheritance is highly unusual for an X-linked trait; normally males cannot be unaffected carriers for an X-linked trait, because they will express whatever genes are present on their single X chromosome. Another oddity is that female carriers possess the gene for fragile X syndrome, but the fragile X chromosome can only be observed in some of these. Furthermore, about one third of the carrier females are mentally retarded, and others have learning disabilities. The daughters of transmitting males (those males with the fragile X gene but who have normal IQ) are rarely retarded, although the sons of these daughters (the grandsons of the transmitting males) may be. None of these characteristics is typical of either an X-linked recessive or an X-linked dominant trait.

Because of its unusual pattern of transmission, the rules of X-linked inheritance cannot be strictly applied to fragile X syndrome. For example, with an ordinary X-linked recessive trait, any unaffected male cannot pass on the trait. Therefore, a normal brother of an affected male would not need to be concerned about passing the trait to his children. However, because some males with fragile X are apparently normal, a healthy brother of an individual with fragile X syndrome still possesses about a 10 percent chance of carrying the gene. None of the normal brother's children would be affected, because his sons would not inherit his X chromosome and daughters of transmitting males are rarely affected. However, each of his daughters would carry his X chromosome and might produce fragile X sons. Therefore, it is advisable for anyone with a close relative who has fragile X syndrome to seek genetic counseling. The risks of inheriting the disorder when a family member has fragile X depend upon the relationship to the affected person, how severely that individual is affected, and whether their X chromosome shows the fragile site. Prenatal testing for fragile X syndrome is available through amniocentesis.

GALACTOSEMIA. Galactosemia represents a group of hereditary disorders in which a sugar called *galactose* is not broken down. In one form of the disease, an enzyme with the name of *galactose-1-phosphate uridyl transferase* is defective. When this enzyme does not function, vomiting and intestinal problems typically start a few days after birth, as the infant begins to drink milk (a source of galactose). If untreated, the infant fails to thrive, suffers from liver disease, develops cataracts, becomes mentally retarded, and eventually dies. Fortunately, these symptoms can be reduced by placing the infant on a galactose-free diet.

A less severe form of galactosemia results from a deficiency of a different enzyme called *galactokinase*. Here the primary symptom is the development of cataracts. Several additional variants of the disease have been reported.

All types of galactosemia are inherited as autosomal recessive disorders, which means that two copies of the gene for galactosemia are required to produce the disease. If two normal parents have a child with galactosemia, both parents must be carriers for a galactosemia gene, and each additional child they produce will have a one in four chance of having the disease. If one parent has galactosemia, he or she will only produce children with galactosemia if the other parent is a carrier or also has the disease, both of which are unlikely unless the two parents are related; thus, few people with galactosemia give birth to children with the disorder. Prenatal diagnosis for galactosemia can be carried out on cells obtained through amniocentesis or chorionic villus sampling.

GLAUCOMA.   The front portion of the human eye is filled with a fluid called the *aqueous humor*, which is constantly being produced by special structures within the eye. Normally, excess aqueous humor drains from the eye through a small channel, but in individuals with glaucoma this channel becomes blocked. Because the fluid does not drain properly, pressure builds up within the eye. The elevated pressure may damage tiny blood vessels that nourish the back of the eye. When these blood vessels become damaged, the cells in the eye are deprived of oxygen and food, and they slowly die; consequently, vision is diminished. Peripheral vision is lost first, and later central vision is affected. If untreated, glaucoma may ultimately lead to blindness.

There are several different types of glaucoma. The most common form is termed *chronic simple glaucoma* or *primary open-angle type glaucoma*. This type appears most commonly in middle age to late life, and it affects about 2 percent of the population over the age of 40. Outwardly, the eye appears normal, but increased pressure within the eye can be detected with a special instrument. Symptoms of the disorder include mild headaches and blurred vision. Most people with this type of glaucoma respond well to treatment with medicated eye drops.

Chronic simple glaucoma tends to run in families. About 50 percent of the people with this disorder have other family members who are also affected. The pattern of inheritance is not well understood, but in most families the disorder is probably inherited as a multifactorial trait, meaning that multiple genes and environmental factors are involved; with a multifactorial trait, no simple pattern of inheritance is observed. If one parent has chronic simple glaucoma, the chance of a child eventually developing glaucoma is 4 to 16 percent.

A second form of glaucoma, *angle-closure glaucoma*, occurs suddenly and is characterized by severe pain and loss of vision. This form is thought to be related to defects in the anatomy of the eye. The inheritance is not well understood, but it is probably also multifactorial. When a parent has angle-closure glaucoma, the risk of a child developing the disorder is approximately 2 to 6 percent.

Glaucoma occasionally occurs in newborns; this rare condition is called *congenital glaucoma*. Congenital glaucoma arises with a frequency of about 1 in 10,000 births; it is genetically distinct from glaucoma that occurs in adults. In some families, this disorder is inherited as an autosomal recessive trait. In these families, if a couple has one child with congenital glaucoma, the chance that future children will be affected is about one in four. If a parent has congenital glaucoma, the chance of producing an affected child is less than one percent. In other families, congenital glaucoma may be inherited as a multifactorial trait. Congenital glaucoma can also be produced by certain drugs and is associated with some genetic syndromes.

GLUCOSE-6-PHOSPHATE DEHYDROGENASE DEFICIENCY.

Glucose-6-phosphate dehydrogenase is an enzyme that plays an important role in supplying energy to the red blood cells. A number of genetic variants of this enzyme occur in humans; some of these produce no ill effects, some cause relatively mild symptoms, and others produce serious problems. Even in those with severe deficiency of the enzyme, problems do not occur until the patient is stressed, usually by certain drugs, an infection, or contact with a particular kind of bean called fava beans.

In individuals with mild glucose-6-phosphate dehydrogenase deficiency, taking certain drugs causes destruction of the red blood cells. The urine turns black from the breakdown of the red blood cells, and the person may feel weak and experience some back pain. These symptoms typically disappear within a week, even if the person continues to take the drug. When a person possesses the more severe form of the disorder, drugs, infection, or fava beans also induce red blood cell destruction, and more serious complications frequently arise.

Glucose-6-phosphate dehydrogenase deficiency is rare among northern Europeans, but it occurs commonly in some Africans, in people living around the Mediterranean, and in Orientals. The disorder is inherited as an X-linked recessive trait. Because it is X-linked recessive, males require only a single copy of the gene to have the disorder, whereas females must inherit two copies to have the disorder; thus, glucose-6-phosphate dehydrogenase deficiency occurs almost exclusively among males. When a male has this disorder, he will pass the defective gene on to all his daughters, who will be normal carriers as long as they receive a normal gene from their mother. None of an affected male's sons will inherit the disease from him, because each son receives his father's Y chromosome and not his X. When the mother is a carrier and the father is normal, on the average half of the sons will have glucose-6-phosphate dehydrogenase deficiency and all of the daughters will be normal, although half of the daughters (on the average) will carry the defective gene.

GRAVES' DISEASE. See Thyroid disease.

HAIR COLOR. Hair color is one of the most frequently cited examples of a simple hereditary trait and is widely used to illustrate how heredity works. There is little doubt that genes strongly influence hair color; this fact has been obvious to people for centuries. However, the inheritance of hair color is more complex than most people realize, and even today the genetic basis of hair color in humans is not completely understood.

A major difficulty in studying the inheritance of hair color is the multitude of colors and shades that human hair can assume. People are frequently categorized as blonds, brunettes, and red heads, but these are actually vague terms that lump together people with many different shades of hair color. For example, a blond person might have very light brown hair, golden-colored hair, or almost white hair. A red-haired person might be strawberry blond or carrot orange. A brunette might be brown or jet black. Another problem is that hair color may change during one's lifetime: Many blond babies later develop brown hair. With this much variability, it is certain that hair color is not a simple genetic trait involving a single locus. Hair color is probably multifactorial, with a number of genes and even some environmental factors contributing to the trait. (See Chapter 4.)

Even though multiple genes and environmental factors undoubtedly contribute to hair color in humans, a few genes appear to play a major role; others probably add only minor refinements. It is the influence and inheritance of these major genes that give hair color the appearance of a simple genetic trait. For example, in many families strikingly blond hair is inherited as a trait that is recessive to dark hair. Each person inherits two copies of the gene for hair color—one from their mother and one from their father. If blond hair is recessive, then a blond-haired individual must carry two blond genes (in technical terms two blond alleles). When a person has even a single gene for dark hair, their hair will be dark. So, two dark-haired parents might produce a blond-haired child, if both parents carried a recessive gene for blond in addition to their dominant gene for dark hair. In such families, we would actually expect that on the average one out of four of the children would have blond hair and three out of four would have dark hair. If, on the other hand, both parents were blond, then all their children should be blond, because blond individuals only possess blond genes. However, dark-haired babies have been born to two blond-haired parents, indicating that the inheritance of blond hair is not always so simple.

Red hair is another example where a major gene appears to largely influence the trait, although other genes may modify the type of red hair. The pair of genes that affects whether or not one has red hair appears to be separate from the pair that influences blond hair. One pair of genes (one locus) apparently determines whether one has dark hair or blond hair, and another pair (a second locus) determines whether one has red hair. To keep this straight, the blond locus will be called B, and the red locus R. Most geneticists believe that red hair is recessive, which means that one has red hair only if two genes for red are present at the R locus. However, the presence of red hair is also affected by what alleles are present at the B locus. If one has black hair or dark brown hair as a consequence of the genes at the B locus, then the red won't show. This phenomenon—genes at one locus influencing how the genes at another locus are expressed—is what geneticists call *epistasis*. Red hair may be recessive to nonred hair and epistatic to dark hair.

It should be emphasized, once again, that other genes are involved in the determination of hair color. In many families blond is recessive to dark hair and red hair is recessive to nonred hair, but this is not always the case. Try as they might, geneticists cannot seem to make hair color fit a simple pattern of inheritance.

HAIRY EARS. Although rare in North Americans, hairy ears is a common trait among males in some parts of India, Ceylon, and Israel. In these regions, the frequency of hairy ears may reach as high as 70 percent of all adult males. The expression of the trait is quite variable; in some, both ears are covered with bushy hair, but in others only a few hairs are present on the outer ear. Similarly, the hairs may become obvious imme-

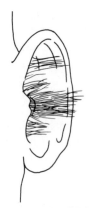

Catalog Figure 7.   Hairy ears.

diately after puberty, or the trait may not be expressed until old age. This variation in the amount of hair and the age of onset makes study of this trait difficult. For example, suppose a man dies at age 45 without hairy ears; did he lack the trait or did he just not live long enough to express it?

Hairy ears is one of the few traits in humans that is potentially Y-linked, meaning that it may be encoded by a gene on the Y chromosome. The Y chromosome appears to contain little genetic information other than the gene that determines maleness (see Sex determinism). However, in a number of families that have been studied, hairy ears is inherited in a manner that is entirely consistent with a Y-linked trait. Y-linked traits should occur only in males, because females do not possess a Y chromosome. Also, a father who has a Y-linked trait should pass the trait on to all his sons, because all sons receive their Y chromosome from their father. However, in some families with hairy ears, not all sons of an affected father have the trait. This might appear to rule out Y-linked inheritance. On the other hand, this observation can also be accounted for by assuming that the trait is Y-linked, but not all males with the gene for hairy ears express it (in technical terms, the gene has incomplete penetrance), or the trait might have eventually been expressed in all the sons, had they lived long enough.

Some investigators have suggested that hairy ears is not Y-linked at all, but is inherited as an autosomal dominant trait that is expressed only in males. In technical genetic terms, such a trait is *sex-limited* (see Chapter 3) to males. In fact, many pedigrees are consistent with both Y-linked inheritance and autosomal dominant sex-limited inheritance; distinguishing between these two types of inheritance can be very difficult. At present, the available pedigrees more closely resemble a Y-linked mode of inheritance with incomplete penetrance, but other types of inheritance such as sex-limited autosomal dominance cannot be excluded.

HANDEDNESS. In all human cultures, over 90 percent of the population exhibit a definite favoring of the right hand, what is called *right-handedness*. A minority favor the left hand (*left-handedness*), and a few have no marked preference of hand use, which is termed *ambidextrous*. Humans are the only known animals in which most individuals are right-handed. The reason for this preference is obscure, but a majority of humans have favored the right hand since the beginnings of human civilization. Study of hand preference depicted in ancient artwork demonstrates that 90 percent of the human race has been right-handed for over 5,000 years.

Psychologists have long been aware of the fact that handedness is related to the organization of information processing in the brain. The upper portion of the brain is divided into right and left halves, termed the *right cerebral hemisphere* and the *left cerebral hemisphere*. In the vast majority of individuals, the left side controls language, whereas the right side controls perception of space. This is only true, however, for right-handed people. In 99 percent of right-handed individuals, the left side of the brain controls language. However, only about 60 percent of left-handed people have language control on the left side. How these basic differences in brain function arise is not known, nor is it understood why handedness is related to the asymmetry of brain function. What is clear is that behavioral asymmetries such as handedness develop at a very early age—most two-to-five-day-old babies show a pronounced tendency to deviate their eyes to the right, and by eight months of age a majority of babies display a preference for use of the right hand.

Many factors affect handedness. There is no doubt that learning and culture can influence which hand is used for common activities like writing with the left hand was less than 3 percent, but the number States has increased in recent times. In 1932, the frequency of individuals writing with the left hand was less than three percent, but the number increased to 11 percent by 1972. This trend is almost certainly due to the relaxation of cultural pressure to be right-handed.

In addition to these cultural and environmental influences on handedness, there are genetic factors that predispose people in the direction of right-handedness or left-handedness. Many studies have shown that left-handedness tends to run in families; children are more likely to be left-handed if one or both parents are left-handed. Research indicates that this relationship only holds for the child's biological parents; there is no resemblance between handedness of children and their stepparents, suggesting that the tendency for left-handedness is inherited and not learned from the parents. Handedness is not, however, inherited in a simple way. The heredity of handedness is most likely multifactorial, meaning that multiple genes and environmental factors influence the trait.

HASHIMOTO'S DISEASE. See Thyroid disease.

HEARING LOSS. See Deafness and hearing loss.

HEART DISEASE. See Cardiovascular diseases.

HEIGHT. Height is one of the first things that one notices about other people. Ask a friend to describe someone they know; invariably their description will include something about height. Height plays a role in who is picked for a spouse—tall women tend to marry tall men and short men tend to marry short women, although there are plenty of exceptions.

Adult height is determined largely by growth during childhood and adolescence. Most people do not reach their final adult height until after age 17, so human height is influenced by growth that occurs over an extended period of time. The rate of growth from conception to maturity is not even, but tends to speed up and slow down during different developmental stages. For example, growth is rapid during the first two years of life. Following this period of rapid growth in infancy, growth continues at a slower pace until puberty, when growth accelerates once again for several years. After this adolescent growth spurt, growth gradually slows and eventually ceases when the final adult height is reached. Different factors influence the process of growth at different ages.

A universal observation is that children resemble their parents in relative height: Tall parents tend to have tall children, and short parents tend to have short children. This similarity in height between parents and their offspring need not be genetic; it might arise from environmental factors that are common to members of the same family. A number of studies indicate, however, that genes do play an important role in determining height at all ages, and much of the variation in height among people is due to heredity.

One of the strongest indications that genes influence height is the observation that identical twins are very similar in height, even when reared apart. Identical twins seldom differ in height by more than an inch, except when one of the twins has been sick with a serious disease during childhood. On the other hand, nonidentical twins may be quite different in height even when reared in the same environment, which is consistent with the fact that they share only 50 percent of the same genes.

Although genes clearly influence human height, it is equally certain that environmental factors also make a contribution. In North America and Europe, humans have been increasing in height—at a rate of about 1 inch per generation—during the past 100 years; experts agree that this secular trend in adult height results from better diet and health care. This trend has reversed itself in some countries during years of famine, war, or disease epidemics. Numerous studies also document the fact that people of upper socioeconomic classes tend to be taller than those living in poverty. All these observations indicate the potential importance of environmental factors in height.

How heredity determines height is still poorly understood. For most individuals, the inheritance of height can best be described as multifactorial, meaning that both genes and environmental factors are involved. (See Chapter 4 for a discussion of multifactorial inheritance.) Much of the "normal" variation that is seen in height is probably influenced by a large number of genes, each of which has a small effect. These genes determine one's potential stature, but the degree to which this potential is realized depends on the influence of environmental factors such as diet, health, protection from cold, and physical exertion.

Heritability is a parameter that geneticists use to represent the proportion of the differences in a multifactorial trait that results from genetic differences among individuals; heritability gives an estimate of the proportion of variation in a trait that is genetic. Estimates of heritability for adult height vary from study to study, but the estimates frequently range from 0.5 to 0.8, indicating that genes are quite important in stature, accounting for as much as 80 percent of the differences in height. It is important to keep in mind, however, that most estimates of heritability have been based on studies of Americans and northern Europeans. In other societies, environmental influences on height—diet and health care, for example—may vary more from one family to another, and thus more of the differences in height may be determined by these non-hereditary factors. (See Chapter 4 for a full discussion of heritability.)

Although many genes undoubtedly contribute to height, some individual genes can make a dramatic difference in height. For example, there are individual genes that prevent the bones in the arms and legs from developing normally; such genes produce a person that is dwarfed. Many chromosome abnormalities and genetic syndromes also lower height. Genetic defects in the enzymes that break down food—the so-called inborn errors of metabolism—frequently retard growth and produce short stature. Some of these defects are discussed under the headings Short stature and Dwarfism. Genes with a major impact on height are rare, however, and most of the variation in height observed among humans has a multifactorial basis.

HEMOPHILIA. Clotting is a complex and wonderful thing. When blood vessels are severed and fluids begin to pour out, a cascade of reactions swing into motion, ultimately producing a self-sealing blood clot. More than 13 different factors are involved in the clotting reaction, each factor affecting another. For example, factor XII is converted to factor XIIa, which then converts factor XI to factor XIa, which then converts factor IX to factor IXa, and so on. Eventually, a substance called *fibrin* is activated; fibrin molecules stick together to form a gel, which then stops the flow of blood.

Hemophilia is a hereditary disease in which the clotting process is defective; sometimes this disorder is termed *bleeder's disease*. Because defects may occur at a number of different places in the complex set of clotting reactions, there are a number of different types of hemophilia. Most of these are rare. Here, three of the more common hemophilias, classic hemophilia, von Willebrand's disease, and Christmas disease, will be discussed.

Classic Hemophilia. Classic hemophilia, also termed *hemophilia A*, results from an abnormal or missing clotting factor VIII. This disease occurs in about 1 out of every 10,000 white males. It is inherited as an X-linked recessive disorder. Individuals with classic hemophilia bleed excessively, although the severity varies from family to family. Bleeding episodes may appear at birth, but they typically increase in frequency after infancy, as the child becomes more active and prone to injury. Bleeding often occurs spontaneously, particularly into joints such as the elbows, knees, and ankles. Joint bleeding produces considerable pain and swelling; it frequently erodes the bones, crippling the hemophiliac.

Because classic hemophilia results from an X-linked recessive gene, males must inherit only a single copy of the hemophilia gene to have the disease, as they possess only a single X chromosome. Females, on the other hand, must inherit two copies of the gene, one from each parent, to have the disease; consequently, almost all classic hemophiliacs are male. Females can be carriers, possessing a single hemophilia gene along with a normal gene for clotting factor VIII. Carriers are typically normal, although they may experience slower clotting. If a female is a carrier, half of her sons on the average will have hemophilia, and half of her daughters will be carriers. If the husband has hemophilia, all his daughters will be carriers; none of his sons will be affected. Classic hemophilia can be detected prenatally with a fetal blood sample obtained through fetoscopy or fetal blood sampling. In some families, carrier detection can be carried out through DNA analysis.

Classic hemophilia is treated by giving concentrated preparations of the missing clotting factor during bleeding episodes. Although expensive and cumbersome, the treatment is usually effective. New diagnostic procedures utilizing DNA analysis make prenatal testing available at selective centers.

von Willebrand's Disease. von Willebrand's disease is another bleeding disorder that involves a clotting factor called von Willebrand factor. The symptoms and the inheritance differ from classic hemophilia. Unlike classic hemophilia, which is X-linked, von Willebrand's disease is caused by an autosomal gene; its inheritance is generally considered to be autosomal dominant. Thus, a parent with von Willebrand's disease will pass it on to an average of 50 percent of his or her children. Prenatal diagnosis is possible with fetal blood samples obtained through fetoscopy or fetal blood sampling. The symptoms of the disorder show considerable variation, even within families.

Christmas Disease. Christmas disease, also termed *hemophilia B*, results from an abnormal or missing factor IX. The symptoms of this clotting disorder are the same as those for classic hemophilia: excessive bleeding, pain, swelling, bone deformities, and crippling. Also like classic hemophilia, Christmas disease is inherited as an X-linked recessive trait. Thus, primarily males have the disorder. Female carriers pass the disease on to half of their sons on the average, and half of their daughters on the average will be carriers like their mother. If the father has hemophilia, all his daughters will be carriers, and none of his sons will be affected. Prenatal diagnosis is available through analysis of a blood sample obtained with fetoscopy or fetal blood sampling.

HEREDITARY TREMOR. Hereditary tremor is an involuntary shaking of the hands, arms, and head, which typically first appears in middle age but may occur at any age. The tremor usually begins in the hands and arms, and it increases in severity over time. In later stages, it also involves the facial muscles and sometimes the voice. The shaking is more pronounced during activities that involve fine muscle control, such as writing, drinking, or eating. The tremor is exacerbated by fatigue and anxiety, but typically disappears during rest.

A number of diseases and disorders, as well as psychiatric problems and some drugs, may produce a tremor. For example, Parkinson's disease is a brain disorder that produces tremor along with a number of other symptoms. Hereditary tremor, however, is unaccompanied by other symptoms or problems. As the name implies, this trait runs in families; the pattern of inheritance is usually autosomal dominant. Most people that have hereditary tremor possess only a single copy of the gene for this trait; in technical terms they are heterozygous. When one parent has the trait and is heterozygous, each child has a 50 percent chance of inheriting the tremor. If both parents have hereditary tremor and both are heterozygous, each child has a 75 percent chance of inheriting the tremor. In the rare event that one parent carries two copies of the tremor gene—the individual is a homozygote—all the children will inherit the tremor.

HIGH BLOOD PRESSURE. See Cardiovascular diseases.

HUNTER SYNDROME. Hunter syndrome is a genetic disease resulting from a deficiency of an enzyme termed *iduronate sulfatase*. The normal function of this enzyme is to break down larger molecules called *mucopolysaccharides*. When this enzyme is missing, mucopolysaccharides accumulate in the body tissues, and a number of abnormalities result. Symptoms of the disorder include stiff joints, stunted growth, course facial features, and enlarged liver and spleen. Deafness and loss of vision are common. Mental deterioration frequently occurs with age. Heart problems develop and often cause death, but some patients with this disorder are long lived.

Patients with Hunter syndrome vary tremendously in the severity of their symptoms; it is likely that several different mutations cause this disease and account for some of this variation. Hunter syndrome is inherited as an X-linked recessive disease. If parents have one child with Hunter syndrome, then the mother may be a carrier for the Hunter gene;

alternatively, the disease in the affected child might have resulted from a new mutation in one of the mother's egg cells. However, if the couple has a second child with Hunter syndrome, or if the mother has a brother with Hunter syndrome, she is almost certainly a carrier and her sons will have a 50 percent probability of inheriting the disease. Prenatal diagnosis by amniocentesis or chorionic villus sampling is available for Hunter syndrome.

HUNTINGTON DISEASE. Huntington disease is a devastating neurological disorder, initially appearing in middle age, which leads to a slow, steady disintegration of the brain. For most people with the disorder, the first signs appear between the ages of 30 and 45, but a few individuals experience symptoms in childhood and in others the disease is not obvious until old age.

Huntington disease is caused by an autosomal dominant gene. New mutations rarely arise; thus, virtually all affected individuals inherit the gene from one of their parents. (However, some parents may die of other causes before the symptoms of Huntington disease appear, so not all people with the disorder have a parent who had Huntington disease.) Because Huntington disease occurs relatively late in life, many affected individuals bear children before they are aware that they have the disorder. As a result, the disease is easily transmitted from one generation to the next. Of the tens of thousands of people worldwide who have Huntington disease, almost all may be related, at least distantly, to a common ancestor who first had the disorder several hundred years ago.

In 1872, George Huntington first fully described the symptoms of the disease, and others who followed gave the disorder his name. The symptoms appear slowly and are subtle. An early sign is marked change in personality. The affected person may become depressed and be hard to get along with; he or she is frequently obstinate or moody and may exhibit erratic, inappropriate behavior. Because such personality changes are common and have many potential causes, the disease often goes unrecognized at this stage. More obvious symptoms follow; these include jerky, involuntary movements called *choreic movements.* The choreic movements typically first appear in the arms, neck, and face. Although mild in the beginning, they progress to facial grimaces, hesitant speech, and irregular trunk movements. Individuals with the disorder develop a clumsy, shuffling walk; their speech becomes indistinct, and emotional disturbance may occur. Others frequently mistake these symptoms for drunkenness. Later, walking becomes impossible and swallowing difficult. The disease may lead to insanity. Although these are typical symptoms, the course of the disease varies greatly from one affected person to another.

On the average, death in a person with Huntington disease occurs 17 years after the onset of symptoms, usually from infection. However, some patients may live as long as 30 years after being diagnosed with the disease. In advanced cases, nerve cells in the brain die, and the brain may actually decrease in weight by as much as 20 to 30 percent. There is no treatment available for halting the steady advance of this disease.

As mentioned previously, Huntington disease is caused by an autosomal dominant gene. An individual with the disorder thus has a 50 percent chance of passing the disease on to each of his or her children. However, because the symptoms do not begin until middle age, children with a Huntington disease parent may not learn whether they carry the Huntington gene for many years. This uncertainty, coupled with the terrible course of the disease, is frequently unnerving to the families involved. Until recently, there has been no means of determining which family members have inherited the disorder. However, in 1983 geneticists established that the gene causing Huntington disease is located near the end of the short arm of chromosome 4; this was determined using DNA analysis and the largest known family with Huntington disease, consisting of over 7,000 individuals, including 100 with the disease, living on the shores of Lake Maracaibo in Venezuela. Several genetic markers close to the Huntington gene have been isolated and now allow for predictive testing of those who carry the disease gene. (See Chapter 6 for a discussion of genetic diagnosis using DNA techniques.) At the time of this writing, the Huntington gene itself has not been found, so the predictive test is not 100 percent accurate. Also, the genetic markers vary from family to family, so DNA from other family members must be available to do the test, and the test cannot provide information on the inheritance of Huntington disease for all families. These problems will disappear when the Huntington disease gene is found. However, there may be serious problems in providing predictive information to people at risk for developing Huntington disease. Information about whether one will develop the disease in later life may be useful in making future plans and in deciding whether to have children. Those who learn that they are free of the disease may be greatly comforted by the news. However, for those who receive a positive test result—news that they carry the gene and will die of a slow incurable disease—the information may be devastating. Also, many legal and social questions surround predictive testing; for example, will diagnosis affect employment and insurability? Currently, pilot studies, which provide predictive testing along with genetic counseling for some individuals at risk for the disorder, are being conducted at selective medical centers in the United States (see Chapter 1). The outcome of these experimental programs will determine the future of genetic diagnosis for all those with the potential of inheriting Huntington disease.

HURLER SYNDROME. Hurler syndrome is a grave disease resulting from the absence of an enzyme, α-L-iduronidase. Normally, this enzyme helps to degrade large molecules with long sugar chains called mucopolysaccharides. Because this enzyme is deficient in a child with Hurler syndrome, partially degraded mucopolysaccharides accumulate, producing a wide array of symptoms. Infants with this disorder are born normal, but their condition deteriorates after one year of age. By the age of two or three years their head becomes enlarged, and the facial features become coarse. Other symptoms include stunted growth, numerous bone deformities, stiff joints, enlargement of the liver and spleen, and deafness. The cornea, a clear protective layer that covers the eye, clouds over. Heart problems develop, and mental retardation occurs. Most patients with the disorder die before the age of ten. Hurler syndrome is a rare condition, occurring in approximately 1 in 100,000 births. It is inherited as an autosomal recessive trait. As a recessive trait, two copies of the Hurler gene are required to produce the disease. If parents have one child with Hurler syndrome, each additional child they conceive has a 25 percent chance of developing the disorder. Hurler syndrome can be detected with prenatal diagnosis by amniocentesis.

HYPERTENSION. See Cardiovascular diseases.

HYPOSPADIAS. Hypospadias is a relatively common birth defect (about 1 in 1,000 live births) involving the penis. Normally, the urethra (the tube that carries urine from the bladder) opens at the tip of the penis, but in males with hypospadias the opening is on the underside of the penis. In mild forms of hypospadias, the urethral opening may be just below the normal site and may be barely obvious; in more severe cases it opens further back along the shaft of the penis. Fortunately, hypospadias is correctable by surgery, which usually is carried out at an early age.

Genetically speaking, hypospadias is a heterogeneous trait. This means that it may arise from several different causes. Most commonly, hypospadias is multifactorial, involving the interaction of several genes and environmental factors. Heritability of the trait is estimated at around 0.70, indicating that 70 percent of the variation in presence or absence of hypospadias results from genetic differences. If one male child has hypospadias, there is about a 10 percent chance of subsequent brothers having it; if the father has hypospadias, there is also about a 10 percent chance that each male child will have it.

Occasionally, hypospadias is not inherited in a multifactorial fashion. In a few families, hypospadias appears to be inherited as an autosomal dominant trait; here a father with hypospadias would have a 50 percent chance of passing it on to his sons. In other families, the inheritance may be autosomal recessive, which would mean if one child is affected, each additional male child would have a 25 percent chance of inheriting it. There are also certain rare genetic syndromes in which hypospadias appears as one of a constellation of birth defects. For example, the telecanthus–hypospadias (BBB) syndrome is characterized by widely spaced eyes, a wide high nose bridge, hypospadias, and mental retardation. This syndrome is most likely inherited as an X-linked trait.

Hypospadias can also arise as a consequence of general problems in sexual development. The normal development of male sex structures, including formation of the penis, results from male hormones produced by the testes of a fetus. Occasionally, male hormones may be abnormally produced in a female fetus, causing the development of male characteristics in an individual that is genetically female. The male traits of these genetic females are often not complete, and hypospadias may be present. Several studies also suggest that female sex hormones taken by the mother during the first three months of pregnancy may interfere with normal male development and may increase the likelihood of producing a child with hypospadias.

For reasons that are not clear, the incidence of hypospadias varies from country to country and even among regions within countries. For example, the incidence of hypospadias in the midwestern section of the United States is almost ten times higher than in other parts of the country. Also puzzling is a reported increase in the incidence of hypospadias over the past few years.

INTELLIGENCE. There is no doubt that genes influence human intelligence. Evidence for this fact comes from a number of genetic disorders that produce mental retardation. For example, PKU (phenylketonuria) is a genetic disease caused by a defective enzyme called phenylalanine hydroxylase; if untreated, PKU produces profound mental retardation. PKU is inherited as a simple autosomal recessive trait; thus, children who inherit two defective copies of the gene coding for phenylalanine hydroxylase have profound deficiencies of intelligence, unless the disease is treated. Many genetic diseases—Tay-Sachs disease, galactosemia, fragile X syndrome, Down syndrome, and numerous others—also cause low intelligence. Thus, genes clearly play a role in the development of the human nervous system and ultimately affect intelligence. Although there is no question that genes influence mental development, much controversy still surrounds the question of to what extent genes determine the differences that occur within the "normal range" of intelligence. For example, do genes affect grades earned in school? Are some people better at arithmetic or spelling because of their genes? How much of one's intelligence is set at birth by the genes he or she possesses and how much can be improved by a stimulating environment?

Nowhere is the study of genetics more controversial than when it attempts to examine the role of heredity in intelligence. One problem in trying to determine the influence of genes on intelligence is how to define and measure intelligence. The most widely used indicator for general intelligence is the Stanford-Binet IQ test and variations of this test that give IQ scores. IQ stands for intelligence quotient and it is a standardized measure of mental age compared to chronological age. To obtain IQ, an individual's mental age—as determined by the IQ test—is divided by chronological age and multiplied by 100. For example, suppose Jack is ten years old, and an IQ test indicates that he can perform mental tasks normally expected of an 11-year-old. Jack's IQ would be computed as $11/10 \times 100 = 110$. Because of the way it is computed, normal IQ at any age is 100.

Experts disagree on exactly what IQ measures, and whether IQ tests are culturally biased. In spite of this controversy, IQ is a good predictor of scholastic achievement in school, which is what the test was originally designed to measure. Also, IQ scores measured on the same individual tend to remain relatively stable over time. Thus, many genetic studies have focused on the heredity of IQ.

A tremendous number of studies have examined the influence of genes on variation in IQ. These studies include research on family members, children whose parents are blood relatives, twins, adopted individuals, and many other groups. The results overwhelmingly demonstrate that variation in IQ is influenced by genes. These studies also demonstrate that environment plays a role in determining IQ. For example, comparison of identical twins and nonidentical twins consistently shows that identical twins are more similar in their IQ than are nonidentical twins; this is what we expect if genes help to determine individual differences in IQ, because identical twins have exactly the same genes, whereas nonidentical twins have only 50 percent of the same genes. At the same time, these studies demonstrate that identical twins frequently differ somewhat in IQ. Because they have exactly the same genes, differences in the IQ of identical twins must have an environmental cause. Thus, both genes and environment contribute to the differences in IQ.

Adoption studies also indicate that genes influence the differences that occur in IQ; the IQ of adopted-away children is closer to that of their biological parents than it is to the IQ of their foster parents. Heritability of IQ—the extent to which variation in IQ results from differences in genes—has been estimated by various studies to be between 50 and 80 percent; these values indicate that at least half of the differences in IQ are heritable. But it should not be forgotten that the heritability estimates also mean that up to 50 percent of the variation in IQ cannot be accounted for by differences in genes and therefore must be environmental in origin.

Some experts criticize IQ tests because they doubt that intelligence is a single trait; they suggest that what is called *intelligence* is actually a composite of many specific mental abilities. A number of tests of specific mental abilities such as verbal ability, spatial ability, abstract reasoning, memory, and mathematical ability have been devised, and much research has focused on the heredity of specific mental abilities measured by these tests. Once again, twins studies, family studies, and adoption studies provide evidence that genes do influence these specific mental abilities.

Although much evidence supports the idea that both genes and environment influence intelligence, how intelligence is inherited is not clearly understood. No "smart" gene has been identified, and high intelligence does not exhibit any simple pattern of intelligence. Almost certainly many genes affect intelligence, and genetic differences interact with differences in the environment. This type of trait is best described as multifactorial, meaning that multiple factors—both genetic and non-genetic—influence intelligence in complex ways.

KLINEFELTER SYNDROME. Klinefelter syndrome arises from abnormalities of the sex chromosomes, occurring in individuals who possess at least two X chromosomes and a Y chromosome (XXY). Because the male-determining gene is on the Y chromosome, these individuals develop male characteristics. There are no obvious features of Klinefelter syndrome in infancy or childhood, unless the chromosomes are examined for some other reason; most males with the disorder are not recognized until puberty. Indeed, some affected individuals do not learn that they possess an extra X chromosome until they seek treatment for sterility after many years of marriage.

Although male in appearance, individuals with Klinefelter syndrome have abnormalities of the testes and distinctive physical traits that become apparent at puberty. Affected individuals tend to be taller than normal; their tallness results primarily from abnormally long legs. Most Klinefelter males possess normal intelligence, although a small percentage may have mild retardation. Usually, the penis is of normal size or is only slightly reduced. The testes are small, but this is frequently apparent only upon close examination. Many individuals with the disorder exhibit some breast enlargement. Facial and pubic hair are frequently scant; typically a male with Klinefelter syndrome shaves only once or twice a week. Almost all patients with Klinefelter syndrome are sterile, although a few have fathered children. The sterility does not preclude sexual fulfillment; men with Klinefelter syndrome experience erection and ejaculation, and many lead normal married lives.

This disorder occurs in about 1 in 1,000 male newborns. Most Klinefelter syndrome patients are XXY, but a few possess additional X's, being XXXY or even XXXXY. About 10 percent of the individuals with Klinefelter are mosaics, which means that some cells in the body are XY and other cells are XXY. Hormone treatments are sometimes used to enhance the male traits; they increase penis size, reduce breast development, and increase the sex urge. However, the sterility associated with Klinefelter syndrome cannot be altered. Prenatal testing for Klinefelter syndrome is possible by examining the fetal chromosomes in tissue obtained from amniocentesis or chorionic villus sampling.

LACTOSE TOLERANCE. See Milk tolerance.

LEFT-HANDED. See Handedness.

LENGTH OF LIFE. The influence of heredity on length of life is not well understood. Genes might affect longevity in two different ways. First, genes may affect the probability of dying prematurely from a variety of causes. For example, individuals with certain genes might be less susceptible to heart disease; because heart disease is a leading killer among middle-age adults, people with these genes would have less heart disease and would tend to live longer, on the average, than those without the genes. Second, genes might affect the aging process itself, so that individuals in certain families might be more likely to live to very old age, into their eighties and nineties.

A number of studies, some dating back to the 1800s, have examined the question of whether genes influence longevity in humans. Many of the older studies, however, contain biases and cannot be objectively used to evaluate the contribution of heredity to length of life. Separating the influence of heredity and environment on this trait is a difficult task. Personal habits, life-style, education, economic status, and numerous other environmental factors undoubtedly affect health and longevity; relatives share many of these nonhereditary factors, in addition to genes. To separate the hereditary and environmental components of life span, geneticists have turned to adoption studies.

In one recently published study, geneticists investigated over 900 adopted people who were born in Denmark between 1924 and 1926. Almost all the adoptees included in the study were separated from their biological parents at birth, and all were raised by unrelated foster parents. The study showed that when at least one biological parent died of natural (nonviolent) causes before the age of 50, the mortality rate in their adopted-away offspring increased; it was twice the rate of those adoptees whose biological parents lived past the age of 50. In contrast, the premature death of a foster parent was not related to the overall mortality rate of the adoptees. If the biological parent died of an infection before the age of 50, the probability that the adoptee would die from infection was five times greater. Once again, no association was observed between the death of a foster parent from infection and the mortality rate of the adoptee. These findings indicate that hereditary factors do influence premature death from natural causes, particularly from infection.

LESCH-NYHAN SYNDROME. One of the most bizarre of all genetic disorders is Lesch-Nyhan syndrome. Children with this biochemical defect exhibit compulsive aggression and a tendency toward self-mutilation. They bite their lips, tongues, and fingers, often producing disfiguring injuries. They may throw themselves from the bed, bang their head against the wall, or stick their fingers into the spokes of their wheelchair. Although this behavior is typical for patients with Lesch-Nyhan syndrome, considerable variation occurs from patient to patient.

Individuals with Lesch-Nyhan disease appear normal at birth. One of the first indications of the disease, usually noted by mothers, is the presence of orange-colored "sand" in the diapers. The orange sand is actually crystals of uric acid, which is excreted in high quantities in the urine. By three to four months of age, developmental retardation becomes apparent; for example, the child with Lesch-Nyhan syndrome may not be able to hold its head up. Uncontrollable muscle spasms and mental retardation usually follow. Most of the patients are short and underweight.

Lesch-Nyhan syndrome results from a deficiency of an enzyme called hypoxanthine-guanine phosphoribosyl transferase, which is abbreviated HPRT. This enzyme plays a role in recycling some of the components of DNA, but how the absence of this enzyme produces the behavioral characteristics of the disorder is not known. Lesch-Nyhan disease is very rare, occurring in only about 1 in 100,000 infants.

The disease is an X-linked recessive disorder and exhibits typical X-linked transmission (see Chapter 3). Like many X-linked recessive disorders, Lesch-Nyhan syndrome occurs only in males. Because males have a single X chromosome, if they inherit a single copy of the gene for Lesch-Nyhan syndrome, they will have the disease. On the other hand, females have two X chromosomes, and thus a female would have to inherit two copies of the gene for Lesch-Nyhan syndrome—one from the mother and one from the father—to have the disease. If a father carried a gene for Lesch-Nyhan syndrome on his X chromosome, he would have the disease and would be unable to reproduce; thus, females are not affected.

When a couple has a boy with Lesch-Nyhan disease, the woman may be a carrier; alternatively, the child may have inherited a new mutation that arose during the formation of the egg which contributed his X chromosome. If the female is a carrier, each of her sons has a 50 percent chance of developing the disease. If the child inherited a new mutation, the chance of additional children in the family having the disease is very low. The gene that causes Lesch-Nyhan disease, a defective HPRT gene, is located on the long arm of the X chromosome. Prenatal testing for Lesch-Nyhan disease is possible with amniocentesis or chorionic villus sampling.

MANIC DEPRESSION. Manic depression is a mental illness characterized by extreme mood swings. The disorder is also termed *bipolar illness*. People with manic depression oscillate between periods of intense activity—termed *mania*—and periods of hopelessness termed *depression*.

While in the manic phase, they are frequently euphoric or may be highly irritable. They seem filled with energy and cannot sit still. This increased activity is frequently accompanied by poor judgment; for example, a manic person may go on a shopping spree and purchase a large number of unneeded items. During mania, the person often feels as though thoughts are racing through his or her head and talks incessantly. He or she is easily distracted. Conversations flip rapidly from one subject to another with no logical connection. In moments of extreme mania, the person may experience delusions of grandeur or persecution.

Following the manic phase, many patients with this disorder fall into a period of low depression (see Depression). They feel worthless and despondent. They become withdrawn and have difficulty finding the motivation to complete even simple tasks. Insomnia and loss of appetite are common. A significant number of people suffering from manic depression attempt suicide while depressed.

The mood swings associated with manic depression often appear to occur spontaneously, without any obvious external cause. Extended periods may separate the manic and depressed stages. Experts estimate that manic depression affects one to two percent of the population, and over 1 million Americans have this disease. Once debilitating, the disease can now be successfully treated in many patients with long-term drug therapy.

Manic-depressive illness has a strong genetic influence. Numerous studies show that this disease tends to run in families. Twin and adoption studies also indicate that genes are involved in the disorder. For example, when one identical twin has manic depression, the chance that the other twin will also develop the disorder is about 80 percent. However, if a nonidentical twin has manic depression, the chance that the other twin will develop the disorder is only 20 percent. This is the expected result if genes influence manic depression, because identical twins possess 100 percent of the same genes, whereas nonidentical twins share only 50 percent of the same genes. Among adopted individuals with manic depression, 28 percent of their biological parents also have the disease, whereas only 2 percent of the biological parents of adoptees without manic depression are affected; these facts indicate that genes play a role in the disorder.

For many years geneticists have argued over the mode of inheritance for manic depressive illness. Some geneticists favor a simple mode of inheritance, such as autosomal dominant or X-linked dominant. Others have suggested that the disease displays a complex pattern of inheritance, resulting from the interaction of many genes and perhaps environmental factors as well. Recently, several extended families have been identified in which the disease does display a simple pattern of inheritance. For example, manic depression occurs among the Old Order Amish, an isolated group of people descended from about 50 couples who immigrated to Pennsylvania in the 1700s. In the Amish, manic depression is inherited as an autosomal dominant trait, which means that a single copy of the gene produces the disease. Thus, a person with manic-depressive illness would have a 50 percent chance of passing the gene responsible for the disorder on to each offspring. However, in the Amish, the gene displays incomplete penetrance, meaning that not all those who inherit the gene develop the disease; roughly 50 percent of those with the gene will eventually experience manic depression. This suggests that environmental factors and/or other genes are also involved. Studying the DNA of Amish families, scientists have recently established that the gene responsible for their manic depression is located near the tip of the short arm of chromosome 11.

Researchers have identified other families in which manic-depressive illness also appears to be caused by a dominant gene. Several families from Iceland exhibit a dominant pattern of inheritance for the disease, but in this group no evidence could be found that the offending gene is located on chromosome 11. Likewise, in a study of three North American families with manic depression, scientists could detect no association between genes on chromosome 11 and the gene causing manic depression. In yet another study, geneticists found that manic depression in several families from Israel was caused by a gene on the X chromosome. Taken together, these studies indicate that manic depression may be caused by several different genes, located on different chromosomes. The mode of inheritance may vary among different families, depending on which genes are involved. Thus, no single pattern of inheritance for manic-depressive illness is observed. What is certain is that heredity plays a critical role in most cases of manic-depressive illness.

From statistics gathered on a large number of patients with manic depression, empiric risk figures (see Chapter 4) have been calculated. These calculations indicate that, on the average, when a person has manic-depressive illness, his or her children have an eight percent chance of becoming manic-depressive, versus a one to two percent chance for the children of parents without the disorder. Furthermore, another 12 percent of the children of a manic-depressive parent will develop depression alone (see Depression), indicating that manic depression and depression are genetically related.

Also see Depression.

MARFAN SYNDROME. Marfan syndrome is a genetic disease of connective tissue. Because connective tissue is found extensively throughout the body, Marfan syndrome affects a number of different organs and produces a diverse set of symptoms; symptoms involving the heart, bones, blood vessels, and eyes are the most serious.

Most individuals with Marfan syndrome are tall and thin, with unusually long arms and legs. The fingers and toes are also exceptionally long. The ribs do not grow properly, and as a result, the sternum (breast bone) is often deformed, being displaced either inward or outward. Joints are frequently loose. Eye problems also occur in people with Marfan syndrome. The most dangerous symptoms involve defects in the heart and blood vessels. Frequently, the valves of the heart function improperly, with the result that blood does not flow efficiently through the heart. This forces the heart to pump harder, which may eventually lead to heart failure. The major vessel leaving the heart—the aorta—is often enlarged and weak in individuals with Marfan syndrome; this weakness may cause the aorta to split or rupture, leading to sudden death. Numerous cases of sudden death have occurred in young people with Marfan syndrome while they were playing sports or when they were involved in relatively minor car accidents.

Marfan syndrome is a rare disorder; experts estimate that only about four to six out of every 100,000 people are affected. However, the symptoms vary from one person to the next, and many cases may go unnoticed; therefore, the true incidence of the disorder is difficult to ascertain. The underlying biochemical defect that produces the diverse symptoms of Marfan syndrome is unknown, but it most likely involves a defect in one of the components of connective tissue. The disorder is inherited as an autosomal dominant trait. Because Marfan syndrome is rare, virtually all people with the disorder are heterozygous, carrying a single copy of the disease gene. Thus, when one parent has Marfan syndrome, each child has a 50 percent chance of inheriting the disease. In the unlikely event that both parents have the disease, each child would possess a 75 percent chance of inheriting it.

MENSTRUAL PAIN. Most women experience some cramping and discomfort with their menstrual period. The severity of this discomfort varies considerably. In some women, the severity of menstrual pain limits normal activities and may require medical treatment; in medical terminology this is called *primary dysmenorrhea*. Primary dysmenorrhea is the leading cause of work absence among young women.

Menstrual pain tends to be similar among female relatives. Twin studies suggest that the severity of menstrual pain is influenced by genes, but nongenetic factors are also important. One study reported heritability values of 0.22 for amount of flow, 0.38 for the severity of pain, and 0.36 for the degree to which menstrual pain limits normal activity. (Heritability represents the proportion of the differences among individuals that results from genetic differences; see Chapter 4). Although these findings suggest that the severity of menstrual pain has some genetic basis, the trait is not inherited in a simple manner. Severe menstrual pain is probably multifactorial, resulting from the combination of many genes and environmental factors.

MENTAL RETARDATION. Mental retardation is characterized by subnormal intelligence and associated deficiencies in behavior that first appear during childhood. Individuals with subnormal intelligence are those possessing an IQ below 70. (IQ, or intelligence quotient, measures general intelligence in a standardized way. Average IQ is 100, and about 95 percent of the general population has an IQ ranging from 70 to 130. See Intelligence for more information on the genetics of IQ.) Mental retardation has an incidence of about 3 percent in the general population, while three to five individuals in every 1,000 are severely retarded.

A large number of genetic and nongenetic factors cause mental retardation. Genetic deficiencies causing retardation include abnormal numbers of chromosomes and defects in the structure of chromosomes. Other genetic influences involve defective enzymes, which are usually inherited as simple genetic traits (autosomal recessive, autosomal dominant, or X-linked factors). Multiple genetic factors that display no simple pattern of inheritance may also produce mental retardation. Environmental conditions are another major cause of mental retardation; these include some infectious diseases, drugs and alcohol taken during pregnancy, problems during delivery, injuries before and after birth, toxic substances, and a host of other factors. In many cases, the specific cause of retardation can never be established. Estimates of the proportion of individuals with mental retardation resulting from genetic factors vary widely. One study suggested that chromosomal abnormalities caused 15 percent of the cases of mental retardation, single genes with a simple pattern of inheritance produced another 17 percent, and about six percent of the cases involved more than one gene. The causes of the other 62 percent were environmental or could not be determined.

Defects in hundreds of different genes are capable of producing mental retardation, but most of these are quite rare. Frequently, multiple genes interact to produce mild retardation (IQ between 50 and 70). Because individuals with mild retardation often reproduce, the genes causing their mental deficiencies are transmitted to the next generation; therefore, mild retardation tends to run in families. On the other hand, severely retarded individuals (those with IQ below 35) rarely reproduce; consequently, most severely retarded children arise from new mutations and are born to normal parents. The single most common genetic cause of mental retardation is Down syndrome, which results from the presence of an extra chromosome. The second leading genetic cause is the fragile X syndrome, a still poorly understood genetic disorder caused by a gene on the X chromosome. This disorder occurs primarily among males. Some other genetic causes of mental retardation include phenylketonuria, Tay-Sachs disease, Lesch-Nyhan disease, Hunter syndrome, and Hurler syndrome.

For more information, see Down syndrome, Fragile X syndrome, Hunter syndrome, Hurler sydrome, Lesch-Nyhan disease, Phenylketonuria, and Tay-Sachs disease.

MIDDIGITAL HAIR. Middigital hair is a common characteristic that is primarily inherited as an autosomal dominant trait. Each finger consists of three segments: a segment that connects the finger to the palm of the hand, a middle segment, and a short, terminal segment containing the fingernail. These three segments are separated by folds of skin covering the joints between the bones of the fingers. In some people, hair grows on the middle segment of one or more fingers; this trait is termed *middigital hair*. Sometimes, the hairs are relatively long and easily observed; at other times, the hairs may be short or missing, but if the trait is present, close examination should reveal the presence of hair follicles (small pits from which the hairs grow).

The occurrence of middigital hair varies widely among different racial groups. For example, about 75 percent of North American whites have middigital hair, but in certain native American Indian tribes, the frequency may be as low as 25 percent. And among Eskimos, middigital hair is almost totally absent, occurring in less than 2 percent of the population.

Middigital hair seems to be inherited as an autosomal dominant trait, at least in most families. This means that only a single copy of the gene for middigital hair is required for the trait to be expressed. If the gene for middigital hair is symbolized with the letter H, and the gene for the

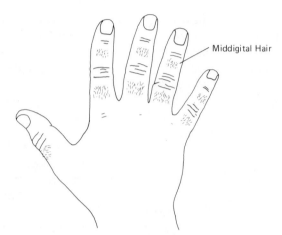

Catalog Figure 8.   Middigital hair.

absence of hair with a small *h*, then those with genotypes *HH* and *Hh* will exhibit middigital hair, whereas those with genotype *hh* will have no middigital hair. Because the absence of middigital hair occurs only in people with the genotype *hh*, two parents without middigital hair (*hh* X *hh*) should produce only children without middigital hair. However, in a few families, two parents without middigital hair produce a child with middigital hair; this suggests that the trait is not always inherited in a simple dominant fashion. Furthermore, surveys frequently reveal that middigital hair is more common in males than females, and the trait sometimes changes with age. These observations indicate that non-genetic factors can affect the trait, and the inheritance of middigital hair is probably more complex than is frequently thought.

MILK TOLERANCE. Mammals are the only animals that possess mammary glands and produce milk for their offspring. Most mammals only consume milk, however, when young. In fact, most adult mammals cannot completely digest milk, and it frequently makes them sick.

Nutritionally, one of the most important components of milk is a sugar called *lactose*. Large amounts of lactose are found in milk, and much of the energy a young mammal needs for its growth and development comes from the lactose in milk. Mammals cannot, however, use lactose directly, for lactose cannot pass through the intestine and into the body.

The lactose in milk must first be broken down into simple sugars; this breakdown or digestion of lactose is carried out by a special enzyme called *lactase*. (Lactose and lactase are easily confused because of their similar spelling; lactose is the sugar and lactase is the enzyme that breaks down this sugar.) Fortunately, young mammals have plenty of lactase in their intestine, and, thus, they can readily digest lactose in milk. However, as mammals grow older, the amount of the enzyme in their intestine decreases. By the time they reach adult age, most mammals have very little enzyme. If they drink milk, the lactose within the milk is not fully digested. Undigested lactose often upsets normal bowel movements, absorbs water that causes diarrhea, and produces gas and abdominal pain. This rarely creates a problem in nature, because after they are weaned, most mammals never have the opportunity to drink milk.

The one exception to the rule that adult mammals cannot digest lactose is humans. Actually, most humans in the world are not an exception; like other mammals, they cannot digest the lactose in fresh milk as adults. The exception applies specifically to Caucasians with European ancestry and a few smaller ethnic groups that can digest the lactose in milk as adults. People in these groups have a unique genetic trait—in some respects, a genetic abnormality—that causes the lactase enzyme to persist after childhood. Because levels of lactase in their intestine remain high throughout adult life, these people are able to digest the lactose in milk, and many of them consume large amounts of fresh milk as adults. The majority of the world's population, however, lacks persistence of lactase, and they are unable to digest the lactose in milk after childhood. Many of these people experience intestinal pain, gas, and diarrhea if they drink large amounts of fresh milk, although some apparently do drink milk without discomfort.

The persistence of lactase activity into adulthood, and thus the ability to tolerate large amounts of fresh milk as an adult, is a trait determined by an autosomal dominant gene. Let the capital letter L represent the gene causing lactase persistence, and the small letter l represent the alternative gene that causes a decrease in lactase activity after childhood. Each person has two genes—their genotype—that determine their ability to digest lactose as an adult. If someone possesses LL or Ll, she has persistence of lactase and can drink fresh milk comfortably as an adult. If someone else possesses two normal genes, ll, his lactase activity in adulthood is low and he may not be able to drink fresh milk as an adult. These genes only affect the ability to digest lactose as an adult; with a few rare exceptions, all humans have high lactase activity and can consume fresh milk in infancy and childhood.

The frequency of the lactase persistence trait differs among various ethnic groups. For example, less than 25 percent of people in most parts of Africa, the Middle East, India, Southeast Asia, China, and Japan have persistence of lactase activity in adulthood. However, 77 percent of French, 85 percent of Germans, 95 percent of Danes, and 99 percent of Swedes can digest lactose as adults. In the United States, over 90 percent of adult Caucasians with a northern European ancestry have the capacity to digest large amounts of lactose. On the other hand, only about 35 percent of black adults in the United States have this trait.

The differences that exist in the ability of humans to digest lactose are not widely recognized; this general lack of knowledge about lactose and milk intolerance has several reasons. First, fresh milk simply is not available in many parts of the world, and thus few people experience problems in digesting milk. Even where milk is available, many people are unaware that they cannot digest it. Apparently, many of those without lactase activity frequently develop an aversion to drinking large amounts of milk; they simply know that they do not like milk, although many are unaware of the fact that drinking it may make them sick. In addition, even those without lactase activity may be able to drink moderate amounts of milk without obvious discomfort. The symptoms associated with drinking milk in those who cannot digest lactose vary greatly. Some experience diarrhea, gas, and abdominal pain after drinking only a small amount of milk; in others, relatively large amounts of milk may be consumed without discomfort. Thus, tolerance to milk is influenced by genetic differences in lactase persistence, but the association between lactose tolerance and milk tolerance is not perfect. Finally, people in many parts of the world who lack the ability to digest fresh milk utilize dairy products in their diet by modifying the milk so that the lactose content is reduced. For example, when milk sours, bacteria in the milk break down the lactose to simpler sugars, and the sour milk can then be digested by adults without lactase activity.

Because the ability to digest lactose as an adult is a dominant trait, and the inability to digest it is recessive, two parents who lack lactase ($ll \times ll$) can only produce offspring who lack this enzyme as adults. On the other hand, two parents who are lactose tolerant may produce some offspring with and some offspring without lactose tolerance as adults. For example, the two lactose-tolerant parents might be Ll and Ll; they would produce one-quarter LL, one-half Ll, and one-quarter ll offspring on the average. Because of the variability in response to milk drinking, however, the presence or absence of lactose tolerance is very difficult to determine without special blood or breath tests.

MOLES. Common moles are small pigmented spots or lumps found on the skin; typically they exhibit an oval or round shape and are uniformly tan or brown. Most adult Caucasians possess at least a few common moles. Some geneticists have proposed that the presence of moles is inherited as an autosomal dominant trait; however, common moles are found so frequently that their inheritance is difficult to confirm. On the other hand, large moles present at birth (often called *birthmarks*), do show a tendency to be inherited.

In a few families, individuals possess large numbers of peculiar moles called *dysplastic nevi*. These moles are absent at birth, typically first appearing and increasing in number at puberty. Dysplastic nevi are often larger and more numerous than common moles; unlike common moles, they tend to be a haphazard mixture of colors and they have margins that fade into the adjacent normal skin. Dysplastic nevi are inherited as an autosomal dominant trait, and they may be precursors to a type of malignant skin cancer called a *melanoma*. Recently, geneticists have discovered that the gene causing dysplastic nevi is located on the short arm of chromosome 1. When one parent has dysplastic nevi and is heterozygous (homozygotes are rare), each child has a 50 percent chance of developing dysplastic nevi.

MUSCULAR DYSTROPHY. Muscular dystrophy is a disease in which the muscles progressively weaken and slowly waste away. There are several different forms of muscular dystrophy; all are inherited disorders. The most common of the muscular dystrophies is called *Duchenne muscular dystrophy*. This disease affects males almost exclusively. A boy with Duchenne muscular dystrophy appears normal at birth, but he usually begins to experience problems with muscle weakness at about age three. Early symptoms are stumbling, difficulty climbing stairs, and difficulty getting up from the floor. The calf muscles of affected boys look larger than normal, and many individuals have a tendency to walk on their toes. The muscles in the arms and legs become progressively weaker over time; most affected individuals are confined to a wheelchair by the age of 11. About one third of those with the disease have some mental retardation. Most boys with Duchenne muscular dystrophy die before the age of 20, usually as a result of respiratory or heart failure.

Within the past few years, the biochemical defect that causes Duchenne muscular dystrophy has been traced to a protein called *dystrophin*. Dystrophin is found in all normal muscle cells. Its exact function is unclear at the present time, but individuals with Duchenne muscular dystrophy lack dystrophin in their muscles. The gene that normally codes for dystrophin is huge, encompassing about two million nucleotides of DNA. Geneticists have determined that this gene resides on the short arm of the X chromosome.

Because the dystrophin gene is located on the X chromosome, Duchenne muscular dystrophy is inherited as an X-linked recessive disease. Females have two X chromosomes; therefore, females who inherit a defective copy of the dystrophin gene on one X chromosome still possess a normal copy of the gene on their other X chromosome, and this normal copy produces enough dystrophin to prevent the disease. Women with one normal copy and one defective copy of the dystrophin gene are said to be carriers; they do not have muscular dystrophy (although a small number may show some muscle wasting), but they do have the capacity to transmit the defective copy of the dystrophin gene to their offspring. In contrast to the situation in females, males possess only a single X chromosome; if they inherit a defective copy of the dystrophin gene on their single X, they do not produce dystrophin and they will have muscular dystrophy.

When a woman is a carrier, 50 percent of her sons on the average will develop Duchenne muscular dystrophy. Furthermore, about 50 percent of her daughters will be carriers, with the potential to pass the defective gene on to their sons. Males who have Duchenne muscular dystrophy rarely live long enough to produce children, and thus they almost never pass the defective gene to their children. Unaffected sons of a female carrier cannot pass on the disease, because if they carried the gene for Duchenne muscular dystrophy, they would have the disorder. Sometimes, the disease may occur in a child as a result of a new mutation in one of the reproductive cells that gave rise to the child; when this is the case, the mother of the affected son will not be a carrier, and the chance of future sons having the disorder is very low. However, if more than one son has the disease, or if the mother's brother, her uncle on her mother's side of the family, or a grandson has the disease, then the mother is almost certainly a carrier, and any additional sons she conceives will have a 50 percent chance of developing Duchenne muscular dystrophy. Her daughters are also at risk for passing the gene on to their sons.

Recent advances in molecular genetics have now made prenatal diagnosis and detection of carriers possible for some families. These tests are still somewhat experimental and available only at special genetics centers.

A second form of muscular dystrophy is *Becker muscular dystrophy*. The symptoms of Becker muscular dystrophy are similar to those for Duchenne muscular dystrophy, but the disease develops more slowly. Muscle weakness usually first appears in the early teens, and most individuals with this disorder can walk until age 25 or older. Like Duchenne muscular dystrophy, Becker muscular dystrophy is caused by a defect in the gene that codes for dystrophin, but the nature of the defect differs. Because Becker muscular dystrophy is also due to a defective gene on the X chromosome, its transmission is essentially the same as that for Duchenne muscular dystrophy. One difference is that males with Becker muscular dystrophy frequently live long enough to reproduce and may pass on the gene for the disease; because the gene is located on the X chromosome, affected males cannot transmit it to their sons, but all their daughters will be carriers.

There are a number of other types of muscular dystrophy. Some of these are inherited as X-linked disorders; others are autosomal recessive or autosomal dominant disorders. All of these are rare.

NEARSIGHTEDNESS. Nearsightedness occurs when a person can see nearby objects clearly but has difficulty seeing objects at a distance. This common eye problem is also termed *myopia*. In a normal eye, light enters the eye through the pupil, which is the black disk in the center of the eye, and passes through the lens, which sits just behind the pupil. As light passes through the lens, it is focused into an image on the back of the eyeball, much as a projector focuses a picture on a movie screen. The image falls on special sensors located within a layer of cells called the *retina;* these sensors send information about the image to the brain, where the information is then reconstructed into the visual picture that we see.

In a normal eye, the lens focuses the light exactly on the retina. However, in people with myopia the image is focused in front of the retina, and, thus, the picture falling on the retina is out of focus. The same phenomenon would occur if you focused a picture from a projector on a movie screen and then moved the screen backward several feet; the picture that was once clear would now become blurred. Most nearsightedness occurs because the eyeball is too long, although it can arise for other reasons, such as an abnormal curvature of the eye. Fortunately, nearsightedness is easily corrected with eyeglasses or contact lens, which bend the light before it enters the lens and move the image backward onto the retina.

Nearsightedness is very common in modern society; about one out of every four people has this problem. Nearsightedness usually develops in childhood or early adolescence and it rarely gets worse after the age of 30.

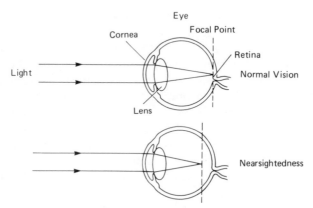

Catalog Figure 9.   Normally light passing through the eye focuses on the retina. In nearsightedness, the light coming through the lens focuses in front of the retina and thus appears out of focus.

For years, scientists have argued about the causes of nearsightedness. Some have emphasized the importance of environmental factors in this disorder. They point out that people with more education have higher incidences of nearsightedness, suggesting that reading and other close work associated with schooling may cause myopia. Some studies in animals also suggest that environmental factors play a role in near-sightedness. On the other hand, geneticists have noted that nearsighted-ness frequently runs in families. Studies of twins indicate that near-sightedness has a strong genetic component. In a few families, myopia may be inherited as a simple genetic trait, with either an autosomal dominant or autosomal recessive pattern of inheritance. However, in most families myopia is multifactorial, resulting from a complex interac-tion of many genes and environmental factors; thus, it does not usually exhibit a simple pattern of inheritance. Nearsightedness also occurs along with other physical defects in some genetic syndromes and genetic diseases. For example, individuals with Marfan syndrome are frequently nearsighted. When part of a syndrome or genetic disease, nearsighted-ness will follow the pattern of inheritance of the disease or syndrome. However, these genetic causes are responsible for only a small fraction of the cases of nearsightedness.

NEURAL TUBE DEFECTS. The nervous system is the commu-nications network of the body, consisting of the brain, spinal cord, and nerves. About three weeks after conception, the nervous system begins development as a hollow tube of neural tissue that runs down the back of the embryo. Eventually this tube enlarges at one end to form the brain; here, the neural tube is closed off and protected by the bones of the skull. At the other end, the neural tube is enclosed by rings of bone—the vertebrae—and this forms the spinal column. Within the spinal column runs the spinal cord. Many nerves branch off the spinal cord, passing to different parts of the body.

Neural tube defects are deformities that occur when the neural tube fails to close completely during development. If the tube fails to close at the head, the skull bones do not develop, and part of the brain is missing. This is called *anencephaly*. Infants born with this defect die soon after birth. If the tube fails to close at the other end, the vertebrae do not completely fuse, and the spinal cord and a protective sac that surrounds the cord may protrude from the back. This condition is referred to as *spina bifida*. Symptoms associated with spina bifida vary depending on how much of the spinal cord lies outside the vertebrae: If only the protective sac protrudes, the condition is less severe than if the cord and associated nerves protrude. Some cases of spina bifida can be surgically corrected, but this is always a serious birth defect.

The incidence of neural tube defects in the United States is about one or two affected children born for every 1,000 live births. These disorders are more common among females. Most cases of neural tube defects are thought to be multifactorial, resulting from the influence of both genetic and environmental causes. Occasionally, neural tube defects may occur as a part of a genetic syndrome, such as Meckel's syndrome, which is characterized by neural tube defects, cleft palate, extra fingers, and other birth defects. In many cases, such syndromes have simple modes of inheritance; Meckel's syndrome, for example, is inherited as an autosomal recessive trait.

Spina bifida and anencephaly appear to arise from the same set of factors; if a couple has a child with anencephaly, they are not only more likely to produce another child with anencephaly, but they are also at greater risk for producing a child with spina bifida. When a couple has one child with a neural tube defect, the chance of producing another child with one of these deformities is about 3 to 5 percent. When one of the parents has a neural tube defect, the chance of producing an affected child is also about 3 to 5 percent. Neural tube defects can be detected prenatally by examining the α-fetoprotein levels in the amniotic fluid with amniocentesis. High levels of α-fetoprotein in the mother's blood during pregnancy sometimes indicate that the fetus has a neural tube defect; however, many other factors may also elevate α-fetoprotein in the mother's blood, so follow-up tests (ultrasound and amniocentesis) are required to confirm the diagnosis (see Chapter 6).

Recent studies suggest that taking vitamins at the time of conception may lower the chances of producing a child with a neural tube defect in women at high risk. Whether taking vitamins has any beneficial effects for women who are not at high risk is not yet known.

NEUROFIBROMATOSIS. Neurofibromatosis is a genetic disease that causes multiple tumors in the tissue of the nervous system. Physicians have identified several different types of neurofibromatosis. The most common type was first described by Friedrich von Recklinghausen in 1882 and today is known as *Recklinghausen neurofibromatosis*, or *neurofibromatosis 1*. About 90 percent of all patients with neurofibromatosis have neurofibromatosis 1; this includes about 100,000 people in the United States. The discussion here will focus on neurofibromatosis 1.

Neurofibromatosis occurs in about 1 out of every 3,000 individuals. People with the disorder vary greatly in their symptoms: Some are only mildly affected and the disease may go unnoticed for many years; others experience multiple, disfiguring tumors; still others are mentally retarded. The name *neurofibromatosis* refers to the hallmark of the disease: multiple tumors that occur along the nerves. Tumors may also arise in the skin and a variety of organs as well. Another common characteristic of those with the disease is the presence of medium brown patches, called café-au-lait spots, on the skin. An additional feature is abnormal growth of bones and other tissues that can, in severe cases, produce disfiguring and disabling deformities. Many individuals with neurofibromatosis have some mental impairment; about 2 to 5 percent are mentally retarded.

Neurofibromatosis 1 is caused by an autosomal dominant gene. Affected individuals usually possess one copy of the neurofibromatosis gene. Therefore, if one parent has neurofibromatosis, each child has a 50 percent chance of inheriting the disease. Normally, a person who is free of an autosomal dominant trait cannot transmit the disease to his or her children. However, some people with the neurofibromatosis gene are so mildly affected that the disease is overlooked; the children of these mildly affected individuals would still possess a 50 percent chance of developing neurofibromatosis, and they can be severely affected. Also, for unknown reasons, the mutation rate of the neurofibromatosis gene appears to be much higher than usual. As a result, almost 50 percent of all cases result from new mutations that took place in the reproductive cells of normal parents. Geneticists have recently established that the gene causing neurofibromatosis 1 is located on the long arm of chromosome 17.

NEVUS. See Moles.

NIGHT TERRORS. See Sleepwalking.

OBESITY. See Weight.

OSTEOGENESIS IMPERFECTA. Osteogenesis imperfecta is a group of genetic disorders characterized by brittle bones. Some people with this disease are only mildly affected; in others, the bones are so fragile that the baby is born literally crumpled with multiple bone fractures. Osteogenesis imperfecta results from genetic defects in a substance called *collagen*.

Collagen is the most abundant protein in the human body. Occurring almost everywhere, it provides much of the scaffolding that supports the organs and tissues. For example, it is found in skin, bone, the tendons that connect the muscles to the bones, teeth, and the walls of blood vessels. Weight for weight, collagen is as strong as steel. Its incredible strength derives from a complex molecular structure, which consists of three protein chains that are wrapped around each other like the strands of a rope. A number of different varieties of collagen exist, differing in the types of chains that make up the molecule.

The manner in which our body manufactures collagen is even more complex than the molecule itself. A number of different steps are involved, and these take place in several different parts of the cell. Defects may occur at any one of a number of points in the process of collagen synthesis; consequently, there are a large number of different hereditary disorders that involve defective collagen.

The most obvious characteristic of osteogenesis imperfecta is brittle bones—bones that break easily. Numerous skeletal deformities also occur; these are produced by repeated fractures and abnormal bone growth. In severe cases, even the simple weight of the body may cause the bones to break. Bone fractures and deformities often lead to short stature. The teeth may also be affected, appearing gray in color, brittle, and misshapen. Deafness is common, and the whites of the eyes may remain blue in color after infancy. (The whites of the eyes are frequently blue even in healthy babies, but the blue color disappears with age.)

Much variability occurs in the symptoms of people with osteogenesis imperfecta. Some of this variability results from a number of different genetic defects producing osteogenesis imperfecta—what is termed *genetic heterogeneity*. Four types of osteogenesis imperfecta that make up the majority of cases will be discussed. Keep in mind that other forms of the disease also occur, and the symptoms may vary considerably even with each type.

Type I. In this form of osteogenesis imperfecta, broken bones may occur at any time, but fractures are rarely present at birth; most broken bones occur after the first year of life. The whites of the eyes are blue after infancy. In about 50 percent of the cases, hearing loss occurs with age. This type of osteogenesis imperfecta is thought to be inherited as an autosomal dominant trait. As in other autosomal dominant traits, when one parent has this type of osteogenesis imperfecta, each child has a 50 percent chance of inheriting the disease.

Types II and III. These types of osteogenesis imperfecta are severe. Multiple bone fractures occur at birth; frequently the child does not live through the birthing process. If the child survives, many bone deformities occur, and individuals are usually dwarfed. The whites of the eyes may or may not be blue in color. In some families osteogenesis imperfecta types II and III are inherited as autosomal recessive traits, but in other families the inheritance is thought to be autosomal dominant.

When the disease is inherited as an autosomal recessive trait, both parents of a child with osteogenesis imperfecta are usually normal, but both are carriers for the disease-causing gene. A child who inherits two copies of the gene—one from each parent—will have the disease. Each additional child conceived by this couple has a one in four chance of also inheriting two copies of the gene and having osteogenesis imperfecta. When a parent has one of these types of osteogenesis imperfecta, his or her children will only have the disease if the other parent is a carrier for the disease-causing gene, which is unlikely because the disease is rare; thus, children of affected parents are almost always normal. In those families where these forms of osteogenesis imperfecta are inherited as autosomal dominant traits, a parent with the disorder has a 50 percent chance of passing the disease on to each of his or her children.

Type IV. This type of osteogenesis imperfecta is usually mild; brittle bones are not a problem until after birth. Tooth development may be defective, and the whites of the eyes are normal in color. Sometimes dwarfing occurs because of multiple fractures. This form is inherited as an autosomal dominant disorder, and a parent with this type of osteogenesis imperfecta has a 50 percent chance of passing the disease on to each child.

Some forms of osteogenesis imperfecta can be detected prenatally with ultrasound or X-rays. Within the past few years, geneticists have learned much about the molecular basis of collagen formation and how genetic defects in this process lead to osteogenesis imperfecta. This work has revealed that several different genes are involved in producing collagen. Detailed study of these genes reveal that they are extraordinarily large, and mutations can arise in a number of different places and in several ways. Individuals with osteogenesis imperfecta do not all have the same mutation; in fact, the number of genetic defects occurring among those individuals with the disease is probably quite large; this genetic variation appears to account for much of the variability observed in the symptoms of osteogenesis imperfecta.

OTITIS MEDIA. See Ear infection.

PATAU SYNDROME (Trisomy 13). Patau syndrome is a severe chromosome abnormality characterized by mental retardation, a small head, small eyes, deafness, extra fingers, and numerous other defects. Individuals with Patau syndrome possess three copies of chromosome 13; hence, the condition is also called *trisomy 13*. Fewer than 15 percent of the infants born with this disorder live beyond the first year. The incidence of Patau syndrome is not precisely known but lies somewhere between 1 in 4,000 and 1 in 10,000 births.

As with many chromosome abnormalities, Patau syndrome usually results from a random accident during the process of chromosome division. Thus, most parents who produce a child with this disorder are not likely to have other children with it. However, occasionally extra copies of chromosome 13 may occur in a child because one of the parents has a chromosome problem. For example, a copy of chromosome 13 may be attached to another chromosome in one of the parents, a condition known as a *translocation*. When a parent has a translocation, the parent's chromosomes may not divide properly when reproductive cells are produced, and each child will have a greater than normal chance of getting an extra copy of chromosome 13. Some of the normal children of such parents may be carriers, and their children will also have a higher probability of inheriting an extra copy of chromosome 13. Patau syndrome can be detected prenatally by chromosome analysis carried out on fetal tissue obtained with amniocentesis or chorionic villus sampling.

PERSONALITY. A number of studies have examined the question of whether personality traits have a genetic basis. These have included twin studies and adoption studies. Some of the more recent investigations examined large numbers of individuals and utilized sophisticated statistical techniques. Although the results vary somewhat from study to study, a growing consensus is that personality traits are hereditary, at least to some extent. Even when adopted into foster homes at birth, people seem to display personalities similar to those of their biological parents. Heritabilities for personality traits typically range from 0.4 to 0.50, indicating that 40 to 50 percent of the variation in these traits results from genetic differences. (See Chapter 4 for a discussion of heritability.) It should not be forgotten that the other 50 to 60 percent of the variation results from nonhereditary influences—personality is certainly not all genetic! A surprising finding of many recent studies, however, is that the common family environment appears to have relatively little effect on the development of personality. In other words, if family members resemble each other in personality, it is because they share genes and not because they share the same home environment. This is supported by the fact that individuals adopted into foster homes show little overall similarity to the personality traits of their foster parents (no similarity greater than that expected on a chance basis).

PHENYLKETONURIA (PKU). In 1934, a Norwegian physician and biochemist named Folling discovered that some retarded children gave off an odd, musty odor. Upon investigating, he discovered that the odor emanated from their urine, which contained an abnormal substance called phenylpyruvic acid. This observation led to the discovery of the genetic disease called phenylketonuria, abbreviated PKU.

More than any other disorder, PKU illustrates the benefits of screening for genetic diseases. If untreated, PKU produces severe mental retardation—96 to 98 percent of all untreated PKU patients exhibit an IQ less than 50. (For comparison, normal IQ averages 100.) Other features of PKU include eczema, a musty odor, light skin color, and decreased growth. These symptoms can be avoided if the disease is detected soon after birth and treatment is started immediately. Before the benefits of early treatment were recognized, PKU was a major cause of severe mental retardation. Today, because of widespread screening for PKU among newborns, most patients are treated, and few develop retardation.

PKU arises because of a genetic defect in the gene that codes for phenylalanine hydroxylase, which is an enzyme that helps to metabolize the amino acid phenylalanine. Phenylalanine is normally present in the proteins that are eaten, and it is an essential amino acid, meaning that the body must have it to grow and function properly. Too much phenylalanine during infancy and childhood—the period during which the brain is developing—can produce mental retardation. Thus, the amount of phenylalanine in the body is critical: Too little inhibits growth and development; too much causes brain damage. Fortunately, the body carefully regulates the amount of phenylalanine by converting it to another substance called tyrosine. This conversion of phenylalanine to tyrosine is carried out by the enzyme phenylalanine hydroxylase. In a person with PKU, this enzyme is defective. Consequently, phenylalanine is not converted to tyrosine, the amino acid builds up in body tissues, and, in a way not yet fully understood, the increase in phenylalanine produces mental retardation.

Before birth, a mother's own enzyme keeps the level of phenylalanine low in a PKU fetus. Therefore, a baby with PKU is born normal. After birth, however, when the infant starts to consume milk (a source of phenylalanine), the level of phenylalanine rises, and the increase causes damage as the brain develops. Fortunately, the disease can be treated by putting the child on a low-phenylalanine diet. Because phenylalanine is essential for proper growth and development, it cannot be eliminated entirely; blood levels of phenylalanine must be closely monitored throughout childhood. Phenylalanine apparently produces brain damage only as long as the brain is growing and developing. How long the child must remain on the low-phenylalanine diet to avoid mental problems is still controversial. Previously, the special diet was often discontinued around the ages of four to six, but now many experts suggest that it be continued until eight to ten years of age or even longer.

Classic PKU is inherited as an autosomal recessive trait. This means that two copies of the gene must be inherited—one from each parent—to have the disease. In most cases, both parents of a child with PKU are normal, but they both carry one copy of the recessive PKU gene. If two normal parents have one child with PKU, then both parents are carriers and each additional child they produce will have a one in four chance of developing the disease. The disease can be detected prenatally.

The gene that causes PKU is situated on chromosome 12. Some variants of this disease, called *hyperphenylalaninemias*, are also inherited as autosomal recessive disorders. PKU arises most frequently among Caucasians, particularly among those of Celtic origin (people from England, Scotland, and Ireland). The incidence among Caucasians in the United States is about 1 in 11,000.

The treatment of PKU has been so successful that many patients with the disease are now reaching reproductive age. Because PKU is an autosomal recessive disease, a person with PKU will produce a PKU child only if their spouse also has the disorder or is a carrier for the PKU gene, both of which are unlikely events. Special problems arise in the pregnancy of a PKU mother. When the mother has PKU, her blood levels of phenylalanine will be abnormally high, and the unborn child will be exposed to high phenylalanine during its development in the womb. This can cause mental retardation, even though the child does not have PKU. High levels of phenylalanine in the mother also result in miscarriages, low birth weight, and birth defects. Fortunately these problems can be avoided if the mother adheres to a low-phenylalanine diet throughout conception and pregnancy.

PHENYLTHIOCARBAMIDE (PTC) TASTER. The ability to taste a chemical called phenylthiocarbamide (PTC) is an inherited trait. To the majority of people, even weak concentrations of PTC taste quite bitter. Others, however, find the substance tasteless (unless it is present in relatively high concentrations). Thus, people can be classified as *tasters* or *nontasters*. About 70 percent of North American Caucasians are tasters. Genetic studies suggest that the ability to taste low concentrations of PTC is inherited as an autosomal dominant trait. Let the gene for the ability to taste PTC be represented with the capital letter T, and the gene for the inability to taste PTC be represented with the little letter t. Because the taster trait is dominant, individuals with either one (Tt) or two (TT) copies of the taster gene would have the ability to taste PTC. Nontasters could only possess nontaster genes (tt). Thus, two nontaster parents ($tt \times tt$) would produce only nontaster children (tt). Because tasters may possess both taster and nontaster genes (TT or Tt), they may produce both taster and nontaster children. Although this simple genetic system appears to explain the inheritance of the taster trait in many families, the presence of a few individuals with intermediate tasting ability and the slightly higher incidence of the taster trait in females suggest that other factors may also be involved.

PHYSICAL FITNESS. Physical fitness varies tremendously among people, but family members are frequently alike in standardized tests of endurance and strength. This familial resemblance might be due to heredity; alternatively, it could result from shared life-styles and other environmental factors common to members of the same family. A number of studies have examined the influence of genes on physical fitness. These studies point to heredity as one factor contributing to physical fitness, but the studies differ in their conclusions about the relative contributions of genetic and environmental factors. Variation in these findings probably reflects differences in the type of physical fitness measured, the group studied, or the method of genetic analysis used. One recent study conducted on 375 French Quebec families obtained the following heritabilities (the proportion of the measured variation in the trait that can be accounted for by genetic differences; see Chapter 4): For submaximal power output, heritability $= 0$; for reaction time, heritability $= 0.20$; for muscular endurance, heritability $= 0.21$; for muscular strength, heritability $= 0.30$; and for movement time, heritability $= 0$. In another study of eastern European twins, heritability for the 60-meter dash was estimated to be 0.85, heritability for the long jump was 0.74, and heritability for the shotput was 0.71. These are just a few of the dozens of heritability estimates that have been calculated for fitness traits; other studies exist that provide different heritability estimates for these fitness tests. Although differing in the heritability estimates obtained, most studies indicate that genes moderately influence individual differences in physical fitness. Geneticists generally assume that when genes influence fitness traits, the inheritance is multifactorial, meaning that many genes and environmental factors play a role in determining the fitness trait.

POLYDACTYLY. See Fingers, extra.

PREMATURE BIRTH. Premature birth is a common complication of pregnancy, but a costly one in terms of lives and dollars. Although the survival of premature babies in the United States has increased dramatically during the past ten years, many preterm babies still die. For those that do survive, the cost of treatment in a U.S. hospital is frequently $20,000 to $80,000 for each preterm infant. An estimated 200,000 premature babies are born in the United States each year.

A number of environmental factors have been shown to influence a mother's chances of giving birth to a preterm infant, including smoking, excessive work, the mother's age and weight, socioeconomic status, infections in the mother during pregnancy, and medications. Several studies have also demonstrated that many women give birth to more than one premature baby. For example, in one study 22 percent of the women who gave birth to a preterm infant had given birth to a previous preterm child, whereas among those women who gave birth to a term baby (not premature), only about one percent had given birth to a previous preterm baby. Some investigators have interpreted this observation to mean that genes influence premature birth. However, this conclusion is not warranted, because similar environmental factors acting on the mother may affect both pregnancies. At this time, it is not known whether producing premature infants has a hereditary basis.

PSEUDOHERMAPHRODITISM. See Sex determinism.

PSORIASIS. Psoriasis is a relatively common skin disease characterized by small pink eruptions that group together to produce red patches. These eruptions heal over, forming grayish white scales. Most commonly, psoriasis occurs on the scalp, the elbows, the knees, or the buttocks; sometimes the nails, eyebrows, underarms, and pubic region are also involved. The disease typically affects those between the ages of 10 and 40, but it may strike at any age. For most people with psoriasis, the condition is mild, though annoying; only rarely does it develop into a serious, disabling disease.

Psoriasis occurs in about two to four percent of the Caucasian population. It is much less frequent among blacks. The cause is unknown, but genes seem to be involved. Twin studies show that when one identical twin has psoriasis, the other twin is more likely to also have it than when one nonidentical twin has the disease, which is the expected result if genes contribute to the disorder. In some families, psoriasis appears to be inherited as an autosomal dominant trait. However, in other families, the inheritance is more complicated; in these families the inheritance is most likely multifactorial, meaning that multiple genes and nongenetic factors are involved. Individuals with certain HLA alleles—genes involved in coding for the immune system—are more likely to develop psoriasis than individuals without these alleles, but why this relationship exists between the HLA genes and psoriasis is not clear.

PTOSIS. See Eyelid, droopy.

READING DISABILITY (Dyslexia). Most children begin to read around the age of six, and after two to three years of schooling, the majority have mastered the basic skills of reading. However, a number of children exhibit significant problems in learning to read; their reading disability interferes with all other aspects of their education. Many factors may contribute to reading problems. In some cases, vision or hearing is impaired, and, if uncorrected, these defects may impede the learning process. In other cases, mental retardation, emotional disturbances, or other behavioral problems interfere with mastering the skill of reading. Sometimes cultural or home environments inhibit reading. All of these factors may contribute to reading problems, but a number of children with normal intelligence have difficulty reading in the absence of any such factors. These children are said to have reading disability or dyslexia.

A major difficulty in understanding reading disability is that reading skills, like most mental activities, vary tremendously from one person to the next. Thus, it is difficult to know whether a slow reader has a special problem or whether he or she is simply at the low end of the normal range of reading ability. No simple test exists for identifying those with reading disabilities, and even reading experts disagree on exactly how to define reading disability.

In a literate society, reading disability can be a major handicap. Poor reading limits educational opportunities and employment, it influences social acceptance, and it may affect the quality of life. Reported incidences of reading disability vary, depending on how the disorder is defined, but 10 to 15 percent of school-age children have serious reading problems. For unknown reasons, three to four times as many males have reading disability as females. The high incidence of reading disability and the limitations it imposes in today's society make this disorder a major social, educational, and mental health problem.

As early as 1905, geneticists suggested that reading disability was inherited, and studies have consistently shown that the disorder runs in families. A large proportion of children with reading disability have a close relative who is also reading impaired. Twin studies also strongly support a genetic basis to this disorder. When one identical twin has reading disability, the other twin has it about 90 percent of the time. On the other hand, when one nonidentical twin has reading disability, the other twin is affected only about 30 percent of the time. Because identical twins possess the same genes, whereas nonidentical twins possess only 50 percent of the same genes, identical twins should be more similar if genes influence reading disability. One recent study estimated that as much as 30 percent of variation in reading disability is inherited. This finding suggests that environmental factors are also important, perhaps accounting for 70 percent of reading deficits.

Although considerable evidence suggests that reading disability is partially genetic, the pattern of inheritance is not known. In most families, the disorder does not exhibit a simple pattern of inheritance; it is more likely determined by a complex interaction of many genes and nongenetic factors. A number of geneticists believe that several different types of reading disability exist, and the pattern of inheritance may be different for the different types. Consistent with this idea, reading disability appears to be inherited as an autosomal dominant trait in a small number of families. In these families, about 50 percent of the children of a parent with reading disability also have reading problems. Evidence tentatively suggests that a gene on chromosome 15 may cause reading disability in these select families. However, in most families, the transmission of reading disability is not consistent with an autosomal dominant mode of inheritance, and it is more likely to be caused by the interaction of genetic and environmental factors.

RED HAIR. See Hair color.

RHEUMATOID ARTHRITIS. Rheumatoid arthritis is a disease caused by inflammation and swelling within the joints. Most commonly, the small joints in the fingers and toes are affected, but rheumatoid arthritis may affect the wrists, knees, ankles, or even the neck. During an attack of arthritis, the inflamed joints become red, swollen, stiff, and painful to move.

Rheumatoid arthritis affects about one percent of the population; women are affected more often than men. The disease usually first appears between the ages of 35 and 45, but it may strike people of any age. The symptoms tend to come and go, and rheumatoid arthritis is frequently a chronic, lifelong disease. In a few cases, the joints and associated bones may deteriorate from inflammation, producing permanent crippling.

Rheumatoid arthritis in adults is thought to be an autoimmune disease. (A juvenile form of the disease appears to have different causes.) In an autoimmune disease, the immune system—the body's defense system that normally attacks foreign substances such as bacteria and viruses—somehow becomes confused about what is foreign and what is part of the body; it mistakenly attacks the body's own tissue. In the case of rheumatoid arthritis, membranes within the joints are attacked, and the immune reaction that follows produces swelling and inflammation.

Physicians have long noted that rheumatoid arthritis may occur in several members of the same family. Although heredity appears to be involved, the disease does not follow any simple pattern of inheritance. Rheumatoid arthritis tends to be associated with certain genes that play a role in the ability of the immune system to recognize self and nonself. These genes are part of a large complex of genetic information called the HLA system. Individuals with rheumatoid arthritis are more likely to have particular alleles in the HLA system than are unaffected individuals. For example, one study found that 70 percent of the individuals with rheumatoid arthritis possess the HLA-DR4 allele, whereas only 28 percent of people without the disease have this allele. It appears that possessing particular alleles in the HLA system predisposes one to the disease, although not all those with the predisposing alleles develop arthritis. Clearly, other factors are involved in stimulating the autoimmune response, but the identity of these factors and how they act is not known.

SCHIZOPHRENIA. Schizophrenia, which literally means "split mind," is often thought of as a mental disease characterized by split personality. However, schizophrenia produces a variety of different symptoms, none of which are present in all schizophrenics. Consequently, experts have difficulty agreeing on how to diagnose the disease. There is a good possibility that schizophrenia is not a single disease, but consists of several distinct disorders that have been lumped together because they produce symptoms that superficially appear similar.

Schizophrenia is most commonly defined as disorganization of thought and feeling, often with a gradual withdrawal from reality. People with schizophrenia frequently exhibit disorganized speech; for example, their remarks may jump from subject to subject with no obvious connection. Clear, logical thinking becomes increasingly difficult. Auditory hallucinations, usually in the form of voices, are common. For example, a person with schizophrenia might believe that voices are broadcasting his or her thoughts over the television. Delusions and paranoia also occur. A person with schizophrenia might be convinced, for example, that aliens from space are controlling his or her body.

The symptoms of schizophrenia usually first appear in late adolescence or early adult life. For many of those with schizophrenia, the disease is lifelong. There may be remissions, during which normality returns, but attacks of schizophrenic behavior often recur. However, some patients do recover completely from schizophrenia. Experts believe that about one percent of the general population in the United States has schizophrenia; thus 1.5 to 2 million people in the United States alone suffer from this debilitating disease.

A large number of studies, conducted over many years, have consistently demonstrated that schizophrenia tends to run in families. If one parent has schizophrenia, his or her child has about a ten percent chance of developing the disease. If both parents have schizophrenia, each of their children has about a 40 percent chance of becoming schizophrenic. The observation that schizophrenia runs in families does not prove that the disease is hereditary; multiple members of the same family might be schizophrenic because of predisposing environmental factors that they share. However, adoption and twin studies have demonstrated unequivocally that genes influence schizophrenia. For example, in one early adoption study, geneticists examined a group of 47 adults whose biological mothers had been hospitalized for schizophrenia. Because their mothers were mentally ill, these 47 individuals had been put up for adoption as infants and had grown up with nonschizophrenic foster parents. When examined as adults, five of the adoptees were diagnosed as having schizophrenia. On the other hand, no individuals in a control group of adoptees with nonschizophrenic biological parents later developed the disease. These results strongly implicate genes in the development of schizophrenia. Other adoption studies have produced similar results.

Twin studies also support the conclusion that schizophrenia is heritable. For example, if one identical twin has schizophrenia, there is about a 40 percent chance that the other twin will also have the disorder. However, if one nonidentical twin has schizophrenia, the other twin will develop the disease only about 10 percent of the time. Because identical twins have the same genes whereas nonidentical twins share an average of 50 percent of the same genes, more similarity between identical twins is expected when genes influence a trait. Although twin studies emphasize the importance of genetic factors in schizophrenia, they also emphasize the importance of nongenetic factors in this disease: 60 percent of the time that one identical twin has the disorder, the other twin is normal, which can only be explained by nongenetic influences on schizophrenia.

In spite of strong evidence that genes predispose some individuals to schizophrenia, the exact mode of inheritance is not known. Most cases of schizophrenia do not exhibit a simple pattern of inheritance. Geneticists have proposed three major theories to explain the tendency of schizophrenia to run in families. Some suggest that schizophrenia results from a major gene that produces a predisposition to the disorder. This gene would be inherited in a simple way—perhaps as an autosomal dominant trait. However, not everyone who inherited the gene would develop schizophrenia; other genes and/or environmental factors would play a role in determining which of those with the schizophrenia gene would actually develop the disease. In technical terms, proponents of this theory say that schizophrenia is determined by a major gene with incomplete penetrance. (See Chapter 3 for a discussion of penetrance.) Other geneticists have suggested that schizophrenia arises from the interaction of many genes and environmental factors; technically the disease would be called multifactorial. A third possibility is that schizophrenia is not a single disease, but several separate diseases that only appear similar. Under this theory, called *genetic heterogeneity,* no single pattern of inheritance would be seen for all cases; different types of schizophrenia might exhibit different patterns of inheritance. Several recent studies provide support for the idea that different genes may be involved in the symptoms of schizophrenia. Researchers examined several families in Iceland and in England in which a large number of family members have the disorder. In these families, schizophrenia appeared to be inherited as an autosomal dominant trait. Close examination of DNA from these families indicated that the gene that conferred a predisposition to schizophrenia was located on chromosome 5. However, other researchers examining families from Sweden, Scotland, and Utah could detect no association between schizophrenia and the chromosome 5 gene. These findings suggest that more than one gene may predispose to schizophrenia.

SEX DETERMINISM. In humans, sex is determined by a special pair of chromosomes, appropriately termed the *sex chromosomes.* Females possess two large, X-shaped chromosomes, whereas males possess a single X chromosome and a much smaller chromosome called the Y chromosome. Like all pairs of chromosomes, the sex chromosomes separate when sperm cells and egg cells are formed, one sex chromosome going into each of these reproductive cells. Because females possess two X chromosomes, each egg cell receives one X. Males, on the other hand, possess an X and a Y, so a sperm may receive an X chromosome or a Y chromosome. Chance determines which chromosome any particular sperm acquires, so approximately 50 percent of the sperm acquire an X and 50 percent acquire a Y. At the moment of conception one sperm unites with a single egg and the sex of the offspring is set, determined by which sex chromosome the sperm provides. If the sperm donates an X chromosome, the newly created embryo possesses two X's, one from the egg and one from the sperm. The resulting child will be female. Alternatively, if the sperm carries a Y chromosome, the embryo is endowed with an X and a Y, so the child will be male.

Most of the Y chromosome carries no genetically useful information. However, near the end of the short arm of this chromosome lies a gene that is responsible for the development of male characteristics. This gene is called the *testis determining factor* (TDF) *gene.* Exactly what the TDF gene codes for is not known, but this single gene is the ultimate source of all the anatomical, physiological, and behavioral differences that separate men and women. Other genes on the X and Y chromosomes, as well as numerous genes on the nonsex chromosomes, help determine fertility and code for various male and female features, but the TDF gene is the master switch that controls and activates all other genetic contributors to sex.

When the egg and sperm fuse in the act of fertilization, the sex chromosomes determine the genetic sex of the offspring. However, there are no immediate consequences of this sex determination; initially, both XX and XY embryos develop in an identical manner. Sex-neutral gonads develop within the embryo; they contain tissues with the capacity to become either testes or ovaries. The precursors to both male and female sex ducts also form. At this point the embryo is asexual, capable of becoming either male or female.

In male embryos, a Y chromosome has been inherited from the father; this chromosome contains the TDF gene. About eight weeks after fertilization, the TDF gene somehow triggers the neutral gonad to begin developing into a male testis. As the inner cells of the gonad assume characteristics of a testis, they start producing the male hormone—testosterone. Testosterone stimulates numerous additional changes in the embryo that eventually lead to male anatomy: The male sex ducts grow; the prostate gland and other male glands develop; a scrotum and a penis form; certain parts of the brain that control sexual behavior are altered. Simultaneously, the testis produces a second substance that causes destruction of the female sex ducts. Later, at puberty, testosterone again exerts a strong influence on male development by stimulating male traits, such as facial and pubic hair, a deepening voice, musculature, and the male sex drive.

If a Y chromosome is absent, female structures spontaneously begin to develop by 12 weeks following conception. The gonad develops into an ovary, and the male sex ducts degenerate. Female reproductive structures such as the Fallopian tubes, uterus, and vagina develop. The external female genitals grow. During puberty, female hormones produced by the ovary and the absence of male hormones induce the development of female traits—breast enlargement, growth of the female genitals, pubic hair, and female body shape.

In rare instances, the normal process of sex determination goes awry, and individuals with abnormal or ambiguous sex may result. For example, abnormal numbers of sex chromosomes result in individuals with sexual abnormalities such as *Turner syndrome* (possessing a single X chromosome) and *Klinefelter syndrome* (most commonly possessing XXY). (See Turner syndrome and Klinefelter syndrome). Another rare disorder of the sex chromosomes involves *XX males*, which are individuals with male characteristics in the absence of a Y chromosome. Recent research has determined that at least some of the XX males possess a small part of the Y chromosome, containing the TDF gene, attached to one of their X chromosomes. Conversely, there are rare XY individuals that develop as females. These *XY females* possess a Y chromosome in which the TDF gene is missing, and thus they fail to develop male traits in spite of a Y chromosome.

Another disorder of sexual development, called *androgen insensitivity syndrome*, results in XY individuals—chromosomally male—who produce testosterone, but develop externally as females. Superficially, these individuals appear completely female, with full breasts, a vagina, and a normal female physic. However, the vagina ends blindly, there are no ovaries, uterus, or Fallopian tubes, and testes are present within the abdomen. Because no ovary or uterus is present, these women do not menstruate and are sterile. Androgen insensitivity syndrome results from a genetic defect in a receptor that normally allows the cell to bind testosterone. Because this receptor is defective, testosterone has no effect.

Hermaphrodites—individuals that are both man and woman—have been of part of legends for thousands of years. A *true hermaphrodite* possesses both ovaries and testes. This condition is rare, but a number of hermaphrodites have been reported by physicians. Hermaphrodites can arise in several different ways; some hermaphrodites are XX, some are XY, and still others contain a mixture of XX and XY cells. The reason for the development of both reproductive organs in many of these individuals is unknown and baffling. The external genitals in most cases are sexually ambiguous; about two thirds are raised as females, the other third as males. A few true hermaphrodites have become pregnant.

Female pseudohermaphrodites are chromosomally female (XX) individuals who develop some masculinized traits. The external genitals are variable in appearance, but frequently the clitoris is enlarged and the vagina small. In extreme cases, the external sex may be superficially male. A number of different factors can produce female pseudohermaphroditism, including genetic defects in enzymes that manufacture hormones, abnormal growth of certain glands, and some hormones and drugs taken during pregnancy. *Male pseudohermaphroditism*, in which XY individuals have ambiguous genitals or inadequate masculinization, also occurs; as in female pseudohermaphroditism, there are many potential causes.

SHORT STATURE. In this catalog account, the genetics of proportionate short stature will be discussed, which includes causes of shortness in which the different parts of the body are in normal proportions. Many genetic disorders produce shortness in which the body parts are disproportioned; for example, the head and trunk may be of normal size, but the arms and legs short; these conditions are discussed under Dwarfism. Normal variation in height is discussed under the heading Height.

Normal variation in human height is multifactorial in nature, arising from a complex interaction of numerous genes and environmental factors such as diet and health (see Height). Many individuals are short simply because they are at the lower end of this normal range of variation in height. Most of these individuals come from short parents, and they inherit a tendency to be short, but their pattern of growth is usual in all respects. In contrast to those with normal short stature, a few people are short because they have abnormal patterns of growth.

Abnormally short stature can be caused by many different factors. Although genetic abnormalities of bone development may lead to shortness, most of these conditions produce disproportionate short stature or dwarfism. Most proportionate short stature—the focus of the discussion here—results from other causes. For example, many chromosomal abnormalities such as Down syndrome and Turner syndrome produce retardation of growth and lead to short stature. Genetic defects in enzymes that are important for growth and development, such as phenylkentonuria, cystic fibrosis, and Hurler syndrome, may slow the growth process during childhood and produce children with short stature. A number of genetic syndromes also cause short stature along with other deformities. All of these are genetic causes of short stature; in these conditions the inheritance of short stature will follow the pattern of inheritance characteristic of the genetic defect.

Growth in childhood and during puberty is regulated by hormones, and hormonal deficiencies may also produce short stature. Some, but not all, hormonal disorders are hereditary. Stunted growth can also arise from malnutrition, chronic disease during childhood, and even severe emotional deprivation, which are environmental causes.

Parents are frequently concerned because their children appear short compared to their peers. In such situations, it is important for the parents to recognize that children grow at different rates, and a tremendous amount of normal variation in stature occurs at all ages. The vast majority of these "short" children are within the normal range of height and are growing normally. When one suspects that a child is growing abnormally, a specialist in genetics or endocrinology should be consulted. Pinpointing the exact cause of abnormal growth or short stature can be quite difficult and may require careful measurements or special tests.

SICKLE CELL DISEASE (Sickle Cell Anemia). Hemoglobin is the substance found in red blood cells that transports oxygen and imparts to blood its crimson color; sickle cell disease occurs when this molecule is defective. Stuffed with hemoglobin, each red blood cell is normally disk shaped; these cells are capable of passing through very small blood vessels, carrying oxygen to all parts of the body. In a person with sickle cell disease—also called *sickle cell anemia*—the hemoglobin is genetically altered. Upon exposure to low levels of oxygen, this altered form of hemoglobin induces the red blood cell to change shape or to "sickle," which means that the cell bends into a distorted shape that resembles a sickle. The sickled cells tend to pile up and block the small vessels of the circulatory system. Consequently, oxygen is not delivered to the tissue where sickling occurs, resulting in severe pain and tissue destruction. In addition, the sickled red blood cells are fragile and easily break apart, leading to anemia. Children with sickle cell disease are also susceptible to infections.

Sickle cell disease is most common among people of African descent, occurring with a frequency of one out of every 625 births of American blacks. The disease is inherited as an autosomal recessive disorder. Thus, a child with sickle cell disease possesses two copies of the sickle cell gene, one inherited from each parent. When a couple has a child with sickle cell disease, each additional child they conceive has a one in four chance of having the disease. Carriers of the sickle cell gene are sometimes said to have *sickle cell trait*; these individuals do not have sickle cell disease and are physiologically normal, but they can pass on the sickle cell gene to their offspring. About one in every ten American blacks is a carrier of the sickle cell gene.

Carrier testing is available for detecting those individuals that carry the gene for sickle cell disease. Prenatal testing is also available and can be done with DNA diagnostic procedures on fetal cells obtained through amniocentesis or chorionic villus sampling (see Chapter 6).

There are several different mutations that produce sickle cell disease. The gene that codes for normal hemoglobin is abbreviated *A*, and the most widespread mutation that produces sickle cell hemoglobin is abbreviated *S*. As discussed in Chapter 2, each individual possesses two genes (their genotype) coding for the trait, so a person could possess *AA* (normal), *AS* (normal carrier), or *SS* (sickle cell disease). Another sickle cell mutation is *C*; this gene is found in about three percent of American blacks. Individuals with the genotypes *SC* and *CC* have a less severe form of sickle cell disease. A number of other variants of hemoglobin are also found in low frequency.

The *S* gene that causes sickle cell disease occurs in high frequency throughout tropical Africa; its high frequency in American blacks is a consequence of their African ancestry. The gene is also found in the Middle East. In those areas of Africa and the Middle East where the sickle cell gene is common, malaria is also common. The sickle cell gene has reached high frequency among the peoples of these regions because it confers resistance to malaria when present in a single copy; in other words, individuals with the genotype *AS* are at an advantage because they are less likely to suffer the debilitating effects of malarial disease. Because these individuals are healthier and leave more offspring than those with the *AA* genotype, who are susceptible to malaria, the frequency of the *S* allele has increased in those areas with malaria.

SLEEPWALKING. Sleepwalking is a rather harmless, but bizarre trait. People that sleepwalk get up from bed while still asleep and walk about. During the period of sleepwalking, they usually have their eyes open, but they are generally unresponsive to other people and to events happening around them. Attempts to talk to a sleepwalker or to influence their actions are usually unsuccessful. Sleepwalking episodes may last only a few minutes or they may go on for some time. It is often quite difficult to awaken the person during their sleepwalking. Once awake, the sleepwalker usually cannot remember sleepwalking. Sleepwalking usually begins in childhood, and it often continues into adulthood.

Some experts believe that sleepwalking is related to another sleep disturbance called *night terrors*. A person that experiences night terrors awakens suddenly from deep sleep. For a few minutes, the person is confused, disoriented, and often screams. Their eyes are open, but it is impossible to communicate with them or to calm them down. Their pulse races, their eyes are fully dilated, and they breathe rapidly; they often sweat profusely. During this period of extreme anxiety and disorientation, it is usually impossible to fully arouse the person. The episode typically lasts a few minutes; once completely awake, the person can only vaguely recall a terrifying dream.

One should not confuse night terrors with ordinary nightmares. Nightmares and other dreams occur during a particular period of sleep termed *rapid eye movement* sleep (REM sleep), so called because the eyes tend to move rapidly at this time. Night terrors occur during non-rapid eye movement sleep. Also, nightmares rarely produce the extreme physical symptoms of fright seen in night terrors—the profuse sweating, the dilation of the pupils, the rapid pulse, and the rapid breathing. (These symptoms may occur to some degree in nightmares, but they are much less pronounced than those seen in night terrors.) Also, nightmares are frequently remembered vividly, but night terrors tend to be recalled only in bits and pieces.

Both sleepwalking and night terrors tend to run in families, and frequently both of these sleep disorders occur in members of the same family. One study found that 80 percent of sleepwalkers had one or more relatives that experienced sleepwalking or had night terrors. For those with night terrors, 96 percent had relatives that either sleepwalked or experienced night terrors. Studies of twins indicate that when one twin sleep walks or has night terrors, the other twin is more likely to also be affected when the twins are identical than when the twins are nonidentical. These findings suggest that sleepwalking and night terrors may have a genetic cause, but the numbers of individuals included in these studies is small, so any conclusions about these disorders must be tentative. No simple pattern of inheritance has been observed.

SPINA BIFIDA. See Neural tube defects.

STATURE. See Dwarfism, Height, and Short stature.

STUTTERING. Stuttering is a speech problem that affects 5 percent of all children at some time during their life. Although many children stammer and hesitate when first learning to speak, stuttering as a speech disorder occurs when the child makes frequent repetitions, or prolongations of sounds and words, that disrupt the normal flow of speech and cause problems for the speaker. Most children that stutter begin stuttering before they reach school age. For the majority of these, stuttering lasts less than a year and presents no reason for concern. In all, about 80 percent of those who stutter stop before they reach their sixteenth birthday. However, for a few individuals the problem is severe and continues into adulthood; in these, stuttering may become a major handicap.

Two characteristics of stuttering have long been obvious: Stuttering occurs more frequently in males than females, and stuttering runs in families. Many studies document the familial nature of this disorder. In one typical survey, 38 percent of the stutterers examined had a relative who also stuttered; in contrast, only one percent of nonstutterers had another family member who stuttered. Other studies indicate that this familial tendency results from a strong hereditary influence on stuttering.

Careful examination of families in which stuttering occurs indicates that stuttering is not inherited as a simple genetic trait. It exhibits none of the typical signs of an autosomal dominant, autosomal recessive, or X-linked condition. Multifactorial inheritance—involving both genes and environmental factors—appears to be the most likely explanation for the transmission of stuttering within a family. Because more males than females are affected with this condition, the genes involved appear to be sex influenced; in other words, predisposing genetic factors in males are more easily expressed as stuttering than in females. Put another way, females must have a stronger genetic predisposition to stutter. Evidence for the presence of such sex-influenced genes is seen in the fact that relatives of a female stutterer are more likely to develop stuttering than the relatives of a male stutterer. For example, 19 percent of the brothers of a male stutterer also stutter, but 23 percent of the brothers of a female stutterer are affected. Presumably, this occurs because females who stutter must have a stronger genetic influence, and thus their relatives have a higher chance of inheriting a predisposition for stuttering.

SYNDACTYLY. See Fingers, webbed.

TALIPES EQUINOVARUS. See Clubfoot.

TASTER. See Phenylthiocarbamide (PTC) taster.

TAY-SACHS DISEASE. In 1887, an American physician named Bernard Sachs described a two-year-old girl who had died of a peculiar neurological disorder. The child had been completely normal at birth. At about two months of age, however, her parents noticed she tended to be listless and rolled her eyes around in a curious way. Her muscles were so weak that she was unable to hold her head up or to move about. As the child grew older, she failed to develop mentally: She never played with toys nor seemed to recognize those around her. After her first year, she became completely blind. Her hearing seemed to be particularly acute; the slightest sound would often startle her. Over time, the child's condition steadily worsened, she quit eating properly and finally died of pneumonia.

Over the next several years, Dr. Sachs encountered additional children with the same condition. He discovered that this disorder had been described several years earlier by an English ophthalmologist, Warren Tay, who had noted that the affected children had a cherry red spot on the back of the eye. As additional cases were discovered, almost all in Jewish people, the condition became known as Tay-Sachs disease.

The disorder appears much as described by Bernard Sachs over 100 years ago. The first symptoms, usually muscle weakness, begin between three and six months of age. One of the first things parents notice is that the child is unable to hold its head up. As described by Sachs, the baby startles easily in response to a sharp noise. Muscle weakness usually prevents the child from walking. After one year of age, the child's mental condition deteriorates rapidly. The parents begin to have difficulty feeding the child; blindness and deafness eventually set in. No therapy is available, and all children with Tay-Sachs disease eventually die, most by the age of three.

Tay-Sachs disease results from a defective enzyme called hexosaminidase A, which normally breaks down a fatty substance found in the brain. Termed G_{M2} ganglioside, small amounts of this fatty substance are normally stored in brain cells and are essential for proper brain function. In an individual with Tay-Sachs disease, the hexosaminidase A enzyme cannot break down G_{M2} ganglioside. Consequently, brain cells become stuffed and swollen with G_{M2} ganglioside, and this excess accumulation produces brain damage.

Tay-Sachs disease is inherited as an autosomal recessive disorder; children only develop the disease if both of their parents carry a defective gene for hexosaminidase A. Because the frequency of the gene for Tay-Sachs disease is so low in the general population, the chance of two parents carrying a defective gene is remote. However, the gene for

Tay-Sachs disease occurs in much higher frequency among Jewish people, particularly the Ashkenazi Jews (those descended from Jews who settled in eastern Europe). Among Ashkenazi Jews in the United States, about 1 in 30 individuals carries a defective gene for Tay-Sachs disease. Thus, if two Ashkenazi Jews marry, there is a higher risk that the offspring will inherit two defective copies of the gene and will have Tay-Sachs disease; indeed about 1 in 3,600 Ashkenazi infants is born with the disorder.

Because of the relatively high incidence of Tay-Sachs disease among the Ashkenazi Jews, special programs have been implemented to screen for carriers of the defective gene. A simple blood test can determine whether an individual is a carrier. If only one partner in a marriage carries a copy of the defective gene, all the offspring will be normal, although half of the children will be carriers. If both partners are carriers, then one in four of the offspring, on the average, will be affected with Tay-Sachs disease. For these couples, prenatal testing for Tay-Sachs disease through amniocentesis or chorionic villus sampling is an option.

Screening programs for Tay-Sachs disease carriers in the Ashkenazi community have been remarkably successful. Testing is now available for Ashkenazi Jews in 73 different cities and 13 countries around the world; the success of this effort is demonstrated by the fact that the incidence of Tay-Sachs disease has declined in recent years. In the United States, for example, between 50 and 100 infants with Tay-Sachs disease were born in 1970 before widespread screening; 80 percent of these were of Jewish ancestry. But in 1980, only 13 new patients were reported in the Jewish community.

The gene that causes Tay-Sachs disease is located on the long arm of chromosome 15. There are a number of other genetic disorders related to Tay-Sachs disease, including Sandhoff's disease and the G_{M1} gangliosidoses. These diseases are also inherited as autosomal recessive disorders; all are rare.

THALASSEMIA. Thalassemia is not a single disease, but rather a series of diseases that involve decreased synthesis of one of the components of hemoglobin. Hemoglobin is the substance found in red blood cells; it transports oxygen from the lungs to all parts of the body and imparts to blood its red color. Hemoglobin in normal adults is made up of four protein chains: two beta chains and two alpha chains. In individuals with thalassemia, one of the chains is missing or is produced in greatly reduced amounts. As a result, abnormal hemoglobin forms in the red blood cells. For example, the individual with alpha thalassemia does not produce sufficient amounts of the alpha chain, and thus many hemoglobin molecules contain four beta chains, instead of the normal two alpha and two beta chains. This situation differs from sickle cell disease (see Sickle cell disease), another of the hereditary anemias. In sickle cell disease, the hemoglobin contains two alpha and two beta chains, but the beta chains produced are abnormal.

A number of types of thalassemia occur; these differ in which hemoglobin chains are affected and whether synthesis of the chain is reduced or completely absent. In *beta thalassemia major*, little or no beta chains are produced. This condition is also termed *Cooley's anemia*. Patients with beta thalassemia major experience severe anemia beginning shortly after birth. They are susceptible to infection, exhibit stunted growth, and develop bone deformities. In later years, heart problems frequently occur, and most individuals with this disease die before the age of 30. Beta thalassemia major occurs when two copies of a defective gene for the beta chain are inherited, one from each parent. Thus this disease is inherited as an autosomal recessive trait. If a couple has one child with beta thalassemia major, both parents must be carriers for the thalassemia gene and each additional child has a one in four chance of having the disease.

Another form of thalassemia is *beta thalassemia minor*. Here, a defect occurs in only one of the two copies of the gene coding for the beta chain of hemoglobin. In most cases, only mild anemia results from beta thalassemia minor, and no medical treatment is required. Both types of beta thalassemia are common among people of the Mediterranean region, as well as people from some parts of Africa and Asia. For example, among people in the United States with Greek and Italian ancestry, approximately 1 in 2,500 to 1 in 800 individuals has beta thalassemia major and about 1 in 25 has beta thalassemia minor.

Alpha thalassemia is yet another form of thalassemia that occurs predominantly in people of Mediterranean, African, and Asian origin. In this disorder, production of the alpha hemoglobin chains is curtailed. The symptoms of alpha thalassemia vary, depending on how many of the alpha genes are defective. Alpha thalassemia is also inherited as a recessive trait, but the genetics of the disorder is complicated because most individuals possess four genes coding for alpha hemoglobin. Several additional types of thalassemia also occur in low frequency.

The thalassemias can be detected prenatally by examining blood samples of the fetus, which can be obtained from fetoscopy or fetal blood sampling. Newer tests that utilize DNA analysis can also detect these diseases on cells obtained from amniocentesis or chorionic villus sampling.

THYROID DISEASE. Located in the neck, the thyroid gland is a small mass of tissue found on either side of the windpipe. It produces thyroid hormones, which play an important role in regulating growth and metabolism. A number of different diseases of the thyroid gland occur, some of which are hereditary and some of which are not. These thyroid diseases can be divided into two major groups: those that cause an overproduction of thyroid hormone, which is termed *hyperthyroidism,* and those that result in an underproduction of thyroid hormones, which is called *hypothyroidism.* In this section, three types of thyroid diseases that have a hereditary basis will be discussed: Graves' disease, which is a common form of hyperthyroidism; cretinism, which involves hypothyroidism in children; and Hashimoto's disease, which is an inflammation of the thyroid gland. It is important to understand that a number of other thyroid diseases also occur, and most of these are *not* hereditary.

Cretinism. This is a condition that results from a deficiency of thyroid hormone in the fetus and in infancy. Deficiency of thyroid hormone profoundly affects a child's physical and mental development; if untreated, thyroid deficiency produces dwarfism and mental retardation. The hormone deficiency of cretinism may be caused by birth defects in the thyroid gland itself—frequently part or all of the thyroid is missing. These deformities exhibit some tendency to run in families, but the genetics is still poorly understood. Treatment is available and consists of giving the child thyroid hormone; if therapy is begun soon after birth, many affected children grow normally and improve in mental ability.
　　Cretinism also arises when a genetic defect occurs in one of several enzymes involved in the synthesis of thyroid hormone. Most of these enzyme disorders are rare and are inherited as autosomal recessive traits.

Hashimoto's Disease. Hashimoto's disease is characterized by an inflammation of the thyroid gland that commonly produces goiter—an enlargement of the thyroid gland. (Other thyroid disorders also produce goiter; most of these are not genetic.) Hashimoto's disease typically strikes women in their thirties and forties, although it can occur in either sex and at any age. Experts believe that Hashimoto's disease is an autoimmune disorder. The immune system—the defense network of the body—functions to rid the body of foreign organisms, such as bacteria and viruses. Normally, the immune system recognizes its own cells and attacks only substances that are foreign. However, for reasons that are poorly understood, occasionally the immune system mistakenly attacks some of the body's own cells. The resulting inflammation and tissue destruction are referred to as an *autoimmune disease*. In Hashimoto's disease, the immune system attacks the thyroid gland, causing it to become inflamed and defective.

A predisposition to Hashimoto's disease can be inherited. Frequently, a patient with Hashimoto's disease has a close relative with the same disorder. However, the disease exhibits no simple pattern of inheritance and most evidence suggests that it is multifactorial in nature (influenced by a combination of genetic and nongenetic factors; see Chapter 4).

Graves' Disease. Graves' disease is a common form of hyperthyroidism, in which the thyroid gland produces too much thyroid hormone. The excess hormone typically causes symptoms of nervousness, weakness, a sensitivity to heat, sweating, overactivity, and weight loss in spite of a healthy appetite. In individuals with Graves' disease, the thyroid gland frequently becomes enlarged and sometimes the eyes bulge. The exact cause of Graves' disease is not known, although it is probably another example of an autoimmune disease. Graves' disease tends to run in families, but the inheritance is poorly understood. Researchers have observed that Graves' disease tends to be associated with certain genetic variants (HLA alleles) of the immune system; however, the significance of this association is not clear at the present time.

TONGUE ROLLING. The ability to roll the tongue into a U-shaped trough is called *tongue rolling*. Some people can roll their tongues, but others cannot. Tongue rolling is often said to be a simple genetic trait, with the ability to roll the tongue dominant over the inability to roll it. However, recent twin studies indicate that this trait is *not* genetically determined.

TURNER SYNDROME. Sex in humans is determined by a special pair of chromosomes, the so-called sex chromosomes. Normally, females possess two X chromosomes, whereas males possess one X and a different sex chromosome called the Y. Occasionally accidents occur in the division of the sex chromosomes, and individuals are produced that possess abnormal numbers or arrangements of these chromosomes. One such disorder is Turner syndrome. In Turner syndrome, a single X chromosome is present. Individuals with this syndrome are female in appearance, but possess some distinctive characteristics including short stature, a low hairline, a broad chest, and folds of skin on the neck. Women with Turner syndrome rarely mature sexually without hormone treatment; typically they do not menstruate, their breast development is slight, and their pubic hair is sparse. Sterility is the rule, although a few women with Turner syndrome have borne children. Most Turner women possess normal intelligence. Height and the development of female traits, such as breast development, can be improved by treatment with hormones, but fertility cannot be restored. When treated, girls with Turner syndrome are fully capable of marriage, sexual fulfillment, and raising a family through adoption.

About 60 percent of the individuals with Turner syndrome have a single X chromosome. Others may be mosaics, possessing some cells with a single X and other cells with two or three X's. In other cases of Turner syndrome, part of one of the X chromosomes may be missing. Most of these chromosome abnormalities arise as random accidents during the process of chromosome division, and it is rare for such accidents to occur in more than one child in the same family.

TWINS. In many animals, each pregnancy produces a litter of offspring. In humans, however, multiple births are uncommon: only 1 in 90 births produces twins, only 1 in 8,000 births produces triplets, and only one in a million births produces quadruplets. Although rare, multiple births have been the subject of human fascination for centuries; they have also been the focus of numerous genetic studies. Human twins come in two types: nonidentical twins and identical twins.

Nonidentical Twins. In a fertile woman, the ovary normally releases a single egg each month. Occasionally, however, two eggs may be released at the same time. If both eggs are fertilized—each by a different sperm—nonidentical twins result. Nonidentical twins are also called *dizygotic twins,* which literally means "from two zygotes." (*Zygote* is a technical term for embryo.) Another term frequently used for nonidentical twins is *fraternal twins.* On the average, nonidentical twins share 50 percent of the same genes, which is the same proportion of genes shared by all brothers and sisters. Nonidentical twins may be the same sex—both boys or both girls—or they can be different sexes—a boy and a girl.

The frequency of nonidentical twins differs among human racial groups. In North American Caucasians, nonidentical twins are born at a rate of about 7 nonidentical twin pairs per 1,000 pregnancies. In Orientals, the rate is about 3 per 1,000. The highest rate of twinning occurs among Nigerians, where 1 in 25 pregnancies (40 per 1,000) produces nonidentical twins. Age of the mother influences the probability of producing nonidentical twins: Up to the age of 37, older women are more likely to produce nonidentical twins, but after age 37, the rate of twinning declines. The age of the father apparently has no effect on the probability of producing twins.

Both genetic and environmental factors affect the conception of nonidentical twins. For nonidentical twins to arise, the mother's ovaries must release two eggs in the same menstrual cycle; thus twinning is really a trait of the mother, not the twins themselves. Any factor that stimulates the release of multiple eggs will increase a woman's chances of producing nonidentical twins. One factor already mentioned—maternal age—influences nonidentical twinning. Some fertility drugs also stimulate the ovary to release multiple eggs; thus these drugs increase the chances of producing twins.

Heredity also plays a role in twinning, and producing nonidentical twins tends to run in families. Genealogical records of the Mormon church show that female twins produce twins at a rate of about 17 per 1,000 pregnancies, compared to an average rate of only 7 per 1,000 among most women in the U.S. population. Male twins, however, do not have more twin offspring than other fathers. Sisters of twins are more likely to have twins, but brothers are not. These facts indicate that producing nonidentical twins is genetic—at least to some extent—but that the tendency to produce nonidentical twins is only expressed in females. Producing twins is not inherited as a simple genetic trait; the transmission appears to be multifactorial, involving multiple genes and environmental factors.

Identical Twins. Identical twins arise from a single egg fertilized by a single sperm, initially producing one embryo. Later, this embryo divides producing two embryos that then develop into two babies. Identical twins are also called *monozygotic twins,* which means "from a single zygote." Because they originated from a single egg and sperm, these twins are genetically identical, sharing 100 percent of the same genes. Identical twins are always the same sex. The splitting of the original embryo appears to be largely a chance event, which is not influenced by maternal age or fertility drugs. In most ethnic groups this event occurs with a frequency of about 4 twin pairs per 1,000 pregnancies. Recent research indicates that the production of identical twins may have a slight tendency to run in families, but any genetic influence on identical twinning is much weaker than that observed for nonidentical twinning.

WEIGHT.   Experts estimate that 25 to 50 percent of all people in affluent societies are overweight, and obesity is one of the most serious health problems of modern culture. Obesity increases the chances of developing heart disease, high blood pressure, and diabetes. It shortens length of life, it can cause psychological problems and, in severe cases, obesity can be an incapacitating handicap.

Obesity frequently runs in the family. Statistics show that when both parents are obese, their children have an 80 percent chance of also being obese. On the other hand, when both parents have normal weight, the chance of their children being obese is less than 15 percent. The similarity of body weight that is observed among members of the same family need not be genetic, however. Because members of a family typically eat together, the types and amounts of foods eaten are often similar for members of the same family. Furthermore, activity patterns, eating habits, and attitudes about exercise may be learned and produce similarity in the body weights of relatives.

A number of genetic studies have examined the role of heredity in body weight and obesity. Most of these studies have concluded that genes affect body weight; however, most also report that environmental factors make an important contribution to body weight, and the relative importance of genes versus environment in determining body weight has been controversial. Some studies conclude that genes are very important in determining weight. Others find that the effect of genes is relatively minor, and environmental factors play a larger role. Many of these studies have methodological problems and cannot completely separate the influence of genes from the effects of environment. However, several recent studies have attracted wide attention, because they examined the role of heredity in body weight and obesity in large numbers of twins and adopted individuals. These studies indicate that genes play an important part in determining individual differences in body weight.

In one study, geneticists examined the body weight of over 13,000 male twins born between 1917 and 1927 and who served in the U.S. armed forces. Because weight is correlated with height, and height is inherited, weight and height values were converted to a body-mass index, which provides an estimate of weight that is independent of height. Body-mass index was examined at the time of induction into the armed forces (at ages 18 to 28) and again approximately 25 years later when the twins were 40 to 50 years of age. Identical twins tended to be much more similar in body-mass index than nonidentical twins, which is exactly the result expected when genes influence a trait. (Identical twins share 100 percent of the same genes, whereas nonidentical twins share an average of only 50 percent of their genes; thus, if genes influence a trait, identical twins should be more similar to one another than nonidentical twins.) Furthermore, the study estimated that about 80 percent of the differences in body-mass index were produced by genetic factors and that this difference remained relatively stable over the adult lifetime. Other twin studies suggest that approximately 80 percent of the variation in obesity among children is genetically determined.

The most convincing evidence for a genetic influence on adult body weight comes from adoption studies. In these studies, the weights of adopted individuals are compared with the weights of their biological parents, with whom they share genes in common, and with the weights of their foster parents, with whom they share a common environment. The largest adoption study ever conducted on body weight examined 540 Danish adults, who were adopted by unrelated foster parents between 1924 and 1947. The adult weights of these adoptees were compared with the adult weights of their biological parents and with the adult weights of their foster parents. The results showed that obese adoptees tended to have heavy biological parents, and thin adoptees tended to have thin biological parents. There was no relationship between the weights of the adoptees and the weights of their foster parents.

The conclusion from these recent twin and adoption studies is that genes play an important role in determining weight in adult humans. However, caution must be used in applying these conclusions too widely. One study was conducted on American males who served in the armed services and the other study examined Danish adoptees. The results indicated that *in these groups* genes are important in determining weight, but the situation may differ for other groups. For example, in less developed countries there may be larger environmental differences in nutrition; some children from upper-income families may receive an excellent diet, whereas those from low-income families may be malnourished. In these societies, environment may be more important and heredity less important in determining differences in adult weight. Other studies have frequently reported that environment plays a much more important role in human weight than that suggested by the recent studies discussed here; this discrepancy may be due to differences in the populations examined or may reflect different methodologies for analyzing the influence of heredity.

Body weight is not inherited in a simple manner. Most likely, this is a multifactorial trait, influenced by multiple genes and environmental factors.

How genes influence body weight is not clear. The genes affecting body weight may act on the basic metabolic rate of the body; in other words, some individuals may burn more calories in normal day-to-day activities than others, and these genetic differences in metabolic rate might affect differences in body weight. Indeed, several recent studies indicate that substantial genetic differences do exist in basic metabolic rate. Another possibility is that genetic factors influence activity patterns, which in turn influence the number of calories burned. A recent study concluded that people do differ genetically in their daily levels of activities. Genes may also affect eating habits or appetite.

However they exert their influence, one should keep in mind that genes alone do not determine body weight. Environment is certainly important. One must eat to gain weight, and starvation and/or physical exertion will reduce weight. Genes may, however, predispose one toward a particular body weight; they may influence one's potential to gain and lose weight. Thus, some individuals may gain weight more easily than others at a given level of food and exercise. However, genes do not automatically determine body weight; ultimately, body weight results from how much one eats and exercises.

WILSON'S DISEASE. Wilson's disease is a rare, but treatable hereditary disorder of copper metabolism. Although the exact biochemical defect that causes Wilson's disease is unknown, copper accumulates in various body tissues, producing liver damage, neurological symptoms, and psychiatric problems. Most individuals with this disorder do not begin to experience symptoms until late childhood or early adult life. Liver disease is one of the first symptoms. Later, neurological problems develop, including problems with muscle movement and muscle coordination. Patients often exhibit personality changes, hysteria, and schizophrenia-like symptoms. The disease can be treated successfully with drugs that remove copper from the body; without treatment, patients with the disorder eventually die. Wilson's disease occurs in about 1 out of every 100,000 births. It is caused by an autosomal recessive gene that appears to reside on chromosome 13. An autosomal recessive disease occurs when an individual inherits two copies of the defective gene; thus, if a couple has one child with Wilson's disease, both parents are carriers of the defective gene, and each additional child they produce will possess a one in four chance of having the disease. If one parent has Wilson's disease, all of their children will be normal unless the other parent is a carrier; this event is unlikely. However, if one parent has the disease and the other parent is a carrier, half of the children will develop Wilson's disease.

Appendix I

CLINICAL GENETIC SERVICES CENTERS IN THE UNITED STATES

The following directory of genetics counseling and diagnosis centers has been made available by the National Center for Education in Maternal and Child Health (*Comprehensive Clinical Genetic Services Centers: A National Directory—1985*). These centers provide comprehensive genetic services to those who need genetic counseling, prenatal diagnosis, or treatment of genetic diseases. The centers are listed alphabetically by state and by city within state. Many centers provide some services at satellite sites in additional cities; information about satellite sites has not been included, but can be obtained from the centers.

Information about these centers was obtained directly from the centers and from state health officials. Inclusion in the directory does not constitute endorsement by the National Center for Education in Maternal and Child Health nor by the author of this book.

ALABAMA

Birmingham

University of Alabama in
  Birmingham Medical Center
University Station
1720 Seventh Avenue South
Birmingham, Alabama 35294

  Laboratory of Medical Genetics
  Phone: (205) 934-4973

Mobile

University of South Alabama College
  of Medicine
U.S.A. Medical Center
Moorer Building
2451 Fillingim Street
Mobile, Alabama 36617

  Department of Medical Genetics
  Phone: (205) 476-6305

ALASKA

Anchorage

Genetics and Birth Defects Clinic
March of Dimes Birth Defects
  Foundation
4600 Shelikof Street
Anchorage, Alaska 99507

  Department of Health and Social
    Services
  Division of Public Health
  Phone: (907) 563-3391

ARIZONA

Tempe

The Genetics Center of
Southwest Biomedical Research
  Institute
123 East University Drive
Tempe, Arizona 85281
  Phone: (602) 894-1104

Tucson

University of Arizona Health Science
  Center
College of Medicine
1401 North Campbell Avenue
Tucson, Arizona 85724

  Department of Obstetrics and
    Gynecology
  Phone: (602) 626-6324

ARKANSAS

Little Rock

University of Arkansas Medical
  Sciences Center
4301 West Markham
Little Rock, Arkansas 72205

  Department of Pediatrics
    Slot 512B
  Phone: (501) 661-5991

CALIFORNIA

Alhambra

The Genetics Institute
1708 West Huntington
Alhambra, California 91801

  Phone: (818) 281-0954

Anaheim

Southern California Permanente
  Medical Group
Anaheim Medical Arts Building
1188 North Euclid
Anaheim, California 92801

  Department of Genetics Services
  Phone: (714) 778-8624 (Kaiser
    members only)

Duarte

City of Hope National Medical
  Center
1500 East Duarte Road
Duarte, California 91010

  Department of Medical Genetics
  Phone: (818) 359-8111, ext. 2631

Fresno

Valley Children's Hospital
3151 North Millbrook
Fresno, California 93703

  Department of Medical Genetics
    and Prenatal Detection
  Phone: (209) 225-3000, ext. 1437

Harbor City

Kaiser-Permanente Medical Center
1100 West Pacific Coast Highway
Harbor City, California 90710

  Department of Pediatrics
  Division of Medical Genetics
  Phone: (213) 517-2898 (Kaiser
    members only)

La Jolla

University of California San Diego
Basic Science Building, M-013-F
La Jolla, California 92093

  Department of Medicine
  Division of Medical Genetics
  Phone: (619) 452-4307/4308

Loma Linda

Loma Linda University Medical
  Center
11234 Anderson Street, Room A-527
Loma Linda, California 92350

  Department of Pediatrics
  Division of Genetics
  Phone: (714) 796-7311, ext. 2838

Los Angeles

Children's Hospital of Los Angeles
4650 Sunset Boulevard
Los Angeles, California 90027

Department of Pediatrics
Division of Medical Genetics
Phone: (213) 699-2238

Kaiser-Permanente Medical Center
6041 Cadillac Avenue
Los Angeles, California 90034

Department of Pediatrics
Division of Medical Genetics
Phone: (213) 857-3493 (Kaiser
members only)

Los Angeles County—University of
Southern California Medical Center
1129 North State Street
Los Angeles, California 90033

Department of Pediatrics
Division of Genetics—Cytogenetics
Laboratory
Phone: (213) 226-3816

Martin Luther King Jr. General
Hospital
12021 South Wilmington Avenue
Los Angeles, California 90059

Department of Pediatrics
Phone: (213) 603-4641

Department of Obstetrics and
Gynecology
Phone: (213) 603-3134

University of California Los Angeles
Center for Health Sciences
Los Angeles, California 90024

Department of Pediatrics
Division of Medical Genetics
Phone: (213) 206-6581

Oakland

Children's Hospital
747 52nd Street
Oakland, California 94609

Medical Genetics Unit
Phone: (415) 428-3550

Kaiser-Permanente Medical Care
Program
280 West MacArthur Boulevard
Oakland, California 94611

Department of Genetics
Phone: (415) 428-5816 (Kaiser
members only)

Orange

University of California at Irvine
Irvine Medical Center
101 City Drive South
Orange, California 92668

Department of Pediatrics
Division of Clinical Genetics and
Developmental Disabilities
Phone: (714) 634-5791

Panorama City

Kaiser-Permanente Medical Center
13652 Cantara Street
Panorama City, California 91402-5497

Department of Pediatrics
Division of Genetic Services
Phone: (818) 908-2650 (Kaiser
members only)

Sacramento

Kaiser-Permanente Medical Care
Program
2025 Morse Avenue
Sacramento, California 95825

Department of Genetics
Phone: (916) 486-6726 (Kaiser
members only)

University of California at Davis
School of Medicine and Medical
Center
4301 X Street
Sacramento, California 95817

Department of Pediatrics
Medical Genetic Services
Phone: (916) 453-3721

San Diego

Children's Hospital and Health
Center San Diego
8001 Frost Street
San Diego, California 92123

Department of Dysmorphology and
Genetics
Birth Defects and Genetic
Counseling Clinic
Phone: (619) 576-5808

San Diego Regional Center for the
Developmentally Disabled
4355 Ruffin Road
San Diego, California 92123
Phone: (619) 576-2961

University Hospital
University of California, San Diego
Medical Center
225 Dickinson Street, H-814
San Diego, California 92103

Department of Pediatrics
Division of Genetics and
Dysmorphology
Phone: (714) 294-6992

San Francisco

University of California San Francisco
Third and Parnassus Avenue
San Francisco, California 94143

Department of Pediatrics   U-100
Division of Medical Genetics
Phone: (415) 666-2757 Genetics
       (415) 666-4080 Prenatal

San Jose

Kaiser-Permanente Medical Care
Program
260 International Circle
San Jose, California 95119

Department of Genetics
Phone: (408) 972-3300 (Kaiser
members only)

Stanford

Stanford University Medical Center
300 Pasteur Drive, Room A335A
Stanford, California 94305

Department of Pediatrics
Birth Defects/Genetics Center
Phone: (415) 497-6858

Torrance

Harbor UCLA Medical Center
1000 West Carson Street
Torrance, California 90509

Department of Pediatrics
Division of Medical Genetics
Phone: (213) 533-3667 Clinic
       (213) 533-3759 Prenatal

COLORADO

Denver

The Children's Hospital
1056 East 19th Avenue
Denver, Colorado 80218

Department of Pediatric Medicine
Division of Genetic Services
Phone: (303) 861-6395

Rose Medical Center
University of Colorado School of
  Medicine
4567 East Ninth Avenue
Denver, Colorado 80220

Department of Genetics
Phone: (303) 320-2955

University of Colorado Health
  Sciences Center
School of Medicine   B-160
4200 East Ninth Avenue
Denver, Colorado 80262

Department of Pediatrics
Genetics Unit
Phone: (303) 394-8742/8777

CONNECTICUT

Farmington

University of Connecticut Health
  Center
School of Medicine
Farmington, Connecticut 06032

Department of Pediatrics
Division of Genetics
Phone: (203) 674-2676

New Haven

Yale University School of Medicine
333 Cedar Street
New Haven, Connecticut 06510

Department of Human Genetics
Genetic Consultation Service
Phone: (203) 785-2660

DELAWARE

Newark

Medical Center of Delaware
Christiana Hospital
P.O. 6001
Newark, Delaware 19718

Department of Pediatrics
Cytogenetics Laboratory
Phone: (302) 733-3530

Wilmington

Alfred I. duPont Institute
P.O. Box 269
Wilmington, Delaware 19899

Department of Medical Genetics
Phone: (302) 651-4234

DISTRICT OF COLUMBIA

Washington

Children's Hospital National Medical
  Center
111 Michigan Avenue, N.W.
Washington, D.C. 20010

Department of Clinical Genetics
Phone: (202) 745-2187

Columbia Hospital for Women
2425 L Street, N.W.
Washington, D.C. 20037

Department of Obstetrics and
  Gynecology
Division of Maternal-Fetal Medicine
Phone: (202) 293-5135

George Washington University
  Medical Center
Wilson Genetics Unit
Ross Hall 455
2300 I Street, N.W.
Washington, D.C. 20037

Department of Obstetrics and
  Gynecology
Phone: (202) 676-4096

Georgetown University Medical
  Center
3800 Reservoir Road, N.W.
Washington, D.C. 20007

Department of Obstetrics and
  Gynecology
Division of Medical Genetics
Phone: (202) 625-7852

Department of Pediatrics
Center for Genetic Counseling and
  Birth Defect Evaluation
Phone: (202) 625-2348

Howard University
College of Medicine
Box 75
520 W Street, N.W.
Washington, D.C. 20059

  Department of Pediatrics and Child
    Health
  Division of Medical Genetics
  Phone: (202) 636-7224

FLORIDA

Gainesville

University of Florida
College of Medicine, Box J-296
J. Hillis Milles Health Center
Gainesville, Florida 32610

  Department of Pediatrics
  Division of Genetics
  Phone: (904) 392-2957

Jacksonville

University Hospital of Jacksonville
655 West 8th Street
Jacksonville, Florida 32209

  Department of Pediatrics
  Division of Genetics
  Phone: (904) 350-6872

Miami

University of Miami
School of Medicine
Miami, Florida 33101

Department of Medicine
Division of Genetic Medicine
P.O. Box 016960
1500 N.W. 12th Avenue
Phone: (305) 547-6652

Department of Pediatrics
Mailman Center for Child
  Development
Division of Endocrinology,
  Genetics and Metabolism
P.O. Box 016820
1601 N.W. 12th Avenue
Phone: (305) 547-6091

Tampa

University of South Florida
College of Medicine
Box 15-G
12901 North 30th Street
Tampa, Florida 33612

  Department of Pediatrics
  Division of Medical Genetics
  Phone: (813) 974-3310

GEORGIA

Atlanta

Emory University School of Medicine
2040 Ridgewood Drive
Atlanta, Georgia 30322

  Department of Pediatrics
  Division of Medical Genetics
  Director: Louis J. Elsas, II, M.D.

Augusta

Human Genetics Institute
Medical College of Georgia
1120 Fifteenth Street   CJ-263
Augusta, Georgia 30912
  Phone: (404) 828-2828

HAWAII

Honolulu

Kapiolani Children's Hospital
University of Hawaii
1319 Punahou Street
Honolulu, Hawaii 96826

   Department of Genetics and
      Pediatrics
   Division of Medical Genetic
      Services
   Phone: (808) 948-6872/6834

IDAHO

Boise

Idaho Department of Health and
   Welfare
2220 Old Penitentiary Road
Boise, Idaho 83712

   Department of Health and Welfare
   Bureau of Laboratories
   Phone: (208) 334-5271

ILLINOIS

Chicago

Children's Memorial Hospital
2300 Children's Plaza
Chicago, Illinois 60614

   Division of Genetics
   Phone: (312) 880-4462

Cook County Children's Hospital
700 South Wood Street
Chicago, Illinois 60612

   Department of Pediatrics
   Division of Genetics and
      Metabolism
   Phone: (312) 633-7768

Illinois Masonic Medical Center
836 West Wellington
Chicago, Illinois 60657

   Department of Pediatrics
   Division of Medical Genetics
   Phone: (312) 975-1600, ext. 5705

Michael Reese Hospital and Medical
   Center
Lakeshore Drive at 31st Street
Chicago, Illinois 60616

   Department of Pathology
   Division of Medical Genetics
   Phone: (312) 791-4436

Mount Sinai Hospital
Medical Center of Chicago
California Avenue at 15th Street
Chicago, Illinois 60608

   Department of Pediatrics
   Division of Genetics
   Phone: (312) 650-6472

Prentice Women's Hospital
Northwestern University Medical
   School
333 East Superior Street
Chicago, Illinois 60611

   Department of Obstetrics and
      Gynecology
   Division of Human Genetics
   Phone: (312) 649-7441

Rush-Presbyterian—St. Luke's
   Medical Center
1753 West Congress Parkway
Chicago, Illinois 60612

   Department of Pediatrics
   Section of Genetics
   Phone: (312) 942-6298

University of Chicago Hospital and
Clinics
Pritzker School of Medicine
South Maryland Avenue
Chicago, Illinois 60637

Department of Obstetrics and
Gynecology
Division of Sciences Division
Phone: (312) 962-6588

Department of Pediatrics—Box 413
Phone: (312) 962-6174

University of Illinois
College of Medicine at Chicago
840 South Wood Street
Chicago, Illinois 60612

Department of Pediatrics
Division of Genetics and
Metabolism
Phone: (312) 996-6714

Evanston

Evanston Hospital
2530 Ridge Avenue
Evanston, Illinois 60201

Department of Pediatrics
Division of Genetics
Phone: (312) 492-6771

Park Ridge

Lutheran General Hospital
1775 Dempster
Park Ridge, Illinois 60068

Department of Pediatrics
Division of Medical Genetics
Phone: (312) 696-7705

Springfield

Southern Illinois University
School of Medicine
P.O. Box 3926
Springfield, Illinois 62708

Department of Pediatrics
Division of Genetics Program
Phone: (217) 782-8460

Urbana

Genetic Counseling Service and
Laboratory
Regional Health Resource Center
1408 West University Avenue
Urbana, Illinois 61801

Phone: (217) 333-8172

INDIANA

Evansville

Tri-State Regional Genetics Services
Center
The Rehabilitation Center, Inc.
3701 Bellemead Avenue
Evansville, Indiana 47715

Phone: (812) 479-1411

Fort Wayne

Northeastern Indiana Genetics
Counseling Center
Parkview Memorial Hospital
2200 Randalia Drive
Fort Wayne, Indiana 46805

Phone: (219) 484-6636, ext. 4146

Indianapolis

Riley Hospital, RR 129
Indiana University School of
Medicine
702 Barnhill Drive
Indianapolis, Indiana 46223

Department of Medical Genetics
Phone: (317) 264-2241

South Bend

North Central Indiana Regional
   Genetics Counseling Center
Memorial Hospital
615 North Michigan Street
South Bend, Indiana 46601

   Phone: (219) 284-7300

IOWA

Iowa City

University of Iowa Hospitals and
   Clinics
Iowa City, Iowa 52242

   Department of Obstetrics and
      Gynecology
   Prenatal Diagnosis Program
   Phone: (319) 356-2631

   Department of Pediatrics
   Division of Medical Genetics
   Phone: (319) 356-2674

   Department of Pediatrics
   Regional Genetic Consultation
      Service
   Phone: (319) 356-2674

KANSAS

Kansas City

University of Kansas Medical Center
39th and Rainbow Boulevard
Kansas City, Kansas 66103

   Department of Medicine—Room
      4023-C
   Division of Metabolism,
      Endocrinology and Genetics
   Phone: (913) 588-6043

Wichita

University of Kansas
School of Medicine—Wichita
1010 North Kansas
Wichita, Kansas 67214

Wesley Medical Center
Prenatal Diagnosis and Genetic Clinic
550 North Hillside
Wichita, Kansas 67214

   Departments of Pediatrics and
      Obstetrics and Gynecology
   Division of Medical Genetics
   Phone: (316) 261-2622 Genetics
      Clinic
      (316) 688-2360 Prenatal

KENTUCKY

Lexington

University of Kentucky School of
   Medicine
800 Rose Street
Lexington, Kentucky 40536

   Department of Pediatrics
   Division of Genetics and
      Dysmorphology
   Phone: (606) 233-5558

Louisville

University of Louisville Medical
   School
334 East Broadway
Louisville, Kentucky 40202

   Department of Pediatrics
   Child Evaluation Center
   Clinical Genetics and
      Dysmorphology Clinic
   Genetic Outreach Clinics
   Phone: (502) 588-5331

LOUISIANA

New Orleans

Louisiana State University Medical
  Center
1542 Tulane Avenue
New Orleans, Louisiana 70112

Department of Pediatrics
Division of Genetics
Phone: (504) 568-6221

Tulane University School of Medicine
1430 Tulane Avenue
New Orleans, Louisiana 70112

The Hayward Genetics Center
Human Genetics Program
Phone: (504) 588-5229

Shreveport

University Hospital
Louisiana State University
School of Medicine
1501 Kings Highway
Shreveport, Louisiana 71130

Department of Pediatrics
Birth Defects Center
Phone: (318) 674-6088

MAINE

Bangor

Eastern Maine Medical Center
489 State Street
Bangor, Maine 04401

Department of Pediatrics
Genetics Program
Phone: (207) 945-7354

Scarborough

Foundation for Blood Research
P.O. Box 428
Scarborough, Maine 04074

Division of Clinical Genetics
Phone: (207) 883-4131

MARYLAND

Baltimore

Johns Hopkins University
School of Medicine
Baltimore, Maryland 21205

Department of Medicine
Division of Medical Genetics
The Moore Clinic
600 North Wolfe Street
Phone: (301) 955-3122

Department of Pediatrics
  CMSC-1004
Division of Pediatric Genetics
601 North Broadway
Phone: (301) 955-3071

Department of Obstetrics and
  Gynecology CMSC-1001
Prenatal Diagnostic Center
601 North Broadway
Phone: (301) 955-3091

University of Maryland School of
  Medicine
655 West Baltimore Street
Baltimore, Maryland 21201

Departments of Obstetrics and
  Gynecology and Pediatrics
Division of Human Genetics
Phone: (301) 528-3480

Bethesda

National Institutes of Health
Building 10, Room 9C-436
Bethesda, Maryland 20205

Inter-Institute Clinical Genetics
  Program
Phone: (301) 496-1380

MASSACHUSETTS

Boston

Boston University Medical Center
80 East Concord Street
Boston, Massachusetts 02118

Department of Pediatrics
Division of Human Services
Phone: (617) 247-5720

Brigham and Women's Hospital
721 Huntington Avenue
Boston, Massachusetts 02115

Department of Medicine
Genetics Clinic
Phone: (617) 583-4500, ext. 279

Children's Hospital Medical Center
300 Longwood Avenue
Boston, Massachusetts 02115

Department of Pediatric Medicine
Genetics Division
Phone: (617) 735-7577, ext. 6394

Massachusetts General Hospital
Boston, Massachusetts 02114

Children's Service
Genetics Unit
Phone: (617) 726-3826/3827/3828

Tufts New England Medical Center
171 Harrison Avenue
Boston, Massachusetts 02111

Department of Pediatrics
Center for Birth Defects and
Genetic Counseling
Phone: (617) 956-5454

Waltham

Eunice Kennedy Shriver Center
200 Trapelo Road
Waltham, Massachusetts 02154

Division of Genetics
Phone: (617) 893-4909

Worcester

University of Massachusetts Medical
Center
55 Lake Avenue North
Worcester, Massachusetts 02105

Department of Pediatrics
Genetics Clinic
Phone: (617) 856-3949

MICHIGAN

Ann Arbor

University of Michigan Medical
School
Ann Arbor, Michigan 48109-0010

Department of Internal Medicine
and Human Genetics
Division of Medical Genetics
Box 015
1137 Catherine Street
Phone: (313) 763-2532

C. S. Mott Children's Hospital
Department of Pediatrics
Section of Pediatric Genetics
D1225 Medical Professional Building
Box 46

Phone: (313) 764-0579

Detroit

Hutzel Hospital
Wayne State University School of
Medicine
4707 St. Antoine Boulevard
Detroit, Michigan 48201

Department of Gynecology and
Obstetrics
Phone: (313) 484-7066

Henry Ford Hospital
2799 West Grand Boulevard
Detroit, Michigan 48202

Medical Genetics and Birth Defects
Center
Phone: (313) 876-3116

Children's Hospital of Michigan
Wayne State University
3901 Beaubien Boulevard
Detroit, Michigan 48201

Department of Pediatrics
Division of Clinical Genetics and
Metabolic Disorders
Phone: (313) 494-4513

East Lansing

Michigan State University
B240 Life Sciences Building
East Lansing, Michigan 48824

Department of Pediatrics and
Human Development
Division of Human Genetics,
Immunology, and Toxicology
Phone: (517) 355-2046

Grand Rapids

Blodgett Memorial Medical Center
1840 Wealthy Street, S.E.
Grand Rapids, Michigan 49506

Genetics/Birth Defects/Neurology
Clinic
Phone: (616) 774-7803

Royal Oak

William Beaumont Hospital
3601 West 13 Mile Road
Royal Oak, Michigan 48072

Department of Anatomic Pathology
Birth Defects and Genetic
Counseling Clinic
Phone: (313) 288-8050

MINNESOTA

Minneapolis

University of Minnesota Hospital
Mayo Memorial Building
Box 485
420 Delaware Street, S.E.
Minneapolis, Minnesota 55455

Department of Medicine
Division of Genetics
Phone: (612) 376-4263

Rochester

Mayo Clinic
200 First Street, S.W.
Rochester, Minnesota 55905

Department of Genetics
Phone: (507) 284-8198

MISSISSIPPI

Biloxi

U.S. Air Force Medical Center
Keesler Air Force Base
Biloxi, Mississippi 39534

Department of Medical Genetics
Phone: (601) 377-6393/6702

Jackson

University of Mississippi Medical
Center
2500 North State Street
Jackson, Mississippi 39216

Department of Preventive Medicine
Division of Medicine Genetics
Phone: (601) 987-5611

MISSOURI

Columbia

University of Missouri Health
Sciences Center
One Hospital Drive
Columbia, Missouri 65212

Department of Child Health
Division of Medical Genetics
Phone: (314) 882-6991

Kansas City

Children's Mercy Hospital
University of Missouri at Kansas City
24th and Gillham Road
Kansas City, Missouri 64108

Genetic Counseling Center
Phone: (816) 234-3291

St. Louis

Cardinal Glennon Children's Hospital
1465 South Grand Boulevard
St. Louis, Missouri 63104

Department of Pediatrics
Genetics Section
Phone: (314) 577-5639

St. Louis

St. Louis Children's Hospital
Washington University Medical
School
500 South King's Highway
St. Louis, Missouri 63110

Department of Pediatrics
Division of Medical Genetics
Phone: (314) 454-6075

Jewish Hospital of St. Louis
Washington University Medical
School
216 South King's Highway
St. Louis, Missouri 63110

Department of Obstetrics and
Gynecology
Division of Genetics
Phone: (314) 454-7700

MONTANA

Helena

Shodair Children's Hospital
P.O. Box 5539
840 Helena Avenue
Helena, Montana 59604

Department of Medical Genetics
Phone: (406) 442-1980, ext. 254

NEBRASKA

Omaha

Clinical Genetics Center
8111 Dodge Street, Suite 248
Omaha, Nebraska 68114

Clinical Genetics Center
Phone: (402) 390-1170

University of Nebraska Medical
Center
Hattie B. Monroe Pavillion
4420 Dewey
Omaha, Nebraska 68105

Meyers Childrens Rehabilitation
Institute
Center for Human Genetics
Phone: (402) 559-5070

NEVADA

Las Vegas

The Genetics Center of
Southwest Biomedical Research
Institute
901 Rancho Lane, Suite 104
Las Vegas, Nevada 89106

Phone: (702) 384-5515

Southern Nevada Mental Retardation
  Services
1300 South Jones Boulevard
Las Vegas, Nevada 89158

  Phone: (702) 870-0220

Sparkes

Northern Nevada Mental Retardation
  Services
605 South 21st Street
Sparkes, Nevada 89431

  Phone: (702) 789-0550

NEW HAMPSHIRE

Hanover

Dartmouth-Hitchcock Medical Center
Dartmouth Medical School
Hanover, New Hampshire 03755

  Department of Maternal and
    Child Health
  Dysmorphology/Genetics Unit
  Phone: (603) 646-5473

NEW JERSEY

Camden

University of Medicine and Dentistry
  of New Jersey
School of Osteopathic Medicine
401 Haddon Avenue
Camden, New Jersey 08103

  Department of Pediatrics
  Division of Genetics
  Phone: (609) 757-7819

Newark

University of Medicine and Dentistry
  of New Jersey
100 Bergen Street, MSB-F534
Newark, New Jersey 07103

  Department of Pediatrics
  Division of Human Genetics
  Phone: (201) 456-4499

New Brunswick

University of Medicine and Dentistry
  of New Jersey
Rutgers Medical School   CN-19
New Brunswick, New Jersey 08903

  Department of Pediatrics
  Division of Medical Genetics
  Phone: (201) 937-7891

NEW MEXICO

Albuquerque

University of New Mexico
  School of Medicine
2701 Frontier, N.E.
Albuquerque, New Mexico 87131

  Department of Obstetrics and
    Gynecology
  Phone: (505) 277-4051

  Department of Pediatrics
  Dysmorphology Unit
  Phone: (505) 277-5551

NEW YORK

Albany

Albany Medical College Hospital
New Scotland Avenue
Albany, New York 12208

  Department of Pediatrics,
    Obstetrics and Gynecology
  Division of Medical Genetics
  Phone: (518) 445-5120

Buffalo

The Buffalo General Hospital
100 High Street
Buffalo, New York 14203

Department of Medicine
Division of Medical Genetics
Phone: (716) 845-2167

The Children's Hospital of Buffalo
219 Bryant Street
Buffalo, New York 14222

Department of Pediatrics
Division of Human Genetics
Phone: (716) 878-7530

East Meadow

Nassau County Medical Center
2201 Hempstead Turnpike
East Meadow, New York 11554

Department of Pediatrics
Division of Medical Genetics
Phone: (516) 542-3391

Manhasset

North Shore University Hospital
Cornell University College of
    Medicine
300 Community Drive
Manhasset, New York 11030

Child Development Center
Division of Genetics
Phone: (516) 562-4610

New York (Bronx)

Albert Einstein Medical Center
Rose Kennedy Center, Room 211
College of Medicine
1410 Pelham Parkway
Bronx, New York 10461

Department of Pediatrics
Genetic Counseling Program
Phone: (212) 430-2510

New York (Brooklyn)

Brookdale Hospital Medical Center
Linden Boulevard at Brookdale Plaza
Brooklyn, New York 11212

Department of Pediatrics
Division of Genetics
Phone: (718) 240-5883

Brooklyn Hospital/Caledonian
    Hospital
121 Dekalb Avenue
Brooklyn, New York 11201

Department of Obstetrics/
    Gynecology and Pediatrics
Division of Genetics
Phone: (718) 403-8032

Downstate Medical Center
450 Clarkson Avenue
Brooklyn, New York 11203

Department of Pediatrics
Division of Clinical Genetics
Phone: (718) 270-1692

Long Island College Hospital
350 Henry Street
Brooklyn, New York 11201

Department of Obstetrics and
    Gynecology
Genetics Center
Phone: (718) 780-1773

New York (Manhattan)

Beth Israel Medical Center
10 Nathan D. Perlman Place
New York, New York 10003

Department of Pediatrics
Division of Medical Genetics
Phone: (212) 420-4179

Columbia-Presbyterian Medical
Center
622 West 168th Street
New York, New York 10032

Division of Genetics
Babies' Hospital
Phone: (212) 694-6731

Department of Obstetrics and
Gynecology
Genetic Counseling Service
Phone: (212) 305-4066

Mt. Sinai Medical Center
Annenberg Building
Fifth Avenue and 100th Street
New York, New York 10029

Department of Pediatrics
Division of Genetics
Phone: (212) 650-6947

New York Hospital
Cornell Medical Center
525 East 68th Street
New York, New York 10021

Genetic Counseling Program
Phone: (212) 472-6825

New York University Medical
Center-Bellevue Hospital
550 First Avenue—MSB 136
New York, New York 10016

Department of Pediatrics
Division of Human Genetics
Phone: (212) 340-5746

New York (Queens)

Queens Hospital Center
LIJHMC
82-68 164th Street
Jamaica, New York 11432

Center for Developmentally
Disabled
Phone: (718) 990-3167

Schneider Children's Hospital of
Long Island Jewish—Hillside
Medical Center
271-16 76th Avenue
New Hyde Park, New York 11042

Department of Pediatrics
Division of Human Genetics
Phone: (718) 470-3010

New York (Staten Island)

New York State Institute for Basic
Research in Developmental
Disabilities
1050 Forest Hill Road
Staten Island, New York 10314

Department of Human Genetics
Phone: (718) 494-5230

Rochester

University of Rochester Medical
Center
Box 777
601 Elmwood Avenue
Rochester, New York 14642

Department of Pediatrics
Division of Genetics and
Dysmorphology
Rochester Regional Genetics
Services Program
Phone: (716) 275-3304

Stony Brook

Health Sciences Center
S.U.N.Y. at Stony Brook
Stony Brook, New York 11794

Department of Obstetrics and
Gynecology Genetics Unit
Phone: (516) 444-2790

Syracuse

Upstate Medical Center
State University of New York
766 Irving Avenue
Syracuse, New York 13210

Department of Pediatrics
Regional Genetics Center
Phone: (315) 473-5834

Thiells

Letchworth Village
Thiells, New York 10984

Regional Medical Genetic Services
and Laboratory
Phone: (914) 947-3487

Valhalla

Westchester County Medical Center
Valhalla, New York 10595

Medical Genetics Unit
Phone: (914) 347-7627

NORTH CAROLINA

Chapel Hill

Genetics Associates of
North Carolina, Inc.
Estes Office Park, Suite 107
104 South Estes Drive
Chapel Hill, North Carolina 27514

Phone: (919) 942-0021

University of North Carolina
at Chapel Hill
School of Medicine
Biological Sciences Research Center
#220H
Chapel Hill, North Carolina 27514

Department of Medicine
Division of Medical Genetics
Phone: (919) 966-2266

Department of Pediatrics
Division of Genetics and
Metabolism
Phone: (919) 966-4202

Charlotte

Charlotte Memorial Hospital and
Medical Center
P.O. Box 32861
Charlotte, North Carolina 28232

Department of Pediatrics
Clinical Genetics Program
Phone: (704) 331-3156

Durham

Duke University Medical Center
Durham, North Carolina 27710

Department of Obstetrics and
Gynecology
Division of Perinatal Medicine
Phone: (919) 684-2876/3604

Department of Pediatrics
Division of Genetics and
Metabolism
Phone: (919) 684-2036

Greenville

East Carolina University
School of Medicine
Greenville, North Carolina 27834

Department of Pediatrics
Division of Medical Genetics
Phone: (919) 757-2525

Winston-Salem

Bowman Gray School of Medicine
300 South Hawthorne Road
Winston-Salem, North Carolina 27103

Department of Pediatrics
Genetic Counseling Program
Phone: (919) 748-4321

NORTH DAKOTA

Grand Forks

University of North Dakota
School of Medicine
501 Columbia Road
Grand Forks, North Dakota 58201

Department of Pediatrics
Division of Medical Genetics
Phone: (701) 777-4277

OHIO

Akron

The Children's Hospital Medical
  Center of Akron
281 Locust Street
Akron, Ohio 44308

Genetics Clinic
Phone: (216) 379-8792

Cincinnati

Cincinnati Center for
  Developmental Disorders
3300 Elland Avenue
Cincinnati, Ohio 45229

Department of Human Genetics
Cincinnati Regional Genetic Center
Phone: (513) 559-4760

Cleveland

Case Western Reserve University
School of Medicine
Wearn Building—Room 150
2058 Abington Road
Cleveland, Ohio 44106

Department of Pediatrics
Genetics Center
Phone: (216) 844-3936

Cleveland Metropolitan General
  Hospital
3395 Scranton Road
Cleveland, Ohio 44109

Department of Pediatrics
Division of Medical Genetics
Phone: (216) 459-4323

Columbus

Children's Hospital
700 Children's Drive
Columbus, Ohio 43205

Genetics Section
Phone: (614) 461-2663

Dayton

Children's Medical Center
One Children's Plaza
Dayton, Ohio 45404

Department of Medical Genetics
  and Birth Defects
Division of Genetics
Phone: (513) 226-8408

Toledo

Medical College of Ohio at Toledo
Toledo, Ohio 43699

Department of Pediatrics
C.S. 10008
Genetics Center
Phone: (419) 381-4435

OKLAHOMA

Oklahoma City

Presbyterian Hospital
Northeast 13th Street at Lincoln
  Boulevard
Oklahoma City, Oklahoma 73104

Genetics Diagnostic Center
Phone: (405) 271-6777

Children's Memorial Hospital
Department of Pediatrics
Division of Genetics,
   Endocrinology and Metabolism
Regional Genetic Diagnosis
   and Counseling Center
940 N.E. 13th Street—P.O. Box 26901
Oklahoma City, Oklahoma 73190

Oklahoma Memorial
Department of Medicine
Division of Genetics
800 N.E. 13th Street
Oklahoma City, Oklahoma 73190

   Phone: (405) 271-3468

Tulsa

Children's Medical Center
5300 East Skelly Drive
Tulsa, Oklahoma 74135

   Regional Genetics Center
   Phone: (918) 664-6600, ext. 268

OREGON

Portland

Emanuel Hospital
2801 North Gantenbein Avenue
Portland, Oregon 97227

   Department of Pediatrics
   Oregon Medical Genetics and
      Birth Defects Center
   Phone: (503) 280-3042

Kaiser-Permanente
Division Medical Office
7705 South East Division Street
Portland, Oregon 97206

   Department of Pediatrics
   Phone: (503) 777-3311, ext. 3210
   (Kaiser members only)

Oregon Health Sciences University
3181 S.W. Sam Jackson Park Road
Portland, Oregon 97201

   Department of Medical Genetics
   L-103
   Phone: (503) 225-8344

PENNSYLVANIA

Hershey

Hershey Medical Center
P.O. Box 850
Hershey, Pennsylvania 17033

   Department of Pediatrics
   Division of Genetics
   Phone: (717) 534-8412

Philadelphia

Children's Hospital of Philadelphia
34th and Civic Center Boulevard
Philadelphia, Pennsylvania 19104

   Clinical Genetics Center
   Phone: (215) 596-9800

Pennsylvania Hospital
8th and Spruce Streets
Philadelphia, Pennsylvania 19107

   Division of Perinatology
   Section of Medical Genetics
   Phone: (215) 829-5633

St. Christopher's Hospital for
   Children
2600 North Lawrence Street
Philadelphia, Pennsylvania 19133

   Department of Pediatrics
   Division of Genetics
   Phone: (215) 427-5290

Thomas Jefferson University
10th Street, Suite 425, Main Building
Philadelphia, Pennsylvania 19107

Department of Medicine
Division of Medical Genetics
Phone: (215) 928-6955

University of Pennsylvania Hospital
3400 Spruce Street
Philadelphia, Pennsylvania 19104

Department of Obstetrics and
Gynecology
Prenatal Genetic Diagnosis
Program
Phone: (215) 662-3232

Pittsburgh

Children's Hospital of Pittsburgh
125 De Soto Street
Pittsburgh, Pennsylvania 15213

Department of Pediatrics
Division of Medical Genetics
Phone: (412) 647-5070

Magee Women's Hospital
Forbes Avenue and Halket Street
Pittsburgh, Pennsylvania 15213

Department of Reproductive
Genetics
Phone: (412) 647-4168

RHODE ISLAND

Providence

Rhode Island Hospital
593 Eddy Street
Providence, Rhode Island 02902

Department of Pediatrics
Genetic Counseling Service
Phone: (401) 227-8361

SOUTH CAROLINA

Charleston

Medical University of South Carolina
171 Ashley Avenue
Charleston, South Carolina 29425

Department of Diagnostic Science
Division of Craniofacial Genetics
Phone: (803) 792-2489

Department of Pediatrics
Division of Medical Genetics
Phone: (803) 792-2620

Columbia

University of South Carolina
School of Medicine
3321 Medical Park Road, Suite 301
Columbia, South Carolina 29203

Department of Obstetrics and
Gynecology
Division of Clinical Genetics
Phone: (803) 765-7316

Greenwood

Greenwood Genetic Center
Gregor Mendel Circle
Greenwood, South Carolina 29646

Phone: (803) 223-9411

SOUTH DAKOTA

Vermillion

University of South Dakota
School of Medicine
Julian Hall, Room 208
Clark and 414 E.
Vermillion, South Dakota 57069

Birth Defects/Genetics Center
Phone: (605) 677-5623

TENNESSEE

Johnson City

Regional Clinical Genetics Center
Suite 400, Professional Building
112 E. Myrtle Street
Johnson City, Tennessee 37614

Department of Pediatrics
Division of Genetics and
Dysmorphology
Phone: (615) 926-3188

Knoxville

University of Tennessee
Memorial Research Center and
Hospital
1924 Alcoa Highway
Knoxville, Tennessee 37920

Birth Defects and Human
Development Center
Phone: (615) 544-9030

Memphis

University of Tennessee
Center for Health Sciences
711 Jefferson Avenue
Memphis, Tennessee 38163

Division of Genetics
Child Development Center,
Room 523
Phone: (901) 528-6595

Nashville

Meharry Medical College
1005 18th Avenue
Nashville, Tennessee 37208

Department of Pediatrics
Division of Medical Genetics
Phone: (615) 327-6786

Vanderbilt University School of
Medicine
Room T-2404 Medical Center North
Nashville, Tennessee 37232

Department of Pediatrics
Phone: (615) 322-7601

TEXAS

Dallas

University of Texas Health Science
Center at Dallas
Southwestern Medical School
5323 Harry Hines Boulevard
Dallas, Texas 75235

Department of Obstetrics/
Gynecology and Pediatrics
Division of Clinical Genetics
Phone: (214) 688-2143

Denton

Texas Department of Mental Health
and Mental Retardation
404 West Oak Street
Denton, Texas 76201

Genetic Screening and
Counseling Service
Phone: (817) 383-3561

Galveston

University of Texas
Medical Branch at Galveston
Child Health Center
Galveston, Texas 77550

Department of Pediatrics
Division of Cytogenetics
Phone: (409) 761-3466

Houston

Texas Children's Hospital
Baylor College of Medicine
6621 Fannin
Houston, Texas 77030

Birth Defects/Genetics Clinic
Phone: (713) 791-4774

University of Texas
  Medical School at Houston
Texas Medical Center
P.O. Box 20708
Houston, Texas 77225

  Department of Pediatrics
  Medical Genetics Program
  Phone: (713) 797-4557

San Antonio

Santa Rosa Medical Center
P.O. Box 7330, Station A
San Antonio, Texas 78285

  Birth Defects Evaluation Center
  Phone: (512) 228-2386

University of Texas Health Science
  Center at San Antonio
7703 Floyd Curl Drive
San Antonio, Texas 78284

  Department of Cellular
    and Structural Biology
  Division of Human Genetics
  Phone: (512) 691-6443

  Department of Pediatric Dentistry
  Division of Clinical Genetics
  Phone: (512) 691-7587

UTAH

Salt Lake City

University of Utah Medical Center
50 North Medical Drive
Salt Lake City, Utah 84132

  Department of Pediatrics
  Division of Medical Genetics
  Phone: (801) 581-8943

VERMONT

Burlington

University of Vermont
College of Medicine
A115 Medical Alumni Building
Burlington, Vermont 05405

  Department of Pediatrics
  Vermont Regional Genetics Center
  Phone: (802) 656-4024

VIRGINIA

Charlottesville

University of Virginia Medical School
P.O. Box 386
Charlottesville, Virginia 22908

  Department of Pediatrics
  Division of Medical Genetics
  Phone: (804) 924-2665

Fairfax

Genetics and IVF Institute
3020 Javier Road
Fairfax, Virginia 22031

  Phone: (703) 698-7355

Norfolk

Eastern Virginia Medical School
P.O. Box 1980, Lewis Hall
Norfolk, Virginia 23501

  Department of Pediatrics
  Division of Genetics
  Phone: (804) 623-1500

Richmond

Medical College of Virginia
Virginia Commonwealth University
P.O. Box 33, MCV Station
Richmond, Virginia 23298

  Department of Human Genetics
  Phone: (804) 786-9632

WASHINGTON

Seattle

Children's Orthopedic Hospital
and Medical Center
University of Washington
4800 Sand Point Way N.E.
P.O. Box C5371
Seattle, Washington 98105

Department of Pediatrics
Division of Medical Genetics
Phone: (206) 526-2056

Swedish Hospital Medical Center
747 Summit Avenue
Seattle, Washington 98104
Attn: Perinatal Medicine

Department of Obstetrics
and Gynecology
Phone: (206) 386-2101

University of Washington
Seattle, Washington 98195

Department of Medicine RG-25
Division of Medical Genetics
Phone: (206) 548-4030

Department of Obstetrics and
Gynecology RH-20
Division of Perinatology
Phone: (206) 543-3753

Spokane

Deaconess Medical Center
West 800 Fifth Avenue
Spokane, Washington, 99210

Inland Empire Genetic
Counseling Service
Phone: (509) 458-7115

Tacoma

Mary Bridge Children's
Health Center
311 South "L" Street
Tacoma, Washington 98405

Genetics Clinic
Phone: (206) 594-1415

Walla Walla

St. Mary Medical Center
401 West Poplar, P.O. Box 1477
Walla Walla, Washington, 99362

Blue Mountain Genetics
Counseling Service
Phone: (509) 946-4611, ext. 378

Yakima

Yakima Valley Memorial Hospital
2811 Tieton Drive
Yakima, Washington 98902

Department of Child
Health Services
Central Washington
Genetics Program
Phone: (509) 575-8160

WEST VIRGINIA

Morgantown

West Virginia University
Medical Center
Morgantown, West Virginia 26500

Department of Pediatrics
Genetics Evaluation and
Counseling Center
Phone: (304) 293-7331/4

WISCONSIN

Madison

University of Wisconsin at Madison
337 Waisman Center
1500 Highland Avenue
Madison, Wisconsin 53705-2280

Department of Medical Genetics
Clinical Genetics Center
Phone: (608) 262-2507

Marshfield

Marshfield Genetics and
   Birth Defects Center
Marshfield Clinic
1000 North Oak Street
Marshfield, Wisconsin 54449

Phone: (715) 387-5089

Milwaukee

Milwaukee Children's Hospital
1700 West Wisconsin Avenue
Milwaukee, Wisconsin 53233

Department of Pediatrics
Birth Defects Center
Phone: (414) 931-4039

Mt. Sinai Medical Center
University of Wisconsin
   Medical School
Milwaukee Clinical Campus
950 North 12th Street
Milwaukee, Wisconsin 53201

Department of Obstetrics and
   Gynecology
Genetics Section
Phone: (414) 289-8236

Wauwatosa

Great Lakes Genetics
2600 North Mayfair Road
Wauwatosa, Wisconsin 53226

Phone: (414) 475-7400

WYOMING

Please contact State Genetic
   Services Coordinator

SATELLITE PROGRAM SITES PROVIDED BY OUT OF STATE CENTERS

Casper, Cheyenne, Riverton,
See Denver, Colorado
   University of Colorado Health
   Sciences Center

Appendix II

STATE GENETIC SERVICES COORDINATORS

State Genetic Services Coordinators can provide information about local genetic services, genetic educational programs, and special clinics and programs concerned with specific genetic disorders. This list has been made available by the National Center for Education in Maternal and Child Health. (*Comprehensive Clinical Genetic Services Centers: A National Directory—1985*).

ALABAMA

Director, Laboratory of Medical
   Genetics
University of Alabama-Birmingham
University Station
Birmingham, Alabama 35294
(202) 934-4973

ALASKA

Chief, Family Health Section
Department of Health & Social
   Services
Health and Welfare Building
Pouch H-6B
Juneau, Alaska 99811
(907) 465-3107

ARIZONA

The Genetics Center of Southwest
   Biomedical Research Institute
123 East University Drive
Tempe, Arizona 85281
(602) 894-1104

ARKANSAS

Genetics Program Coordinator
Department of Pediatrics/512 B
University of Arkansas Medical
   Sciences Campus
4301 West Markham
Little Rock, Arkansas 72205
(501) 661-5994

CALIFORNIA

Chief, Genetic Disease Branch
California State Department of Health
   Services
2151 Berkeley Way, Annex 4
Berkeley, California 94704
(415) 540-2552

COLORADO

Director of Medical Affairs and
   Special Programs
State Departments of Health
4210 East 11th Avenue
Denver, Colorado 80220
(303) 320-6137, Ext. 422

CONNECTICUT

Chief, Maternal and Child Health
   Section
State Department of Health Services
150 Washington Street
Hartford, Connecticut 06106
(203) 566-5601

DELAWARE

Genetics Program Coordinator
Handicapped Children Services
Jesse S. Cooper Memorial Building
P.O. Box 637
Dover, Delaware 19903
(302) 736-4786

DISTRICT OF COLUMBIA

Genetics Program Coordinator
Department of Human Services
Commission of Public Health
Bureau of Maternal and Child Health
1875 Connecticut Avenue, N.W.
Room 804-B
Washington, D.C. 20009
(202) 673-6697

FLORIDA

Genetics Coordinator
Children's Medical Services
Department of Health and
   Rehabilitative Services
1317 Winewood Boulevard
Tallahassee, Florida 32301
(904) 488-6005

GEORGIA

Director of Genetic Services
Community Health Section
Georgia Department of Human
   Resources
878 Peachtree Street, 1st Floor
Atlanta, Georgia 30309
(404) 656-4850

HAWAII

Kapiolani-Children's Medical Center
University of Hawaii
1319 Punahou Street
Honolulu, Hawaii 96826
(808) 948-6834

IDAHO

Genetic Services Coordinator
Bureau of Laboratories
Idaho Department of Health &
   Welfare
2220 Old Penitentiary Road
Boise, Idaho 83712
(208) 334-4778

ILLINOIS

Genetic Program Coordinator
Division of Family Health
Illinois Department of Public Health
535 West Jefferson Street
Springfield, Illinois 62761
(217) 785-4526/782-2736

INDIANA

Chief, Genetic Diseases Section
Division Maternal & Child Health
State Board of Health
1330 West Michigan Street
Box 1964
Indianapolis, Indiana 46206
(317) 633-0805

IOWA

Administrative Coordinator
Birth Defects Institute, Division of
    Maternal and Child Health
State Department of Health
Lucas State Office Building
Des Moines, Iowa 50319
(515) 281-6646

KANSAS

Coordinator of Genetic Services
Crippled & Chronically Ill Children's
    Program
Department of Health and
    Environment
Forbes Field, Building #740
Topeka, Kansas 66620
(913) 862-9360 Ext. 455

KENTUCKY

Department for Health Services
Cabinet for Human Resources
275 East Main Street
Frankfort, Kentucky 40621
(502) 564-4430

LOUISIANA

Genetic Nurse Consultant
Genetic Section
Department of Health and Human
    Services
P.O. Box 60630
New Orleans, Louisiana 70160
(504) 568-5083

MAINE

Program Manager of Genetic
    Diseases
Division of Maternal and Child
    Health
Department of Human Services
State House, Station 11
Augusta, Maine 04333
(207) 289-3311

MARYLAND

Division of Hereditary Disorders
Maryland Department of Health and
    Mental Hygiene
P.O. Box 13528
201 West Preston Street
Baltimore, Maryland 21201
(301) 383-6321/2805

MASSACHUSETTS

Unit Director, Perinatal and Genetic
    Services
Division of Family Health Services
Department of Public Health
150 Tremont Street
Boston, Massachusetts 02111
(617) 727-0944

MICHIGAN

Genetics Program Coordinator
State Department of Public Health
3500 North Logan Street
P.O. Box 30035
Lansing, Michigan 48909
(517) 373-0657

MINNESOTA

Supervisor, Human Genetics Unit
State Department of Health
717 Delaware, S.E.
P.O. Box 9441
Minneapolis, Minnesota 55440
(612) 623-5269

MISSISSIPPI

Genetics Project Director
State Board of Health
P.O. Box 1700
Jackson, Mississippi 39215-1700
(601) 982-6571

MISSOURI

Genetics Program Coordinator
Bureau of Chronic Diseases
State Department of Health
P.O. Box 570
Jefferson City, Missouri 65102
(314) 751-2713

MONTANA

Chairman, Department of Medical
   Genetics
Shodair Children's Hospital
840 Helena Avenue, Box 5539
Helena, Montana 59604
(406) 442-1980

NEBRASKA

Director, Bureau of Medical Services
   and Grants and Birth Defects
   Prevention Program
State Department of Health
P.O. Box 95007
Lincoln, Nebraska 68509
(402) 471-3980

NEVADA

Bureau of Community Health
   Services
Nevada Division of Health
505 East King Street, Room 205
Carson City, Nevada 89710
(702) 885-4885

NEW HAMPSHIRE

Genetics Program Coordinator
Bureau for Handicapped Children
Health and Welfare Building
Hazen Drive
Concord, New Hampshire 03301
(603) 271-4533

NEW JERSEY

Coordinator, Genetic Services
   Program
State Department of Health
120 South Stockton Street
CN 364
Trenton, New Jersey 08625
(609) 984-0775

NEW MEXICO

Chief, Maternal and Child Health
  Bureau
New Mexico Health and
  Environment Department
P.O. Box 968
Santa Fe, New Mexico 87504
(505) 984-0030 Ext. 504

NEW YORK

Executive Assistant to the President
Health Research, Inc.
Empire State Plaza Tower
Albany, New York 12237
(518) 474-1208

NORTH CAROLINA

Director Genetics Program
Division of Health Services
Department of Human Resources
P.O. Box 2091
Raleigh, North Carolina 27602
(919) 733-7437

NORTH DAKOTA

Director, Medical Genetics Division
Department of Pediatrics
University of North Dakota Medical
  School
501 Columbia Road
Grand Forks, North Dakota 58201
(701) 777-4277

OHIO

Genetics Program Coordinator
State Department of Health
P.O. Box 118
246 North High Street
Columbus, Ohio 43216
(614) 466-8804

OKLAHOMA

Genetic Project Coordinator
State Department of Health
1000 Northeast 10th Street
P.O. Box 53551
Oklahoma City, Oklahoma 74152
(405) 271-4471

OREGON

Chairman, Department of Medical
  Genetics
Oregon Health Sciences University
3181 S.W. Sam Jackson Park Road
Portland, Oregon 97201
(503) 225-7703

PENNSYLVANIA

Director, Genetic Diseases Program
Division of Maternal and Child
  Health, Department of Health
P.O. Box 90
Harrisburg, Pennsylvania 17108
(717) 787-7440

PUERTO RICO

Director, Genetic Diseases Screening
   Program
University Children's Hospital
University of Puerto Rico Medical
   School
G.P.O. Box 5067
San Juan, Puerto Rico 00936
(809) 765-2363

RHODE ISLAND

Chief & Medical Director
Division of Family Health
Department of Health
75 Davis Street, Room 302
Providence, Rhode Island 02908
(401) 277-2312

SOUTH CAROLINA

Division of Children's Health and
   Rehabilitative Services
Bureau of Maternal and Child Health
Department of Health and
   Environmental Control
2600 Bull Street
Columbia, South Carolina 29201
(803) 758-5491

SOUTH DAKOTA

Director, Genetics Program
University of South Dakota Medical
   School
Clark & Dakota Streets
Vermillion, South Dakota 57069
(605) 677-5623

TENNESSEE

Director of Center Based Programs
Division of Material and Child Health
Tennessee Department of Health and
   Environment
100 9th Avenue, North
Nashville, Tennessee 37219
(615) 741-7335

TEXAS

Division of Maternal and Child
   Health
State Department of Health
1100 West 49th Street
Austin, Texas 78756
(512) 458-7700

UTAH

State Genetics Program Coordinator
Division of Medical Genetics
University of Utah Medical Center
50 North Medical Drive
Salt Lake City, Utah 84132
(801) 581-8943

VERMONT

Director, Vermont Regional Genetics
University of Vermont
College of Medicine
A115 Medical Alumni Building
Burlington, Vermont 05405
(801) 656-4024

VIRGINIA

Program Administrator for Genetics
Bureau of Maternal and Child
  Health, Department of Health
109 Governor Street
Richmond, Virginia 23219
(804) 786-7367

WASHINGTON

Health Services Administrator
Genetic Services Section
Department of Social and Health
  Services
1704 N.E. 150th Street
Seattle, Washington 98155
(201) 545-6783

WEST VIRGINIA

Director, Genetics Evaluation and
  Counseling Center
West Virginia University Medical
  Center
Morgantown, West Virginia 26506
(304) 293-4451

WISCONSIN

Coordinator, Genetics Services
  Network Project
University of Wisconsin-Madison
104 Genetics Building
445 Henry Mall
Madison, Wisconsin 53706
(608) 263-6355

WYOMING

Director, Family Health Services
Department of Health and Social
  Services
Hathaway Building
Cheyenne, Wyoming 82002
(307) 777-6297

Appendix III

GENETIC RESOURCES

The following organizations provide information, services, and activities for patients of genetic diseases and their parents.

March of Dimes Birth Defects
  Foundation
1275 Mamaroneck Avenue
White Plains, N.Y. 10605
(914) 428-7100

National Center for Education in
  Maternal and Child Health
38th and R Streets, N.W.
Washington, D.C. 20057
(202) 625-8400

National Self-Help Clearinghouse
Graduate School and University
  Center/CUNY
33 West 42nd Street
New York, N.Y.
(212) 840-1259

National Down Syndrome Society
666 Broadway
New York, N.Y. 10012
(212) 460-9330 or (800) 221-4602

Muscular Dystrophy Association
810 Seventh Avenue
New York, N.Y. 10019
(212) 586-0808

National Hemophilia Foundation
Soho Building
110 Greene Street, Room 406
New York, N.Y. 10012
(212) 219-8180

Cystic Fibrosis Association
6931 Arlington Rd.
Bethesda, MD 20814
(301) 984-9418

National Association for Sickle Cell
  Disease, Inc.
4221 Wilshire Boulevard
Suite 360
Los Angeles, CA 90010-3503
(213) 936-7205 or (800) 421-8453

GLOSSARY

acrocentric chromosome A chromosome in which the centromere is near one end.

additive genes Several genes whose effects add together to determine a trait.

adoptees Individuals who have been adopted; those separated from their biological parents and raised by foster parents.

alleles Alternate forms of genes that may occur at a locus.

amniocentesis A procedure for obtaining amniotic fluid for prenatal diagnosis. A sterile needle is inserted through the mother's abdomen into the amniotic sac, and a sample of amniotic fluid containing fetal cells is removed. Amniocentesis is usually carried out during the sixteenth week of pregnancy.

amnion A fluid-filled sac that surrounds the fetus.

amniotic fluid Fluid that surrounds the fetus during pregnancy.

antibody A protein produced by cells of the immune system, which recognizes and destroys foreign substances in the body.

antigen A substance recognized by the immune system.

artificial insemination Placing semen into a woman's vagina artificially, without sexual intercourse.

autosome A nonsex chromosome; any of the chromosomes except the X and the Y.

cancer A growth characterized by the presence of cells that multiply and spread in an uncontrollable manner.

carcinogen A substance that causes cancer.

carriers Individuals that carry one copy of a recessive gene for the trait, but do not themselves have the trait.

centromere A constricted region on the chromosome.

chorion A part of the placenta that is found outside of the amnion.

chorionic villus sampling A procedure for obtaining fetal cells for prenatal diagnosis. Under the guidance of ultrasound, a soft plastic tube is inserted through the vagina and cervix into the uterus; a small piece of the chorion (a part of the placenta consisting of fetal tissue) is then removed by suction. Chorionic villus sampling is usually carried out between the ninth and eleventh weeks of pregnancy.

chromatid   One of two copies of a chromosome that exist after replication of the DNA but before the cell has divided; the two chromatids are held together at the centromere.

chromosome   A structure in the cell consisting of DNA and proteins. Humans have 46 chromosomes.

chromosome abnormality   A chromosome mutation.

chromosome mutation   Any change in the number or structure of a chromosome that can be seen under a microscope. Too many or too few chromosomes may be present, a piece of a chromosome may be missing or duplicated, a piece of a chromosome may be inverted, or a piece of a chromosome may be attached to another chromosome. Because many genes reside on each chromosome, a number of genes are usually affected by a chromosome abnormality, and many traits may be altered simultaneously.

codominance   When both genes are expressed in a heterozygous individual; neither allele is dominant over the other.

complex segregation analysis   Complex mathematical procedures for determining the pattern of inheritance of a trait found among the members of one or more families.

concordant   When two members of a twin pair both have a trait.

congenital   Present at birth.

crossing over   Exchange of genetic material between two homologous chromosomes during meiosis.

deletion   A chromosome mutation in which a piece of one chromosome is missing.

discordant   When one member of a twin pair has a trait, but the other twin lacks the trait.

dizygotic twins   Nonidentical twins, arising from two different eggs fertilized by two different sperm. Also called *fraternal twins*.

DNA   Deoxyribonucleic acid, the chemical compound that carries genetic information.

DNA sequencing   Determining the nucleotide sequence of a piece of DNA.

dominant trait   A trait that is expressed when only a single copy of the gene for the trait is present. This means that when the dominant gene is paired with a different gene, the dominant gene is stronger, and it determines the trait. Thus, in a dominant trait the homozygous individual (possessing two copies of the gene) and the heterozygous individual (possessing only a single copy of the gene) both exhibit the features of the trait.

duplication   A chromosome mutation in which a piece of the chromosome is present in two copies.

egg   The female sex cell. It carries half of the mother's genes and fuses with a sperm at conception.

embryo   The individual that results from the fusion of an egg and a sperm at conception. This term is usually reserved for the early stages of development when human characteristics are lacking, most frequently the period from conception to the eighth week of development. After the eighth week, the term *fetus* is used.

empiric risk   The probability of developing a disease or disorder, based on the proportion of individuals affected in other families.

familial trait   A trait that tends to run in families. It may or may not be influenced by genes.

fertilization   The fusion of an egg and sperm at conception.

fetal blood sampling   A relatively new technique for obtaining a blood sample from the fetus. A long sterile needle is inserted through the mother's abdomen into the uterus. Under the guidance of ultrasound, the needle is directed to a blood vessel in the umbilical cord. The blood vessel is punctured with the needle and a sample of blood is removed.

α-fetoprotein   A substance produced by the fetus during its development in the uterus. Normally, α-fetoprotein is high in the blood of the fetus, moderate in the amniotic fluid, and low in the mother's blood during pregnancy. The levels of α-fetoprotein in amniotic fluid and in the mother's blood are used to help diagnose some birth defects.

fetoscopy   Viewing the fetus with a fiber optic instrument that has been inserted into the uterus.

fetus   The developing baby in the mother's womb. It usually refers to the product of conception from 2 months after fertilization until birth. For the first 2 months, the conception is usually called an *embryo*.

fraternal twins   Nonidentical twins, arising from two different eggs fertilized by two different sperm. Also called *dizygotic twins.*

gene   The fundamental unit of heredity; an inherited factor that determines a trait.

gene therapy   Treating genetic diseases by repairing or transplanting genes.

genetic heterogeneity   Several different genes producing the same trait.

genetic marker   A gene or other DNA sequence that lies close to another gene on the same chromosome.

genetic maternal effect   When the mother's genes determine a trait in the offspring.

genetics   The study of genes and heredity.

genotype   The two genes (alleles) that an individual possesses at a locus.

germ cells   The cells that give rise to eggs and sperm.

germ-line genes   Genes contained in germ cells—those cells that give rise to eggs and sperm. The germ-line genes are the genes that are passed on to future generations.

hemoglobin   A protein found in red blood cells that carries oxygen and gives blood its red color.

heritability   In a group of people, the proportion of variation in a trait that is caused by differences in genes. It is often used in a more restricted sense to mean the proportion of the variation that is due to additive differences in genes.

heterozygous   When the genotype consists of two different genes (alleles).

HLA system   A group of genes located on chromosome 6 that allow the immune system to differentiate between self and nonself.

homologous chromosomes   Two chromosomes that carry information for the same traits and that pair during meiosis. One chromosome of the pair comes from the father and one chromosome of pair comes from the mother.

homozygous   When the genotype consists of two identical genes (alleles).

human genome   One complete set of human genes coding for all genetically determined traits.

identical twins   Twins that arise from a single egg fertilized by a single sperm. Identical twins are genetically identical. Also called *monozygotic twins*.

immune system   Cells that serve as the defense network of the body, destroying potentially harmful, foreign substances that enter the body.

inversion   A chromosome mutation in which a chromosome segment has become inverted; the chromosome breaks in two places, the segment flips over, and then reattaches.

in vitro fertilization   Removing an egg from a woman's ovary, fertilizing it with sperm in a test tube, and then transplanting it into the woman's uterus.

karyotype   A set of chromosomes from one individual.

locus   The place on a chromosome where a gene resides.

meiosis   The process of cell division by which sex cells—eggs and sperm—are produced. During meiosis, the number of chromosomes is reduced by half.

metacentric chromosomes   A chromosome in which the centromere is at or near the center of the chromosome; the centromere divides a metacentric chromosome into two approximately equal halves.

miscarriage   Spontaneous expulsion of the fetus before the twentieth week of pregnancy.

molecular genetics   The branch of genetics that studies the molecular nature of genes.

monozygotic twins   Identical twins, arising from a single egg fertilized by a single sperm.

mosaic   An individual that possesses two different types of cells with regard to chromosome composition.

multifactorial trait   A trait that is influenced by multiple genes and by environmental factors.

mutagen   A substance that causes mutations.

neural tube defect   A birth defect in which the neural tube fails to close during development. Spina bifida and anencephaly are examples of neural tube defects.

nonidentical twins   Twins that arise from two different eggs fertilized by two different sperm. Nonidentical twins share an average of 50 percent of the same genes. Also called *fraternal twins* or *dizygotic twins.*

nucleotides   The repeating units that make up the DNA molecule. DNA nucleotides come in four types, abbreviated A, T, G, and C.

oncogene   A gene that causes cancer.

pedigree   A diagram that illustrates the inheritance of a trait in a family over several generations.

penetrance   The percentage of individuals possessing a gene for a trait that actually express the trait. When penetrance is incomplete, not all individuals who possess the gene display the trait.

phenotype   A trait.

placenta   The structure that forms around a fetus during development in the uterus; it consists of both fetal and maternal tissues. The placenta is expelled as afterbirth following delivery.

polygenic   A trait that is determined by genes at many loci.

prenatal   Before birth.

prenatal diagnosis   Testing for the presence of a disease or disorder in an unborn baby.

primary Down syndrome   Down syndrome arising from a failure of chromosome division, producing a child with three copies of chromosome 21.

probability   Chance expressed as a mathematical ratio; it represents the fraction or percentage of the time that an event will occur.

proband   The individual who prompts the creation of a pedigree.

propositus   Same as the proband; the individual who prompts the creation of a pedigree.

protein   A type of molecule found in all living things. The structure of a protein is determined by the nucleotide sequence of the DNA.

proto-oncogene   A normal gene that can cause cancer if it is altered.

recessive trait   A trait that requires two copies of the gene to be expressed; an individual will express the trait only if he or she inherits a copy from the mother and a copy from the father. When a recessive gene is paired with a dominant gene, the dominant gene tends to hide or suppress the recessive trait, and the trait is therefore absent in heterozygotes.

recombinant DNA   Methods for cutting and joining together DNA segments.

restriction fragment length polymorphisms (RFLPs)   Variable genetic markers detected by cutting the DNA with enzymes that recognize specific DNA sequences.

sex-influenced trait   A trait determined by autosomal genes (not located on the sex chromosomes) that is more commonly expressed in one sex than the other.

sex-limited trait   A trait determined by autosomal genes (not located on the sex chromosomes) that is expressed in only one sex.

sibling   A brother or a sister.

single-locus traits   A trait that is determined by a pair of genes (alleles) at a single locus.

somatic genes   Genes located in nonsex cells (somatic cells).

somatic gene therapy   Correcting or transplanting genes that reside in somatic, or nonsex, cells.

somatic mutation   A genetic alteration occurring in the DNA of nonsex or somatic cells.

sperm   The male sex cell. It fuses with an egg during fertilization and contains half of the genes of the father.

stature   Height.

submetacentric chromosome   A chromosome in which the centromere is displaced toward one end, producing a long and a short arm.

syndrome   A group of symptoms and/or traits that occur together.

testis determining factor gene   A gene located on the Y chromosome that causes a fetus to develop into a male.

translocation   A chromosome mutation in which a piece of one chromosome breaks off and sticks to another chromosome, or when segments are exchanged between two chromosomes.

translocation Down syndrome   Down syndrome that occurs when an extra copy of chromosome 21 is attached (translocated) to another chromosome.

trisomy   A chromosome mutation in which three copies of a chromosome are present.

ultrasonography   Use of sound waves for visualizing tissues and structures within the body.

X-linked trait   A trait determined by a gene located on the X chromosome. Also called a *sex-linked trait*.

Y-linked trait   A trait determined by a gene located on the Y chromosome. Also called a *holandric trait*.

zygote   The product of fertilization.

SUGGESTED
READING

Blatt, R. J. R. 1988. *Prenatal Tests*. New York, Vintage Books.

Cohen, S. N. 1975. The manipulation of genes. *Scientific American* 233: 25–33.

Cummings, M. J. 1988. *Human Heredity: Principles and Issues*. New York, West.

Dunn, L. C. 1965. *A Short History of Genetics*. New York, McGraw-Hill.

Goodman, R. M. 1986. *Planning for a Healthy Baby: A Guide of Genetic and Environmental Risks*. Oxford, Oxford University Press.

Hartle, D. L. 1985. *Our Uncertain Heritage: Genetics and Human Diversity*. 2nd ed. New York, Harper and Row.

Loehlin, J. C., L. Willerman, and J. M. Horn. 1988. Human behavior genetics. *Annual Review of Psychology* 39:101–133.

Mange, A. P., and E. J. Mange. 1990. *Genetics: Human Aspects* 2nd ed. New York, Sinauer.

Milunsky, A. 1989. *Choices, Not Chances*. Boston, Little, Brown.

Nilsson, L. 1976. *A Child Is Born*. New York, Delacorte Press.

Russell, P. J. 1986. *Genetics*. Boston, Little, Brown.

Stine, G. J. 1989. *The New Human Genetics*. Dubuque, Iowa, Wm. C. Brown.

Sutton, H. E. 1988. *An Introduction to Human Genetics*, 4th ed. San Diego, Harcourt Brace Jovanovich.

Suzuki, D., and P. Knudtson. 1989. *Genethics: The Clash between the New Genetics and Human Values*. Cambridge, Massachusetts, Harvard University Press.

Thompson, J. S., and M. W. Thompson. 1986. *Genetics in Medicine*. Philadelphia, Saunders.

Technical Works (written primarily for physicians and/or geneticists)

Berini, R. Y., and E. Kahn. 1987. *Clinical Genetics Handbook*. Oradell, New Jersey, Medical Economics Books.

Bergsma, E. (ed). 1979. *Birth Defects Compendium*, 2nd ed. New York, Alan R. Liss.

Benson, P. F., and A. H. Fensom. 1985. *Genetic Biochemical Disorders*. Oxford, Oxford University Press.

Caskey, C. T. 1987. Disease diagnosis by recombinant DNA method. *Science* 236:1223–1230.

Emery, A. E. H., and D. L. Rimoin (ed). 1983. *Principles and Practice of Medical Genetics*. New York, Churchill Livingstone.

Garver K. L., and S. G. Marchese. 1986. *Genetic Counseling for Clinicians*. New York, Year Book Medical Publishers.

Goodman, R. M., and R. J. Gorlin. 1983. *The Malformed Infant and Child: An Illustrated Guide*. Oxford, Oxford University Press.

Kelly, T. E. 1986. *Clinical Genetics and Genetic Counseling*, 2nd ed. Chicago, Year Book Medical Publishers.

McKusick, V. A. 1988. *Mendelian Inheritance in Man: Catalogs of Autosomal Dominant, Autosomal Recessive, and X-Linked Phenotypes*, 8th ed. Baltimore, Johns Hopkins Press.

Moore, K. L. 1989. *Before We Are Born: Basic Embryology and Birth Defects*, 3rd ed. Philadelphia, Saunders.

Ostrer, H., and J. F. Hejtmancik. 1988. Prenatal diagnosis and carrier detection of genetic diseases by analysis of deoxyribonucleic acid. *Journal of Pediatrics* 112:679–687.

Scriver, C. R., et al. (ed.). 1989. *The Metabolic Basis of Inherited Disease*, 6th ed. New York, McGraw-Hill.

Seibel, M. M. 1988. A new era in reproductive technology: In vitro fertilization, gamete intrafallopian transfer, and donated gametes and embryos. *New England Journal of Medicine* 318:828–834.

Valentine, G. H. 1986. *The Chromosomes and Their Disorders*, 4th ed. London, William Heinemann Medical Books.

Vandenberg, S. G., S. M. Singer, and D. L. Pauls. 1986. *The Heredity of Behavior Disorders in Adults and Children*. New York, Plenum Medical Books Company.

Weaver, D. D. 1989. *Catalog of Prenatally Diagnosed Conditions*. Baltimore, Johns Hopkins Press.

INDEX

Achondroplasia, 206–207
Activity levels, 282
Additive genes, 83–85
Adenosine deaminase, 145
Adenosine deaminase deficiency, 137
Adoption studies, 96–97
Affective disorder (*see* Depression;
    Manic depression)
Aging, 237
Albinism, 2–5, 14, 160–161
Albinos (*see* Albinism)
Alcoholism, 5, 161–163
Alexandra, wife of Tsar Nicholas II, 9
Alexis, son of Tsar Nicholas II, 9–11
Alkaptonuria, 14
Alleles, definition of, 28
    multiple, 34
Allergy, 163–165
    in asthma, 167
Alopecia (*see* Baldness)
Alopecia-mental retardation syn-
    drome, 168
Alzheimer's disease, 165–166
Amish, 240
Amniocentesis, 108–109, 127–128
Amniotic fluid, 108, 127, 131, 134
Androgen insensitivity syndrome,
    267
Anencephaly (*see* Neural tube de-
    fects)
Anorexia nervosa, 166
    associated with bulimia, 177
Antibodies, 172, 174
Antigen, 172–176
    ABO, 33–35, 172–174
    Rh, 174, 176
α-1-Antitrypsin deficiency, 137

Arteries, 185
Arthritis (*see* Rheumatoid arthritis)
Artificial fertilization, 143
Asthma, 167
    with allergy, 164
Atherosclerosis, 182
Attached earlobes (*see* Earlobes)
Autoimmune disease, in diabetes,
    201
    in Graves' disease, 277
    in Hashimoto's disease, 276–277
    in rheumatoid arthritis, 262

Baldness, 64, 168
Barr body (*see* Sex chromatin)
Barry, Joan, 35–37
Becker muscular dystrophy (*see*
    Muscular dystrophy)
Bedwetting, 169
Bilirubin, 175
Biochemical tests, 135
Biotechnology, 17
Bipolar illness (*see* Manic depression)
Birthmark, 247
Birth weight, 169–171
Black hair (*see* Hair color)
Bleeders disease (*see* Hemophilia)
Blindness, 171
    see also Cataracts, Glaucoma,
        Nearsightedness
Blond hair (*see* Hair color)
Blood clotting (*see* Hemophilia)
Blood pressure, 185
    high, 98–99
    diastolic, 185
    systolic, 185